Research on Suicide

Bibliographies and Indexes in Psychology

Psychosocial Research on American Indian and Alaska Native Youth: An Inde
Guide to Recent Dissertations
*Compiled by Spero M. Manson, Norman G. Dinges, Linda M. Grounds, and
Carl A. Kalgren*

Research on Suicide

A Bibliography

Compiled by John L. McIntosh

Bibliographies and Indexes in Psychology, Number 2

Greenwood Press
Westport, Connecticut • London, England

Library of Congress Cataloging in Publication Data

McIntosh, John L.
    Research on suicide.
    (Bibliographies and indexes in psychology, ISSN   0736-
2714 ;   no.   2)
    Bibliography: p.
    Includes index.
    1. Suicide—Bibliography.   2. Suicide—United States—
Bibliography.   I. Title.   II. Series.
Z7615.M38   1985   [HV6545]   016.3622   84-15706
ISBN   0-313-23992-4   (lib. bdg.)

Library of Congress Catalog Card Number: 84-15706
ISBN: 0-313-23992-4
ISSN: 0736-2714

First published in 1985

Greenwood Press
A division of Congressional Information Service, Inc.
88 Post Road West, Westport, Connecticut 06881

Printed in the United States of America

10   9   8   7   6   5   4   3   2   1

CONTENTS

INTRODUCTION

Suicide is a serious mental health problem. It ranks among the top ten causes of death in the United States, with nearly 30,000 Americans killing themselves each year. In addition, between 300,000 and 600,000 people attempt suicide each year and fail. At least five million living Americans have at some time attempted to commit suicide (see Chapter 5 for sources of suicide data). While much has been written about suicide, there remain many more questions than answers, especially regarding suicide prevention. It is hoped that this reference guide will aid further study and ultimately prevention measures.

The literature on suicide possesses several characteristics that make conducting library research of a specific subtopic difficult for those not already familiar with the field. These characteristics include a large, extremely widespread, and multidisciplinary literature; dated, little-known, or relatively inaccessible bibliographies; and a great expansion of research articles and other materials on suicide. These aspects demonstrate the need for a single reference that provides background information and sources of articles, books, and bibliographies for those needing or desiring primary materials. The present reference guide attempts to perform this task.

Writings on suicide appear in such diverse fields as medicine and health, psychology, sociology, social work, anthropology, philosophy, and religion. Journals and books in any and all of these disciplines contain works on suicide. Therefore, the researcher who approaches a library cannot simply consider a single or even a small number of sources. Indexes and abstracts in each of these fields (see sections 1.2 and 1.3) would likely list materials on suicide. The reader might also take note that sections 1-6 of Chapter 10 include references directed to specific gatekeepers (e.g., clergy, law enforcement personnel, medical professionals, military and school personnel, social workers and family therapists) who encounter the suicidal in various settings. Section 7 of Chapter 10 includes references on suicide in art and literature.

While several bibliographies on suicide exist (e.g., Farberow, 1972, reference 1-003; Farberow, Shneidman, & Bouvier, 1961, reference 1-004; Prentice, 1974, reference

1-013; Resnik & Hathorne, 1974, reference 1-014), they are
dated due to the great number of references published
annually. Another difficulty with present suicide
bibliographies is that several are published and distributed
by organizations or individuals without much publicity or
attention except among those already working in the area
(e.g., American Association of Suicidology annotated
bibliographies, reference 1-001; Miller, 1979, reference
1-010). With the exception of the latter bibliographies,
few general bibliographic compilations have appeared in
recent years. These and other bibliographic sources are
listed in section 1.1. Bibliographies on specific subtopics
are listed in the appropriate sections of this reference
guide.

     Although data are unavailable on the number of
references appearing annually on the topic of suicide, some
examples will provide clues as to the great explosion of the
literature. Such great expansion makes exhaustive
bibliographies large, expensive, time-consuming to compile,
and quickly outdated. Farberow's (1972, reference 1-003)
updated version of Farberow, Shneidman, and Bouvier's (1961,
reference 1-004) bibliography for 1847 to 1957 is quite
exhaustive. The 1972 bibliography listed 2,202 references
for 1897 to 1957 and 2,542 for 1958 to 1970. Consider also
suicide among the young, a topic of particular contemporary
research and popular interest. In an extensive review of
the literature to the late 1960s, Seiden (1969, reference
5-212) noted that thirty-five articles on young suicides
appeared from 1900 to 1957, but eighty-seven appeared for
1960 to 1967 alone. Similarly, McIntosh (1981, reference
5-149) collected 107 pages of references on child and
adolescent suicide through 1980 and has compiled over 275
additional citations since that time (through 1983). Even
computers have not solved the problems. The extensive and
widespread literature make general computer searches
expensive and difficult. Searches for specialized
subtopics, on the other hand, often yield few sources from a
single data base or index source (for four sources of
computer searches see section 1.9).

     The increased interest in specific topics and in the
general phenomenon of suicide has led both to many books and
two journals publishing primarily articles on suicide
(Suicide and Life-Threatening Behavior, reference 1-083;
Crisis: International Journal of Suicide- and
Crisis-Studies, reference 1-080) and to several which devote
many pages annually to the topic (e.g., Omega: Journal of
Death and Dying, reference 1-082; Essence: Issues in
Ageing, Dying, and Death, reference 1-081).

Method, Coverage, Arrangement
     This reference guide provides the reader with sources
that should make a literature search and review, or study of
a single topic, easier, more efficient, and more economical
in the expenditure of time and energies. The over 2,300
entries are not all or even most of the references on the
topics presented (with the exception of survivors of

suicide, see Chapter 9). Because the amount of available
literature varies widely for the specific topics, the
comprehensiveness of the coverage here varies greatly. The
references cited are intended to provide basic and useful
materials, research, and writings on the many topics. It is
suggested that the reader consult the indexes and abstracts
listed below and in sections 1.2 and 1.3 as well as
reference lists of recent works to find additional sources.

Because extensive, quality bibliographies exist for the
pre-1970 literature (e.g., Farberow, 1972, reference 1-003),
few references prior to 1970 are listed. The listings are
from works published in English primarily from the mid-1970s
through 1983, with a few early 1984 references included as
well. A large number of indexes and abstract sources (the
most useful are listed in sections 1.2 and 1.3),
bibliographies (see section 1.1), books (see especially
sections 1.4 and 1.6), and periodicals were consulted in
compiling this reference guide.

Annotations have been included for noteworthy citations
or where titles were not self-explanatory. References
containing asterisks (an asterisk [*] precedes the citation
number) are selected sources that this author either
recommends to the reader or that have been especially useful
to the author in personal reading and research. The lack of
such notation does not, however, indicate that a reference
is not useful or is of less merit.

To facilitate the use and increase the usefulness of
this reference guide, abbreviations of titles of books and
journals have been avoided. For some citations a source for
an abstract of the citation is included following the
citation itself. The reader wishing to consult a brief
summary before securing the original source itself should
find these abstract sources most helpful. For these
abstract sources only have abbreviations been used. The
sources and their abbreviations are:

Psychological Abstracts [PA]
Excerpta Medica [EM]
Abstracts for Social Workers [ASW] now called Social Work
      Research and Abstracts [SWRA]
Abstracts in Criminology and Penology [ACP] now called
      Criminology and Penology Abstracts [CPA]

The only other abbreviations used are

USGPO for the United States Government Printing Office
AAS for the American Association of Suicidology
WHO for the World Health Organization.

Acknowledgments

This reference guide is the result of over five years of research and reading into the field of suicidology. I have found the work to be rewarding and stimulating, but mostly enjoyable. It is my hope that this reference guide will encourage and facilitate further investigation and study of suicidal behavior. Although accuracy in citations has been carefully checked, errors have undoubtedly occurred. I accept full responsibility for the citations as they appear here and apologize for any errors and the possible difficulty they produce.

Without a number of individuals this project would not have been compiled. I wish first to thank Dr. John Santos of the University of Notre Dame for his major contributions to my career. John has been my advisor, mentor, colleague, coauthor, and especially friend. Without his encouragement and support it would have been difficult for my studies of suicide to have even begun.

I wish also to thank a number of people and organizations who contributed to this volume: the libraries of the University of Notre Dame, the South Bend Medical Foundation, and particularly Indiana University for their cooperation and help in securing the vast majority of the works listed here; the interlibrary loan office of Indiana University at South Bend, especially Phyllis Lawrence and Sonia Marshalek who processed hundreds of requests for books and articles not contained in local libraries; the reference librarians of IUSB, particularly Donna Harlan and Linda Fleshman; Adina Wrobleski and Karen Dunne Maxim for their encouragement and aid on the topic of survivors of suicide; Sharon Valente and Judith Saunders for the citations they sent me on homosexuals and suicide; the many authors who courteously filled my reprint requests; the faculty and Jan Lootens the secretary of the Psychology Department at Indiana University at South Bend for their support and sympathetic ears over the months of this project; Dave Rotman, Dan Sprunger, and Peggy Rose of the IUSB Computing Center for their assistance at various stages in producing this manuscript; Dr. Edwin Shneidman, Dr. Norman Farberow, and Dr. Robert Litman of the Los Angeles Suicide Prevention Center for their pioneer works and writings on suicide which had a profound effect on my education in suicidology; my colleagues of the American Association of Suicidology for the intellectual stimulation and support they have given me at the six annual meetings I have attended; The Retirement Research Foundation for the research grant they awarded me which enabled me to buy a microcomputer used in both research and in much of the work on this guide; and Mary Sive of Greenwood Press for her patience and helpful suggestions during the manuscript compilation and preparation.

I wish also to thank my parents for their numerous

indirect contributions to my education and the lesson that
something worth doing is worth doing correctly. Finally,
and most importantly, I wish to thank those who have borne
the greatest burden and have indulged me the most during the
life of this endeavor. The patience, understanding, and
love of my wife Charleen and my children Kim and Shawn have
been extremely important to me.

SUICIDE LITERATURE

Even when taking into consideration the over 2300
citations in this reference guide, a clear conclusion must
be drawn: Few aspects or topics in the field of suicidology
have been resolved and further attention and the need for
more research remain for nearly all areas. Based on the
literature presented in this guide, some of the specific
aspects which require resolution follow below.

1) A broadly accepted and utilized definition of "suicide"
   is needed, not only to facilitate communication but for
   researchers, clinicians, and also for demographic,
   epidemiologic and death registration reasons.

2) A general theory of suicide recognizing not just single
   components but rather the multiple facets and factors
   producing suicidal behavior--the social, psychological,
   and biological and their interactions--is needed to
   increase our understanding and hopefully prevention of
   suicide.

3) While some have argued that little remains to be
   discovered by demographic investigations, it seems that
   the determination of the levels and trends of suicidal
   actions among high risk groups which have thus far been
   largely ignored is still warranted and needed. Certainly
   neglected or less researched groups such as racial/ethnic
   minorities, the middle aged and other adults,
   homosexuals, and Viet Nam veterans deserve closer
   scrutiny to discover the extent of suicidal behavior and
   high risk subgroups as well as research focused upon
   explanation and prevention.

4) While official data are readily available and frequently
   criticized, few have studied the extent of the data
   problems or have offered viable alternatives to them. At
   the minimum, clearer evidence as to the nature of the
   bias claimed for official figures is needed.

5) Better, more effective and earlier predictors or

indicators of individual suicide risk are needed, not only in the psychological realm but also in the social and biological.

6) Despite its inherent difficulty, a greater attempt is essential to effect global societal changes or actions that foster well being, mental health, and adaptive coping mechanisms among the populations of the various cultures.

7) Vigorous case finding techniques for discovering the high risk individuals who do not employ crisis intervention services or suicide prevention centers is needed to put such people in contact with these and other mental health services. This should be a priority of prevention activities.

8) More emphasis and continued interest in postvention also seems warranted. We still know little about survivors, their experiences, their grieving process, how they are perceived by society, or how to most effectively help them to deal with their loss.

9) Public education efforts hold great promise for prevention and should be continued and expanded. While strides have been made to improve the dissemination of information, we still do not know how much the general public knows about suicide, what "myths" are incorrectly accepted, what information should particularly be conveyed to combat incorrect information, what the most effective means of public education are regarding the recognition of the suicidal and increasing awareness of the available sources of help with this still taboo topic.

10) Relatedly, effecting attitudinal change and lessening the stigma of suicide so that it can be openly discussed and dealt with seems to be a crucial need.

11) With increased attention to the topic of suicide by the public, research on imitation and suggestion (see e.g., references 5-910--5-930) takes on added significance and needs to be further investigated.

There have been advances in knowledge and understanding in the field of suicidology, in some cases large ones, but innovative approaches and ideas are needed to significantly expand that knowledge base. Few have written specifically to the issue of the future of suicide research and treatment (among those who have are: Comstock, 1979, reference 7-065; Farberow, 1970, 1980, references 6-346.01 and 6-012; McGee, 1974, reference 6-322, pp. 281-300; Resnik & Hathorne's edited Suicide prevention in the 70s, 1973, references 2-004, 4-010b, 5-072, 6-240, 6-325, 7-075; Ringel, 1983, reference 3-017; Welu & Cam, 1972, reference 6-036). Many suggestions for future directions and needs are made in these works and it will necessitate the hard work of dedicated, organized, caring individuals--professionals, paraprofessionals, and the general public--to insure that this unnecessary cause of death and important mental health issue receives the attention it deserves.

This initial chapter provides basic information and overview sources. Contained here are general bibliographies on suicide, indexes, abstract sources, general overview references on suicide, and journals and associations interested in suicidal behavior. Chapters following the initial overview chapter present considerations of a wide range of specific subtopics in suicidology. Each is prefaced by a brief consideration of the research findings for the subtopic(s), followed by a list of bibliographies, if any, and of the critical literature. Citations are numbered consecutively from 1 within each chapter, with the chapter number and a dash preceeding the chapter citation number.

1.1 General Bibliographies on Suicide

1-001   American Association of Suicidology. Annotated suicide bibliographies. Denver: AAS.

> As mentioned in text, a number of topical bibliographies are available individually from AAS (9 were available in 1983). This is similar to Miller (1979, reference 1-010) except that there is no single compilation of the topical bibliographies into one master bibliography. The specific bibliographies will be listed in the appropriate chapters of this reference guide. For information and an order form write to AAS (see the address in Section 1.8).

1-002   Blumenthal, S. J. (1982). Annotated bibliography of suicide research, 1978-1982. Rockville, MD: National Institute of Mental Health, Suicide Research Unit.

> A 233-page annotated bibliography of suicide investigations primarily from 1980 and 1981. No indexes are included and the references are arranged essentially in a chronological fashion.

* 1-003   Farberow, N. L. (1972). Bibliography on suicide and suicide prevention, 1897-1957, 1958-1970. Washington, D.C.: USGPO, DHEW Publication No. (HSM) 72-9080 (Revision of PHS Publication No. 1970, originally published, 1969). [SuDoc Number: HE 20.2417: Su3]

> The most extensive bibliography available to

1970. Subject and author indexes for the more
than 4700 citations are included.

1-004 Farberow, N. L., Shneidman, E. S., & Bouvier,
E. A. (1961). Bibliography on suicide,
1897-1957. In N. L. Farberow & E. S. Shneidman
(Eds.), The cry for help (pp. 325-388). New
York: McGraw-Hill.

The original bibliography that was superceded
by Farberow (1972, reference 1-003) above.
The latter included these 1961 references and
an updating of the bibliographic list. The
1961 reference is categorized into broad
topics (Psychological-General, Sociological,
Medical-Legal, Religious-Philosophical).

1-005 Heinz, L. (1978). Annotated bibliography of
"Suicide": AJPH, 1911-1978, and PHR, 1930-1978.
Suicide and Life-Threatening Behavior, 8,
257-262.

A total of 40 citations from two major public
health journals, American Journal of Public
Health (21 citations) and Public Health
Reports (19 citations), are presented
chronologically and briefly annotated.

1-006 Lester, D. (1970a). Bibliography on suicide:
1968. Crisis Intervention, 2, 55-60.

1-007 Lester, D. (1970b). Bibliography on suicide:
1969. Crisis Intervention, 2, 101-105.

1-008 Lester, D. (1971). Bibliography on suicide: 1970.
Crisis Intervention, 3, 47-52.

These three bibliographies by Lester
(references 1-006--1-008) list references
written in English and published during
1968-1970. The 1969 and 1970 bibliographies
include addenda for the preceding year(s).

1-009 Lester, D., Sell, B. H., & Sell, K. D. (1980).
Suicide: A guide to information sources.
Detroit: Gale Research Company.

A source similar to the current one. Much
more attention is given to index, abstract,
and general sources of information about
suicide and much less to specific references
on specific topics. This is an excellent
source for the researcher/person/librarian
wishing to do an exhaustive search for suicide
information which includes even obscure and
little known sources of references as well as

those sources which include few references on
suicide annually. The guide may be difficult
for those new to the topic and those who have
done little library research. However, this
is a very useful guide to the topic and
references on suicide up to the mid to late
1970s.

1-010   Miller, M. (1979). Master bibliography on suicide.
San Diego, CA: Center for Information on
Suicide.

A topical (40 topics) presentation of
references on suicidal behavior (individual
topics are presented in the chapters of this
reference guide). The bibliographies are
updated regularly and are available from the
Center as a package or as individual
bibliographies (the 1984 catalog lists 30
bibliographies).

1-011   Neuringer, C. (1970, May). Suicide: A selected
bibliography. Books and Libraries at the
University of Kansas, 7(2), 1-8.

A chronological presentation and commentary on
major books published on suicide from 1894 to
1969.

1-012   Poteet, G. H., & Santora, J. C. (1978). Death and
dying: A bibliography, 1950-1974. Supplement
Volume 1, Suicide. Troy, NY: Whitson Publishing
Company.

A topical bibliography on suicide
supplementing a larger bibliography (Poteet,
G. H. (1978). Death and dying: A
bibliography for 1950-1974. Troy, NY:
Whitston.) on death and dying. A mixture of
professional and popular press sources on a
large number of topics. Includes also an
author index.

1-013   Prentice, A. E. (1974). Suicide: A selective
bibliography of over 2,200 items. Metuchen, NJ:
Scarecrow Press.

References, primarily from 1960-1973, are
categorized by type (book, dissertations,
popular press, scientific journals, etc.).
Subject and author indexes are included for
the 2,218 references presented.

1-014   Resnik, H. L. P., & Hathorne, B. C. (1974).
Teaching outlines in suicide studies and crisis
intervention. Bowie, MD: Charles Press.

A guide to teaching about topics in
suicidology which is cross-referenced with
Farberow (1972) reference 1-003 above. Also
provided are ratings of readings as
recommended or optional for each topic.

1-015 Rost, H. (1927). Bibliographie des selbstmords,
mit textlichen einfuhrungen zu jedem kapitel
[Bibliography of suicide, with textual
introductions to each chapter]. Augsburg,
Germany: Hass & Grabherr.

An early bibliography on suicide listing over
3500 references.

1-016 Schermerhorn, R. A. (Ed.). (1964). Psychiatric
index for interdisciplinary research: A guide to
the literature 1950-1961. Washington, D.C.:
USGPO. Section 63, "Suicide," pp. 1041-1047.

Compiles a list of 134 journal articles on
suicide.

1-017 Sharma, P. C. (1979). Suicide: Causes, prevention
and intervention (A selected research guide).
Monticello, IL: Vance Bibliographies, Public
Administration Series Bibliography No. P-201.

A ten page, 130 reference presentation from
1950-1974 of books and periodicals.

1.2 Indexes for References on Suicide

1-018   Current Bibliography of Epidemiology (defunct 1977)

* 1-019   Current Contents, Social and Behavioral Sciences
(weekly)

1-020   Current Index to Journals in Education (monthly)

1-021   Education Index (monthly)

* 1-022   Index Medicus (monthly)

1-023   International Bibliography of the Social
Sciences--Sociology (annually)

1-024   Science Citation Index (quarterly)

* 1-025   Social Science Citation Index (quarterly)

1-026   Social Sciences Index (quarterly)

1.3 Abstract Sources for References on Suicide

1-027   Abstracts on Criminology and Penology (formerly
        Excerpta Criminologica) (bimonthly)

1-028   Biological Abstracts (twice monthly)

1-029   Bulletin of Suicidology (defunct 1971, 8 issues
        published) SuDoc No. HE 20.2413: x/9yy (where x
        = issue number and yy = last two digits of the
        year, e.g., 1968 = 968) Included in this
        periodical was a section of abstracts on the
        suicide literature.

1-030   Dissertation Abstracts International (monthly)

* 1-031   Excerpta Medica: Section 7: Pediatrics; Section
        20: Geriatrics; Section 32: Psychiatry.

* 1-032   Psychological Abstracts (monthly)

1-033   Social Work Research & Abstracts (formerly
        Abstracts for Social Workers) (quarterly)

1-034   Sociological Abstracts (bimonthly)

1.4 General & Overview References on Suicide: Books

1-035   Cavan, R. S. (1965). Suicide. New York: Russell
        & Russell. (Originally published, Chicago:
        University of Chicago, 1926.)

1-036a Choron, J. (1972). Suicide. New York: Charles
        Scribner & Sons.

1-036b Cutter, F. (1983). Suicide prevention triangle.
        Mooro Bay, CA: Triangle Books.

          This book contains much practical information
          on many different aspects of suicide from
          prevention to assessment scales and films. A
          model of suicide prevention analogous to the
          three-part fire prevention model is presented.
          The three situations necessary but
          insufficient alone to produce suicide are
          suggested to be the wish to die, distress, and
          method. While the book is useful, the reader
          may find the numerous misspelled words and
          typographical errors distracting and annoying.

1-037   Dublin, L. I. (1963). Suicide: A sociological and
        statistical study. New York: Ronald Press.

1-038   Dublin, L. I., & Bunzel, B. (1933). To be or not
        to be: A study of suicide. New York: Random
        House.

* 1-039 Durkheim, E. (1951). <u>Suicide: A study in</u>
         <u>sociology</u> (J. A. Spaulding & G. Simpson, Trans.;
         G. Simpson, Ed.). New York: Free Press.
         (Originally published, Paris: Payot, 1897.)

         The work which began the scientific study of
         suicide and presents theoretical notions that
         continue to generate contemporary research and
         discussion (see, e.g., Section 4.3).

  1-040 Grollman, E. A. (1971). <u>Suicide: Prevention,</u>
         <u>intervention, postvention</u>. Boston: Beacon
         Press.

* 1-041 Lester, D. (1972). <u>Why people kill themselves: A</u>
         <u>summary of research on suicidal behavior</u>.
         Springfield, IL: Thomas.

* 1-042 Lester, D. (1983). <u>Why people kill themselves: A</u>
         <u>1980s summary of research findings on suicidal</u>
         <u>behavior</u> (2nd ed.). Springfield, IL: Thomas.

  1-043 Lester, G., & Lester, D. (1971). <u>Suicide: The</u>
         <u>gamble with death</u>. Englewood Cliffs, NJ:
         Prentice-Hall.

  1-044 McCulloch, J. W., & Philip, A. E. (1972). <u>Suicidal</u>
         <u>behavior</u>. New York: Pergamon Press.

  1-045 Stengel, E. (1974). <u>Suicide and attempted suicide</u>
         (rev. ed.). New York: Jason Aronson. (First
         ed., Baltimore: Penquin Books, 1964.) (Chapter
         7, "The suicide attempt as a behaviour pattern
         and its definition" (pp. 67-73), reprinted as
         "The suicide attempt" in E. S. Shneidman
         (Ed.) (1984), <u>Death: Current perspectives</u> (3rd
         ed.) (pp. 387-391). Palo Alto, CA: Mayfield.)

  1-046 Victoroff, V. M. (1983). <u>The suicidal patient:</u>
         <u>Recognition, intervention, management</u>. Oradell,
         NJ: Medial Economics Books.

* 1-047a Wekstein, L. (1979). <u>Handbook of suicidology:</u>
         <u>Principles, problems and practice</u>. New York:
         Brunner/Mazel.

  1-047b World Health Organization. (1968). <u>Prevention of</u>
         <u>suicide</u>. Geneva: WHO, Public Health Papers
         No. 35.

         In addition to prevention, this book focuses
         on education and training programs and
         statistics and research. Tables present
         suicide data for many countries. Also
         included are tables which review research
         findings regarding various correlates to

suicide, e.g., alcoholism, broken homes,
mental disorders.

1.5 General Overview References: Chapters/Journal Articles

1-048   Adam, K. S. (1967). Suicide: A critical review of
the literature. Canadian Psychiatric Association
Journal, 12, 413-420.

1-049a   Backer, B. A., Hannon, N., & Russell, N. A. (1982).
Death and dying: Individuals and institutions
(pp. 205-225). New York: Wiley, Chapter 7,
"Suicide."

* 1-049b DeSpelder, L. A., & Strickland, A. L. (1983). The
last dance: Encountering death and dying
(pp. 343-375). Palo Alto, CA: Mayfield, Chapter
12, "Suicide."

1-049c   Eddy, J. M., & Alles, W. F. (1983). Death
education (pp. 147-183). St. Louis, MO: Mosby,
Chapter 6, "Suicide."

* 1-049d Farberow, N. L. (1977). Suicide. In E. Sagarin &
F. Montanino (Eds.), Deviants: Voluntary actors
in a hostile world (pp. 503-570). Morristown,
NJ: General Learning Press.

History, theories, statistics, and prevention
are the major topics discussed in this
overview chapter.

1-050   Gibbs, J. P. (1966). Suicide. In R. K. Merton &
R. A. Nisbet (Eds.), Contemporary social problems
(2nd ed.) (pp. 281-321). New York: Harcourt,
Brace & World.

1-051   Hankoff, L. D. (1982). Suicide and attempted
suicide. In E. S. Paykel (Ed.), Handbook of
affective disorders (pp. 416-428). New York:
Guilford Press.

1-052   Hipple, J., & Cimbolic, P. (1979). The counselor
and suicidal crisis: Diagnosis and intervention
(pp. 3-14). Springfield, IL: Thomas, Chapter 1,
"An overview of suicide."

1-053   Kastenbaum, R. J. (1981). Death, society, and
human experience (2nd ed.) (pp. 238-270).
St. Louis: C. V. Mosby, Chapter 15, "Suicide."
[1st ed., 1977, pp. 266-298.]

* 1-054 Kastenbaum, R., & Aisenberg, R. (1972). The
psychology of death (pp. 251-287). New York:
Springer, Chapter 11, "Suicide."

1-055   Porterfield, A. L. (1968). The problem of suicide.
        In J. P. Gibbs (Ed.), Suicide (pp. 31-57). New
        York: Harper & Row.

           This chapter includes discussions of the
           definition of suicide, statistics, history,
           religion and suicide, philosophy and suicide,
           social and psychological theories, and
           prevention.

1-056   Resnik, H. L. P. (1980). Suicide. In
        H. I. Kaplan, A. M. Freedman, & B. J. Sandock
        (Eds.), Comprehensive textbook of psychiatry (3rd
        ed.) (pp. 2085-2098). Baltimore: Williams &
        Wilkins.

* 1-057 Shneidman, E. S. (1973). Suicide. In Encyclopedia
        britannica (Volume 21, 14th ed.) (pp. 383-385).
        Chicago: William Benton. (Reprinted in Suicide
        and Life-Threatening Behavior, 1981, 11(4),
        198-220. Reprinted in E. S. Shneidman (Ed.)
        (1980), Death: Current perspectives (2nd ed.)
        (pp. 416-434). Palo Alto, CA: Mayfield
        Publishing. Reprinted in L. D. Hankoff &
        B. Einsidler (Eds.) (1979), Suicide: Theory and
        clinical aspects (pp. 143-163). Littleton, MA:
        PSG Publishing, entitled "An overview:
        Personality, motivation, and behavior theories."
        Reprinted in E. S. Shneidman (Ed.) (1976),
        Suicidology: Contemporary developments
        (pp. 5-22). New York: Grune & Stratton,
        entitled "Introduction: Current over-view of
        suicide." Reprinted as "Suicidal logic" in
        W. S. Sahakian (Ed.) (1979), Psychopathology
        today: The current status of abnormal psychology
        (2nd ed.) (pp. 279-292). Itasca, IL: Peacock.)

1-058   Shneidman, E. S. (1976). An overview of suicide.
        Psychiatric Annals, 6(11), 13-14, 17-18, 21-22,
        29, 31, 35, 39, 43-44, 46-47.

1-059   Snyder, S. H. (1980). Biological aspects of mental
        disorders (pp. 33-44). New York: Oxford
        University Press, Chapter 3, "Suicide."

1-060   Suicide. (1968). In International encyclopedia of
        the social sciences, Volume 15 (pp. 375-396).
        New York: Macmillan Company & The Free Press.

           Three considerations of suicide are presented.

        1-060.01 Douglas, J. D. Social aspects.
                  pp. 375-385.

                     Early writings, the definition of
                     suicide, and official statistics on

suicide as well as major theories
are presented.

1-060.02   Shneidman, E. S. Psychological aspects
(1). pp. 385-390.

Definition, theories, and taxonomies
of suicide are considered.

1-060.03   Farberow, N. L. Psychological aspects
(2). pp. 390-396.

Characteristics of the suicidal
person, prediction, theories, and
factors which contribute to and
lessen the likelihood of suicide are
discussed as is the topic of
survivors.

1.6 Edited Books Considering Many Topics in Suicide

* 1-061   Farberow, N. L., & Shneidman, E. S. (Eds.) (1961).
The cry for help. New York: McGraw-Hill. [18
papers]

* 1-062   Farmer, R. D. T., & Hirsch, S. R. (Eds.) (1980).
The suicide syndrome. London: Croom Helm. [21
papers]

  1-063   Gibbs, J. P. (Eds.) (1968). Suicide. New York:
Harper & Row. [13 papers]

  1-064   Giddens, A. (Ed.) (1971). The sociology of
suicide: A selection of readings. London:
Frank Cass & Co., Ltd. [32 papers]

  1-065   Hafen, B. Q., & Faux, E. J. (1971).
Self-destructive behavior: A national crisis.
Minneapolis, MN: Burgess. [35 papers]

* 1-066   Hankoff, L. D., & Einsidler, B. (Eds.) (1979).
Suicide: Theory and clinical aspects.
Littleton, MA: PSG Publishing. [33 papers]

* 1-067   Hatton, C. L., Valente, S. M., & Rink,
A. (Eds.) (1977). Suicide: Assessment and
intervention. New York:
Appleton-Century-Crofts. [18 papers]

* 1-068   Hatton, C. L., & Valente, S. M. (Eds.) (1984).
Suicide: Assessment and intervention (2nd ed.).
Norwalk, CT: Appleton-Century-Crofts. [15
papers]

* 1-069   Perlin, S. (Ed.) (1975). A handbook for the study

of suicide. New York: Oxford University Press.
[11 papers]

* 1-070 Resnik, H. L. P. (Ed.) (1968). Suicidal behaviors:
Diagnosis and management. Boston: Little,
Brown. [38 papers]

* 1-071 Shneidman, E. S. (Ed.) (1967). Essays in
self-destruction. New York: Science House. [24
papers]

  1-072 Shneidman, E. S. (1969). On the nature of suicide.
San Francisco: Jossey-Bass. [13 papers]

* 1-073 Shneidman, E. S. (Ed.) (1976). Suicidology:
Contemporary developments. New York: Grune &
Stratton. [19 papers]

  1-074 Shneidman, E. S. (1981). Suicide thoughts and
reflections, 1960-1980. New York: Human
Sciences Press. [10 articles]

       A special issue of Suicide and
       Life-Threatening Behavior (11(4)), also
       published separately under this title. This
       collection of articles is representative of
       Shneidman's writing over the 20 year period
       and includes articles which give an overview
       (reference 1-057), and those which cover
       topics such as suicide notes (reference
       9-163), cognitive aspects (reference 5-876),
       and postvention (reference 9-067). Most of
       the articles will be cited in the appropriate
       sections of this reference guide simply as
       appearing in SLTB, 11(4).

* 1-075 Shneidman, E. S., & Farberow, N. L. (Eds.) (1957).
Clues to suicide. New York: McGraw-Hill. [18
papers]

* 1-076 Shneidman, E. S., Farberow, N. L., & Litman,
R. E. (Eds.) (1970). The psychology of suicide.
New York: Science House. [44 papers]

  1-077 Waldenstrom, J., Larsson, T., & Ljungstedt,
N. (Eds.) (1972). Suicide and attempted suicide.
Stockholm: Nordiska Bokhandelns Forlag. [20
papers]

       This is a collection of papers presented at
       the sixth Skandia International Symposia held
       in Stockholm September 28-30, 1971.

  1-078 Wilmotte, J., Mendlewicz, C., & Mendlewicz,
J. (Eds.) (1982). New trends in suicide
prevention. Basel: Karger. (Bibliotheca

Psychiatrica, No. 162.)   [7 papers]

1-079   Wolman, B. B. (Ed.) (1976). Between survival and
        suicide. New York: Gardner Press. [8 papers]

1.7 Journals

1-080   Crisis: International Journal of Suicide- and
        Crisis-Studies. Half-yearly. Published by:
        C. J. Hogrefe, Inc., 525 Eglinton Avenue East,
        Toronto, Ontario, M4P 1N5 Canada. Editor:
        Dr. Raymond Battegay, Psychiatrische
        Universitatsklinik, Kantonsspital, CH-4031 Basel.
        In the United States, Dr. Dan J. Lettieri, Chief,
        Psychosocial Branch, National Institute of Drug
        Abuse, 5600 Fishers Lane, Rockville, MD 20857;
        Dr. Norman L. Farberow, Suicide Prevention
        Center, 1041 S. Menlo Avenue, Los Angeles, CA
        90025, USA; or Dr. Robert E. Litman, 1823
        Sawtelle Blvd., Los Angeles, CA 90025, USA, may
        receive manuscripts for submission.

1-081   Essence: Issues in the Study of Ageing, Dying, and
        Death. 3 issues per year. Published by Atkinson
        College Press, 4700 Keele Street, Downsview,
        Ontario, M3J 2R7 Canada. Editor:
        Dr. S. Fleming, Department of Psychology,
        Atkinson College, 4700 Keele Street, Downsview,
        Ontario, M3J 2R7 Canada.

1-082   Omega: Journal of Death and Dying. Quarterly.
        Published by Baywood Publishing Company, Inc.,
        120 Marine Street, P. O. Box D, Farmingdale, NY
        11735. Editor: Robert J. Kastenbaum, Ph.D.,
        Department of Communications, Stauffer Hall,
        Arizona State University, Tempe, AZ 85281.

1-083   Suicide and Life-Threatening Behavior (formerly
        Life-Threatening Behavior, 1970-1974, 1-4;
        Suicide, 1975, 5). Quarterly. Published by
        Human Sciences Press, 72 Fifth Avenue, New York,
        NY 10011. Editor: Ronald W. Maris, Ph.D.,
        Department of Sociology, University of South
        Carolina, Columbia, SC 29208.

1.8 Professional Associations

1-084   American Association of Suicidology, founded 1967.
        Address: Julie Perlman, MSW, Executive Officer,
        2459 South Ash Street, Denver, CO 80222. Phone:
        (303) 692-0985.

1-085   International Association for Suicide Prevention,
        founded 1965. Address: c/o Charlotte P. Ross,
        Secretary General, Suicide Prevention and Crisis

Center, 1811 Trousdale Drive, Burlingame, CA
94010. Phone: (415) 877-5604.

1-086 National Save-A-Life League, founded 1906.
Address: 815 Second Avenue, Suite 409, New York,
NY 10017. Phone: (212) 736-6191.

1-087 The Samitarians, founded in the U.S. in 1974
(originated in Great Britain). Address: Shirley
Karnovsky, Executive Director, 802 Boylston
Street, Boston, MA 02199. Phone: (617)
247-0220.

1.9 Computer Search Sources

1-088 National Clearinghouse for Mental Health
Information Computer Search. Write to: National
Clearinghouse for Mental Health Information,
Attn: Computer Search, National Institute of
Mental Health, 5600 Fishers Lane, Rockville, MD
20857, or phone: (301) 443-4517.

1-089 National Library of Medicine Computerized Searches.
Write to: National Library of Medicine,
Literature Search Program, Reference Section,
8600 Rockville Pike, Bethesda, MD 20209, or
phone: (301) 496-4000 or (301) 496-4840.
Include your name and address typed on a gummed
label.

1-090 PASAR Computerized Literature Search. Write to:
Psychological Abstracts Information Service, 1200
Seventeenth Street, N.W., Washington, D.C.
20036, or phone: (202) 833-5908 or (800)
336-4980. Forms and guidelines are available in
the back of each Psychological Abstracts monthly
issue.

1-091 Suicide Information and Education Centre (SIEC)
Computer Searches. Write to: SIEC, Suite 201,
723-14 Street, N.W., Calgary, Alberta T2N 2A4
Canada, or phone: (403) 283-3031.

1.10 Forthcoming Works on Suicide

1-092 Death Education, Special Issue on "Suicide," due
Fall 1984.

1-093 Drummond, H. P. (due May 1984). Attempted suicide:
Guidebook for medicine, reference and research.
Annandale, VA: Abbe Publishers Association of
Washington, D.C./Virginia Division. ISBN
0881641324

1-094 Headley, L. A. (Ed.) (due February 1984). Suicide

in Asia and the Near East.   Berkeley: University of California Press.   ISBN 0520048113

1-095   Lester, D. (1984).   Suicide.   In C. S. Widom (Ed.), Sex roles in psychopathology.   New York: Plenum Press.   ISBN 0306414066

1-096   Linzer, N. (Ed.) (due 1984).   Suicide: The will to live vs. the will to die.   New York: Human Sciences Press.   ISBN 0898851564

        This book will include chapters dealing with depression and suicide, intervention, pastoral counseling, children and adolescents, family issues, and survivors of suicide among other topics.

1-097   Soubrier, J. P., & Vedrinne, J. (Eds.) (due mid-1984).   Depression and suicide: Medical, psychological, and socio-cultural aspects (Proceedings of the 11th Congress of the International Association for Suicide Prevention, Paris, France).   Fairview Park, NY: Pergamon Press.

1-098   Weightman, J. M. (due November 1983).   Making sense of the Jonestown suicides: A sociological history of People's Temple.   Lewiston, NY: Mellen.   (Studies in Religion and Society, Volume 7.)   ISBN 0889468710

See also the following "in press" articles: references 5-260, 5-479, 9-002, 9-036, 9-081.

CHAPTER 2
DEFINITIONS AND THE VARIETY OF SELF-DESTRUCTIVE BEHAVIOR

While the term "suicide" is rather recent, the behavior certainly is not (see Chapter 3 on history). The word translates literally from its origin to "to kill oneself." Those who have written and studied the phenomenon of suicide have not defined the term so simply. The definition of the term is more than simply a philosophical question. More practically, how the word is defined has implications and large effects for statistics that are compiled on the official number of suicides, and for researchers, so that there is clear communication regarding what and who is being studied.

Among writers in the field of suicidology there is no single, accepted definition. Definitions employed have often been determined by the theoretical orientation of the individual and the specific phenomena under study. Adding to the confusion and disagreement is the fact that the term suicide refers not to a single action but more broadly to a great many varied behaviors. For example, one can speak of suicidal thoughts, intentions, ideation, gestures, attempts, completions, equivalents. The term has been classified into various schemes as well (e.g., Shneidman's, 1973, reference 2-089, degrees of intention). Other terms such as "cessation", "deliberate self-harm", "life-threatening behavior," and "self-destructive behavior" have been used but the issue thus far has not been resolved.

There has been a tendency to study completed suicides (those in which death occurs) vs. suicide attempts (those in which the act ends non-fatally). Many differences between these two groups (see Section 2.2) have been noted, but controversy remains as to whether information gained via the study of attempters provides insight into completers and vice versa (see e.g., Lester, 1970, reference 2-040 vs. Kreitman et al. 1969, reference 2-039).

Another recently discussed comparison has been that of direct vs. indirect self-destructive behavior (ISDB) (see Farberow, 1980, reference 2-057.01 for such a comparison). While both of these classifications end as surely in death,

in the case of direct suicide death is quick and more
obviously what has traditionally been termed "suicide."
With ISDB, on the other hand, we consider slow forms of
suicide which hasten death but are not clearly what is
usually meant by the word "suicide." Some examples of ISDBs
would include overeating and obesity, smoking, alcoholism
and other drug addiction, risk-taking, accident proneness,
and not performing behaviors that would sustain life and
health (see the articles in Farberow, 1980, reference 2-057,
for consideration of these and other ISDBs).

Thus far, no single term, definition, or taxonomy has
served to sufficiently represent the complex set of
behaviors that have been suggested as suicidal. A standard
set of terms and definitions are greatly needed to advance
the science of suicidology and aid communication and
understanding of the field.

2.1 Definitions, Taxonomies, Classifications

2-001a Atkinson, J. M. (1971). Societal reactions to
       suicide: The role of coroners' definitions. In
       S. Cohen (Ed.), Images of deviance (pp. 165-191).
       London: Penguin Books.

2-001b Atkinson, J. M. (1978). Discovering suicide:
       Studies in the social organization of sudden
       death (pp. 87-109, esp. pp. 89-93, "An official
       definition of suicide"). Pittsburgh: University
       of Pittsburgh Press, Chapter 5, "Registering
       sudden deaths: Official definitions and
       procedures."

2-002 Beauchamp, T. L. (1978). What is suicide? In
       T. L. Beauchamp & S. Perlin (Eds.), Ethical
       issues in death and dying (pp. 97-102).
       Englewood Cliffs, NJ: Prentice-Hall.

2-003 Beck, A. T., & Greenburg, R. (1971, Fall). The
       nosology of suicidal phenomena: Past and future
       perspectives. Bulletin of Suicidology, No. 8,
       pp. 10-17.

* 2-004 Beck, A. T., Davis, J. H., Frederick, C. J.,
       Perlin, S., Pokorny, A. D., Schulman, R. E.,
       Seiden, R. H., & Wittlin, B. J. (1973).
       Classification and nomenclature. In
       H. L. P. Resnik & B. C. Hathorne (Eds.), Suicide
       prevention in the 70s (pp. 7-12). Washington,
       D.C.: USGPO, DHEW Publication No. (HSM) 72-9054.
       SuDoc No. HE 20.2402:Sn3.

2-005 Berman, A. L. (1975). Self-destructive behavior
       and suicide: Epidemiology and taxonomy. In
       A. R. Roberts (Ed.), Self-destructive behavior

(pp. 5-20). Springfield, IL: Thomas.

2-006   Burke, A. W. (1980). Classification of attempted
        suicide from hospital admission data: A
        follow-up study among Asian and West Indian
        patients in Birmingham. International Journal of
        Social Psychiatry, 26, 27-34.

2-007   Daube, D. (1972). The linguistics of suicide.
        Philosophy and Public Affairs, 1, 387-437.
        (Reprinted in Suicide and Life-Threatening
        Behavior, 1977, 7, 132-182.)

        A discussion of the terms used for "suicide"
        in various cultures and languages and their
        connotations is presented.

2-008   DeVries, A. G. (1968). Definition of suicidal
        behaviors. Psychological Reports, 22, 1093-1098.

2-009   Dodds, A. (1970). Attempted suicide: Nomenclature
        [Letter]. British Journal of Psychiatry, 117,
        121.

2-010   Douglas, J. D. (1967). The social meanings of
        suicide (pp. 350-383). Princeton, NJ: Princeton
        University Press, Appendix II, "The formal
        definitions of suicide."

2-011   Douglas, J. D. (1984). Definitions of suicide.   In
        E. S. Shneidman (Ed.), Death: Current
        perspectives (3rd ed.) (pp. 362-368). Palo
        Alto, CA: Mayfield. (Reprinted from 2-010
        above.)

2-012   Frey, R. G. (1981). Suicide and self-inflicted
        death. Philosophy, 56, 193-202.

        Frey argues that suicide does not necessarily
        have to be self-inflicted to be a suicide.

2-013   Hankoff, L. D. (1976). Categories of attempted
        suicide: A longitudinal study. American Journal
        of Public Health, 66, 558-563.

2-014   Hawton, A., Osborn, M., O'Grady, J., & Cole,
        D. (1982). Classification of adolescents who
        take overdoses. British Journal of Psychiatry,
        140, 124-131.

2-015   Henderson, A. S., Hartigan, J., Davidson, J.,
        Lance, G. N., Duncan-Jones, P., Koller, K. M.,
        Ritchie, K., McAuley, H., Williams, C. L., &
        Slaghuis, W. (1977). A typology of parasuicide.
        British Journal of Psychiatry, 131, 631-641.

2-016   Henderson, A. S., & Lance, G. N. (1979).   Types of
        attempted suicide (parasuicide). Acta
        Psychiatrica Scandinavica, 59, 31-39. (Abstract:
        PA, 1980, 63, No. 12132, p. 1351)

2-017   Katschnig, H., Sint, P., & Fuchs-Robetin,
        G. (1980). Suicide and parasuicide:
        Identification of high- and low-risk groups by
        cluster analysis. In R. D. T. Farmer &
        S. R. Hirsch (Eds.), The suicide syndrome
        (pp. 154-166). London: Croom Helm.

2-018   Lester, D. (1972). Why people kill themselves: A
        summary of research findings on suicidal
        behaviors (pp. 13-17). Springfield, IL: Thomas,
        Chapter 2, "Taxonomies of suicidal behavior."

2-019   Lester, D. (1983). Why people kill themselves: A
        1980's summary of research findings on suicidal
        behaviors (2nd ed.) (pp. 148-150). Springfield,
        IL: Thomas, Chapter 23, "Suicidal types."

2-020   Lester, G., & Lester, D. (1971). Suicide: The
        gamble with death (pp. 17-23). Englewood Cliffs,
        NJ: Prentice-Hall, Chapter 3, "Labeling death:
        Taxonomies of dying."

2-021   McIntire, M. S., & Angle, C. R. (1970). The
        taxonomy of suicide as seen in poison control
        centers. Pediatric Clinics of North America, 17,
        697-706.

2-022   Paykel, E. S. (1980). A classification of suicide
        attempters by cluster analysis. In
        R. D. T. Farmer & S. R. Hirsch (Eds.), The
        suicide syndrome (pp. 144-153). London: Croom
        Helm.

2-023   Paykel, E. S., & Rassaby, E. (1978).
        Classifications of suicide attempters by cluster
        analysis. British Journal of Psychiatry, 133,
        45-52.

2-024   Pokorny, A. D. (1974). A scheme for classifying
        suicidal behaviors. In A. T. Beck,
        H. L. P. Resnik, & D. J. Lettieri (Eds.), The
        prediction of suicide (pp. 29-44). Bowie, MD:
        Charles Press.

2-025   Shneidman, E. S. (1968a). Orientation toward
        cessation. Journal of Forensic Sciences, 13,
        33-45.

2-026   Shneidman, E. S. (1968b, July). Classifications of
        suicidal phenomena. Bulletin of Suicidology,
        No. 3, pp. 1-9. (Reprinted in B. Q. Hafen &

E. J. Faux (Eds.) (1972), <u>Self-destructive</u>
<u>behavior: A national crisis</u> (pp. 10-22).
Minneapolis, MN: Burgess.)

2-027   Shneidman, E. S. (1971). "Suicide" and
"suicidology": A brief etymological note.
<u>Life-Threatening Behavior</u>, <u>1</u>, 260-263.

2-028   Shneidman, E. S. (1980). A possible classification
of suicidal acts based on Murray's need system.
<u>Suicide and Life-Threatening Behavior</u>, <u>10</u>,
175-181.

2-029   Shneidman, E. S., Farberow, N. L., & Litman,
R. E. (1961). A taxonomy of death--A
psychological point of view. In N. L. Farberow &
E. S. Shneidman (Eds.), <u>The cry for help</u>
(pp. 129-135). New York: McGraw-Hill.

2-030   Victoroff, V. M. (1983). <u>The suicidal patient:</u>
<u>Recognition, intervention, management</u> (pp. 3-8).
Oradell, NJ: Medical Economics Books, Chapter 1,
"Kinds of suicide."

2-031   Virkkunen, M. (1974). On the difficulty of
defining suicide. <u>Medicine, Science, and the</u>
<u>Law</u>, <u>14</u>, 60-63.

2-032   Wekstein, L. (1979). <u>Handbook of suicidology:</u>
<u>Principles, problems, and practice</u> (pp. 22-37,
esp. pp. 24-35, "Terminologies and definitions of
self-destruction," "Varieties and classifications
of suicidal behavior," "Overview of terminology
and classification"). New York: Brunner/Mazel,
Chapter 2, "Orientations to suicidology."

2-033   Windt, P. Y. (1980). The concept of suicide. In
M. P. Battin & D. J. Mayo (Eds.), <u>Suicide: The</u>
<u>philosophical issues</u> (pp. 39-47). New York:
St. Martin's Press.

2-034   Zubin, J. (1974). Observations on nosological
issues in the classification of suicidal
behavior. In A. T. Beck, H. L. P. Resnik, &
D. J. Lettieri (Eds.), <u>The prediction of suicide</u>
(pp. 3-25). Bowie, MD: Chales Press.

See also Allen (1977, reference 3-001), pp. 8-9, "Definition
of suicide"; McCulloch & Philip (1972, reference 1-044),
pp. 4-5, "The problem of nomenclature"; Porterfield (1968,
reference 1-055); Shneidman (1973, reference 1-057), for
definitions and classification discussion.

See also Shneidman (1963, reference 2-089), for
classificatory schemes of suicide and one's role in their
own death.

See also Giddens (1966, reference 4-016), for a typology of
suicide;   Section 4.4 on Psychological Theories, especially
Shneidman (1976, reference 4-067).

See also Beck et al. (1975, 1976, references 6-040 and
6-045, respectively), for classifications of suicidal
intent.

2.2 Attempted ("Parasuicide") vs. Completed Suicide

* 2-035   Davis, F. B. (1967). The relationship between
            suicide and attempted suicide: A review of the
            literature. Psychiatric Quarterly, 41, 752-765.

  2-036   Dorpat, T. L., & Riley, H. S. (1967). The
            relationship between attempted suicide and
            committed suicide. Comprehensive Psychiatry, 8,
            74-79.

  2-037   Farmer, R. D. T. (1980). The relationship between
            suicide and parasuicide. In R. D. T. Farmer &
            S. R. Hirsch (Eds.), The suicide syndrome
            (pp. 19-37). London: Croom Helm.

  2-038   Kreitman, N. (1977). Parasuicide
            (esp. pp. 158-183). New York: Wiley, Chapter 9,
            "Parasuicide in relation to suicide."

  2-039   Kreitman, N., Philip, A. E., Greer, S., & Bagley,
            C. R. (1969). Parasuicide. British Journal of
            Psychiatry, 115, 746-747.

            These authors argue that attempted suicide is
            not the same or similar behavior to completed
            suicide, and therefore, a new term is
            appropriate, i.e., "parasuicide."

  2-040   Lester, D. (1970). Relation between attempted
            suicide and completed suicide. Psychological
            Reports, 27, 719-722.

            Lester contends the similarity of attempted
            and completed suicides is sufficient for
            meaningful study of attempters to learn
            something about completers.

* 2-041   Lester, D. (1972). Why people kill themselves: A
            summary of research findings on suicidal behavior
            (pp. 314-316). Springfield, IL: Thomas, Chapter
            26, "The attempted suicide and the completed
            suicide."

  2-042   Lester, D., Beck, A. T., & Trexler, L. (1975).
            Extrapolation from attempted suicides to
            completed suicides. Journal of Abnormal

Psychology, 84, 563-566.

2-043   Lester, D., Beck, A. T., & Mitchell, B. (1979).
        Extrapolation from attempted suicides to
        completed suicides: A test. Journal of Abnormal
        Psychology, 88, 78-80.

2-044   Modan, B., & Nissenkorn, I., & Lewkowski,
        S. R. (1970). Comparative epidemiological
        aspects of suicide and attempted suicide in
        Israel. American Journal of Epidemiology, 91,
        393-399.

* 2-045 Morgan, H. G. (1979). Death wishes? The
        understanding and management of deliberate
        self-harm. New York: Wiley.

            Morgan discusses fatal deliberate self-harm
            ("suicide", Part 1, pp. 3-84) and non-fatal
            deliberate self-harm (Part 2, pp. 87-158).
            Their differences are particularly stressed on
            page 97, "Suicide and non-fatal deliberate
            self-harm" and pages 134-137, "The
            relationship between non-fatal deliberate
            self-harm and suicide."

2-046   Schmid, C. F., & Van Arsdol, M. D., Jr. (1955).
        Completed and attempted suicides: A comparative
        analysis. American Sociological Review, 20,
        273-283.

2-047   Segal, B. E., & Humphrey, J. (1970). A comparison
        of suicide victims and suicide attempters in New
        Hampshire. Diseases of the Nervous System, 31,
        830-838.

* 2-048 Shneidman, E. S., & Farberow, N. L. (1961).
        Statistical comparisons between attempted and
        committed suicides. In N. L. Farberow &
        E. S. Shneidman (Eds.), The cry for help
        (pp. 19-47). New York: McGraw-Hill. (Reprinted
        as "Attempted and committed suicides," in
        E. S. Shneidman, N. L. Farberow, & R. E. Litman
        (Eds.) (1970), The psychology of suicide
        (pp. 199-225). New York: Science House.)

2-049   Sletten, I. W., Evenson, R. C., & Brown,
        M. L. (1973). Some results from an automated
        statewide comparison among attempted, committed,
        and nonsuicidal patients. Life-Threatening
        Behavior, 3, 191-197.

2-050   Stengel, E. (1968). Attempted suicides. In
        H. L. P. Resnik (Ed.), Suicidal behaviors:
        Diagnosis and management (pp. 171-189,
        esp. pp. 173-179, "Relationship between suicide

and attempted suicide"). Boston: Little Brown.

See also Piotrowski (1970, reference 6-139), for a
consideration of test differences between attempted and
completed suicides.

See also Kreitman (1981, reference 5-101).

2.3 Indirect Self-Destructive Behavior (ISDB)

2-051   Achte, K. (1979). Some forms of indirect
         self-destruction and their psychopathology. In
         K. Achte & J. Lonnqvist (Eds.), Psychopathology
         of direct and indirect self-destruction
         (Psychiatrica Fennica, Supplementum 1978)
         (pp. 35-40). Helsinki: Psychiatrica Fennica.

2-052   Barrett, G. W., & Franke, R. H. (1970).
         "Psychogenic" death: A reappraisal. Science,
         167, 304-306.

2-053   Braucht, G. N., Loya, F., & Jamieson, K. J. (1980).
         Victims of violent death: A critical review.
         Psychological Bulletin, 87, 309-333.

         The literature on suicide, accidental death,
         homicide, and especially their interrelations
         are assessed.

2-054   deCatanzaro, D. (1981). Suicide and self-damaging
         behavior: A sociobiological perspective
         (pp. 175-190). New York: Academic Press,
         Chapter 15, "Chronic self-abuse, risk-taking, and
         other self-damaging behavior."

2-055   Farberow, N. L. (Ed.) (1968). Proceedings:
         Fourth international conference for suicide
         prevention (Los Angeles, October 1967). Los
         Angeles: Delmar.

         A session on ISDB took place and abstracts for
         5 papers are included.

         2-055.01 Dizmang, L. Self-destructive behavior in
                   children: A suicidal equivalent.
                   pp. 316-320.

         2-055.02 Tabachnick, N., & Litman, R. E.
                   Self-destructiveness in accident.
                   pp. 321-327.

         2-055.03 Cantor, J. Alcoholism as a suicidal
                   equivalent. pp. 328-339.

         2-055.04 Hamburger, E. Homicidal behavior as a
                   suicide equivalent. pp. 340-344.

2-055.05   Farberow, N. L., Stein, K., Hirsch, S.,
           Darbonne, A., & Cutter, F. Indirect
           self-destructive behavior in patients
           with a diagnosis of diabetes.
           pp. 345-355.

2-056   Farberow, N. L. (1979). Research in indirect
        self-destructive behavior. In K. Achte &
        J. Lonnqvist (Eds.), Psychopathology of direct
        and indirect self-destruction (Psychiatria
        Fennica Supplementum 1978) (pp. 21-33).
        Helsinki: Psychiatria Fennica.

* 2-057   Farberow, N. L. (Ed.) (1980). The many faces of
          suicide: Indirect self-destructive behavior.
          New York: McGraw-Hill.

          26 chapters on all different aspects of ISDB
          are included.

2-057.01   Farberow, N. L. Indirect
           self-destructive behavior:
           Classification and characteristics.
           pp. 15-27.

2-057.02   Litman, R. E. Psychodynamics of indirect
           self-destructive behavior. pp. 28-40.

2-057.03   Achte, K. A. The psychopathology of
           indirect self-destruction. pp. 41-56.

2-057.04   Filstead, W. J. Despair and its
           relationship to self-destructive
           behavior. pp. 57-75.

2-057.05   Farberow, N. L. Indirect
           self-destructive behavior in diabetics
           and Buerger's disease patients.
           pp. 79-88.

2-057.06   Goldstein, A. M. The "uncooperative"
           patient: Self-destructive behavior in
           hemodialysis patients. pp. 89-98.

2-057.07   Nehemkis, A. M., & Groot, H. Indirect
           self-destructive behavior in spinal
           cord injury. pp. 99-115.

2-057.08   Ginsparg, S. L. Coronary artery illness
           and indirect self-destructive behavior.
           pp. 116-135.

2-057.09   Frederick, C. J. Drug abuse as indirect
           self-destructive behavior.
           pp. 139-155. (Reprinted in
           E. S. Shneidman (Ed.) (1980), Death:

Current perspectives (2nd ed.)
(pp. 520-530). Palo Alto, CA:
Mayfield.)

2-057.10   Ungerleider, J. T. Compulsive addictive
           behavior: Drugs and violence.
           pp. 156-169.

2-057.11   Smart, R. G. Drug abuse among
           adolescents and self-destructive
           behavior. pp. 170-186.

2-057.12   Stanton, M. D., & Coleman, S. B. The
           participatory aspects of indirect
           self-destructive behavior: The addict
           family as a model. pp. 187-203.

2-057.13   Connelly, J. C. Alcoholism as indirect
           self-destructive behavior.
           pp. 207-219.

2-057.14   Burns, M. M. Alcohol abuse among women
           as indirect self-destructive behavior.
           pp. 220-231.

2-057.15   Rowland, C. V., Jr. Hyperobesity as
           indirect self-destructive behavior.
           pp. 232-242.

2-057.16   Lichtenstein, E., & Bernstein, D. A.
           Cigarette smoking as indirect
           self-destructive behavior.
           pp. 243-253.

2-057.17   Simpson, M. A. Self-mutilation as
           indirect self-destructive behavior:
           "Nothing to get so cut up about . . ."
           pp. 257-283. (Reprinted from
           E. S. Shneidman (Ed.) (1976),
           Suicidology: Contemporary developments
           (pp. 286-315). New York: Grune &
           Stratton.)

2-057.18   Selzer, M. L. The accident process and
           drunken driving as indirect
           self-destructive activity.
           pp. 284-299.

2-057.19   Kusyszyn, I. Gambling: An
           existential-humanistic interpretation.
           pp. 300-310.

2-057.20   Toch, H. Self-destructiveness among
           offenders. pp. 313-326.

2-057.21   Hendin, H. The self-destructive roots of

delinquency. pp. 327-340.

2-057.22 James, J. Self-destructive behavior and adaptive strategies in female prostitutes. pp. 341-359.

2-057.23 Geis, G., & Huston, T. L. Altruism, risk-taking, and self-destructiveness: A study of interveners into violent criminal events. pp. 360-372.

2-057.24 Klausner, S. Z. The societal stake in stress-seeking. pp. 375-392.

2-057.25 Delk, J. L. High-risk sports as indirect self-destructive behavior. pp. 393-409.

2-057.26 Blau, T. H. The lure of the deep: Scuba diving as a high-risk sport. pp. 410-427.

2-058 Farberow, N. L., & Nehemkis, A. M. (1979). Indirect self-destructive behavior in patients with Buerger's disease. Journal of Personality Assessment, 43, 86-96.

2-059 Farberow, N. L., Stein, K., Darbonne, A. R., & Hirsch, S. (1970, May). Indirect self-destructive behavior in diabetic patients. Hospital Medicine, 6(5), 123-135.

2-060 Farberow, N. L., Stein, K., Darbonne, A. R., & Hirsch, S. (1970). Self-destructive behavior of uncooperative diabetics. Psychological Reports, 27, 935-946.

2-061 Frederick, C. J. (1972). Drug abuse as self-destructive behavior. Drug Therapy, 2, 49-68.

2-062 Frederick, C. J., Resnik, H. L. P., & Wittlin, B. J. (1973). Self-destructive aspects of hard core addiction. Archives of General Psychiatry, 28, 579-585.

2-063 Gerber, K. E., Nehemkis, A. M., Farberow, N. L., & Williams, J. (1981). Indirect self-destructive behavior in chronic hemodialysis patients. Suicide and Life-Threatening Behavior, 11, 31-42.

2-064 Grimmond, B. B. (1974, August 14). Suicide at the wheel. New Zealand Medical Journal, 80(521), 90-94.

2-065 Huffine, C. L. (1971). Equivocal single-auto

traffic fatalities. Life-Threatening Behavior,
1, 83-95.

2-066 Hutcherson, R. R., & Krueger, D. W. (1980).
Accidents masking suicide attempts. Journal of
Trauma, 20, 800-801.

2-067 Imajo, T. (1983). Suicide by motor vehicle.
Journal of Forensic Sciences, 28, 83-89.

2-068 Jenkins, J., & Sainsbury, P. (1980, October 18).
Single-car road deaths--Disguised suicides?
British Medical Journal, 281(6247), 1041.

2-069 Jury, M., & Jury, D. (1976). Gramp. New York:
Grossman Publishers. (Excerpt reprinted in
Psychology Today, February 1976, pp. 57-63.)

A pictorial account of the life and death of
the authors' grandfather, a retired coal miner
with senile dementia. Quoting from the
Psychology Today excerpt (p. 57): "On
February 11, 1974, Frank Tugend [Gramp], age
81, removed his false teeth and announced that
he was no longer going to eat or drink. Three
weeks later, to the day, he died."

2-070 Kastenbaum, R., & Mishara, B. L. (1971, July).
Premature death and self-injurious behavior in
old age. Geriatrics, 26, 71-81.

2-071 Kiev, A. (1979). The courage to live
(pp. 109-122). New York: Crowell, Chapter 8,
"Self-destructing slowly."

2-072 Knight, B. (1979). Fatal masochism--Accident or
suicide? Medicine, Science, and the Law, 19(2),
118-120.

2-073 Krueger, D. W., & Hutcherson, R. (1978). Suicide
attempts by rock-climbing falls. Suicide and
Life-Threatening Behavior, 8, 41-45.

2-074 Lester, D. (1972). Self-mutilating behavior.
Psychological Bulletin, 78, 119-128.

Lester presents the similarities of
self-mutilating behavior and true suicide.

2-075 Lester, D. (1983). Why people kill themselves: A
1980's summary of research findings on suicidal
behavior (2nd ed) (pp. 151-155). Springfield,
IL: Thomas, Chapter 24, "Other self-destructive
behaviors."

2-076 Lester, D., & Alexander, M. (1971). Suicide and

dangerous sports: Parachuting [Letter]. Journal of the American Medical Association, 215, 485.

2-077   Madison, A. (1978). Suicide and young people (pp. 64-75). New York: Seabury Press, Chapter 6, "Suicide equivalents."

2-078   Maizler, J. S., Solomon, J. R., & Almquist, E. (1983). Psychogenic mortality syndrome: Choosing to die by the institutionalized elderly. Death Education, 6, 353-364.

A literature review of the phenomenon of willing oneself to die among institutionalized elderly is presented.

2-079   McCartney, J. R. (1979). Refusal of treatment: Suicide or competent choice. General Hospital Psychiatry, 1(4), 338-343.

* 2-080   Meerloo, J. A. M. (1968). Hidden suicide. In H. L. P. Resnik (Ed.), Suicidal behaviors: Diagnosis and management (pp. 82-89). Boston: Little Brown.

2-081   Menninger, K. (1938). Man against himself (pp. 77-198, 201-306). New York: Harcourt, Brace & World, Part 3, "Chronic suicide," and Part 4, "Focal suicide."

Menninger's concepts of the many self-destructive behaviors that he called "chronic" and "focal" suicide are examples of ISDB.

2-082   Nelson, F. L., & Farberow, N. L. (1977). Indirect suicide in the elderly chronically ill patient. In K. Achte & J. Lonnqvist (Eds.), Suicide research: Proceedings of the seminars of suicide research by Yrjo Jahnsson Foundation (Psychiatria Fennica Supplementum 1976) (pp. 125-139). Helsinki: Psychiatria Fennica.

2-083   Nelson, F. L., & Farberow, N. L. (1982). The development of an indirect self-destructive behaviour scale for use with chronically ill medical patients. International Journal of Social Psychiatry, 28, 5-14.

2-084   Pokorny, A. D., Smith, J. P., & Finch, J. R. (1972). Vehicular suicides. Life-Threatening Behavior, 2, 105-120.

2-085   Reynolds, D. K., & Nelson, F. L. (1981). Personality, life situation, and life expectancy. Suicide and Life-Threatening Behavior, 11,

99-110.

Among the chronically ill institutionalized
elderly patients who were studied, it was
found that those who died within a year had
higher scores on an observation checklist of
ISDB and a suicide potential scale than did
those who survived.

2-086   Roberts, A. R. (Ed.). (1975). Self-destructive
behavior. Springfield, IL: Thomas.

This book includes a discussion of definitions
which include behaviors classified as ISDB
(see Berman, 1975, reference 2-005) and 4
chapters focusing on specific ISDBs:

2-086.01   Pokorny, A. D.   Self-destruction and the
automobile. pp. 123-137.

2-086.02   Cuskey, W. R., & Edington, B. M.   Drug
abuse as self-destructive behavior.
pp. 138-163.

2-086.03   Hertzman, M., & Bendit, E. A.   Alcoholism
and destructive behavior. pp. 164-187.

2-086.04   Waxler, S. H., & Liska, E. S.   Obesity
and self-destructive behavior.
pp. 188-210.

2-087   Samuels, D. I. (1979). The skilled nursing
facility staff Suicide Awareness Scale (S.A.S.).
Paper presented at the annual meeting of the
Gerontological Society, Washington, D.C.,
November. (Abstract in Resources in Education,
1980, 15, p. 49, ERIC document ED 184 012.)

2-088   Schmidt, C. W., Jr., Shaffer, J. W., Zlotowitz,
H. I., & Fisher, R. S. (1977). Suicide by
vehicular crash. American Journal of Psychiatry,
134, 175-178.

2-089   Shneidman, E. S. (1963). Orientations toward
death: A vital aspect of the study of lives. In
R. W. White (Ed.), The study of lives: Essays on
personality in honor of Henry A. Murray
(pp. 201-227). New York: Atherton Press.
(Reprinted in International Journal of
Psychiatry, 1966, 2, 167-200. Reprinted in
H. L. P. Resnik (Ed.) (1968), Suicidal
behaviors: Diagnosis and management (pp. 19-48).
Boston: Little Brown. Reprinted in
E. S. Shneidman, N. L. Farberow, & R. E. Litman
(Eds.) (1970), The psychology of suicide
(pp. 3-45). New York: Science House. Reprinted

as "Orientations toward death: Subintentioned death and indirect suicide." *Suicide and Life-Threatening Behavior*, 1981, 11(4), 232-253.)

2-090 Shneidman, E. S. (1973). *Deaths of man*. New York: Quandrangle.

In these two references (2-089 and 2-090) and others, Shneidman outlines his concept of cessation and the part one plays in their own death. Frequently this part is "subintentioned," where "the person plays some partial, covert, subliminal or unconscious role in hastening their own demise" (reference 2-090, p. 87).

2-091 Tabachnick, N. (1967). The psychology of fatal accident. In E. S. Shneidman (Ed.), *Essays in self-destruction* (pp. 399-413). New York: Science House.

2-092 Tabachnick, N. (1970, Spring). A theoretical approach to "accident" research. *Bulletin of Suicidology*, No. 6, pp. 18-23. (Reprinted in B. Q. Hafen & E. J. Faux (Eds.) (1972), *Self-destructive behavior: A national crisis* (pp. 85-92). Minneapolis, MN: Burgess.)

2-093 Tabachnick, N. (1973). *Accident or suicide: Destruction by automobile*. Springfield, IL: Thomas.

2-094 Tabachnick, N. (1975). Subintentioned self-destruction in teenagers. *Psychiatric Opinion*, 12, 21-26.

2-095 Tabachnick, N., Litman, R. E., Osman, M., Jones, W. L., Cohn, J., Kasper, A., & Moffat, J. (1966). Comparative psychiatric study of accidental and suicidal death. *Archives of General Psychiatry*, 14, 60-68.

2-096 Wolfgang, M. E. (1968). Suicide by means of victim-precipitated homicide. In H. L. P. Resnik (Ed.), *Suicidal behaviors: Diagnosis and management* (pp. 90-104). Boston: Little Brown.

See also research on mass media coverage of suicides and motor vehicle fatalities (e.g., Phillips, 1977, 1979, references 5-921 and 5-923 respectively, Bollen & Phillips, 1981, reference 5-913, and Bollen, 1983, reference 5-497).

Chapter 3
HISTORICAL BACKGROUND

Suicidal behavior is "probably as ancient as man himself" (Rosen, 1975, p. 3, reference 3-018) and has existed in both institutional (e.g., self-sacrifice for the good of the social group) as well as individual forms (e.g., to express anger and revenge). The word "suicide," however, is a recent one, being first used in 1651 and taken from the Latin words for "self" and "to kill" (Farberow, 1975, reference 3-009). Societies and groups within societies have varied over time from complete condemnation and total disapproval with extreme sanctions against suicide to ambiguity or no clear condemnation and even to encouraging the act.

Philosophers and religions also run the broad range described above with respect to their views of suicide (see also Chapter 8). Legal sanctions have been imposed in some places and times. In general, suicide and attempted suicide are no longer considered criminal acts but such laws do remain in some cultures (and U.S. states, see, e.g., Victoroff, 1983, pp. 229-232, reference 1-046).

Clearly, suicide has not been predominant in only a single culture or time. It has occurred in nearly all places at all times. However, an historical knowledge of suicide "provides perspective for present views" (Rosen, 1975, p. 3, reference 3-018). A similar historical view will point out that suicide is not entirely a medical or psychological phenomenon, but that these in addition to social/cultural factors as well as changes over time are important in explaining and understanding the occurrence of suicidal behavior (see Chapter 4 for theories).

3.1 General References on History

* 3-001   Allen, N. (1977). History and background of
          suicidology. In C. L. Hatton, S. M. Valente, &
          A. Rink (Eds.), Suicide: Assessment and
          intervention (pp. 1-19). New York:

Appleton-Century-Crofts.

3-002   Alvarez, A. (1972). <u>The savage god: A study of</u>
         <u>suicide</u> (pp. 45-75). New York: Random House,
         Part 2, "The background." (Reprinted in
         M. P. Battin & D. J. Mayo (Eds.) (1980),
         <u>Suicide: The philosophical issues</u> (pp. 7-32).
         New York: St. Martins Press.)

3-003   Choron, J. (1968, July). Notes on suicide
         prevention in antiquity. <u>Bulletin of</u>
         <u>Suicidology</u>, No. 4, pp. 46-48.

3-004   Cutter, F. (1983). <u>Art and the wish to die</u>
         (pp. 29-58). Chicago: Nelson-Hall, Chapter 2,
         "A chronology of suicide prevention."

         While this chapter presents the major events
         through history in the prevention of suicide,
         most of this book is historical in nature
         regarding art and suicide: see especially
         Chapters 4, "Pre-Columbian art and
         self-sacrifice" (pp. 83-94); 5, "Self-injury
         themes before the Renaissance" (pp. 95-108);
         6, "Self-injury themes after the Renaissance"
         (pp. 109-130); 7, "Suicide in the Bible"
         (pp. 131-164); 8, "Legendary women who died
         from self-injuries" (pp. 165-196); and 9,
         "Lovers and significant others" (pp. 197-222).

3-005   Davis, P. A. (1983). <u>Suicidal adolescents</u>
         (pp. 3-8). Springfield, IL: Thomas, Chapter 1,
         "The history of social attitudes toward suicide."

3-006   deCatanzaro, D. (1981). <u>Suicide and self-damaging</u>
         <u>behavior: A sociobiological perspective</u>
         (pp. 25-38). New York: Academic Press, Chapter
         3, "Historical and cross-cultural perspective."

3-007   Dublin, L. I. (1963). <u>Suicide: A sociological and</u>
         <u>statistical study</u> (pp. 83-149). New York:
         Ronald Press, Part 3, "The history of suicide."

         Seven chapters are presented: "Suicide among
         primitive peoples"; "Oriental attitudes
         toward suicide"; "Suicide in Jewish history";
         "Suicide in ancient Greece and Rome"; "The
         Christian church and suicide"; "Development
         of modern viewpoints"; "Suicide and the law."

* 3-008 Farberow, N. L. (1972). Cultural history of
         suicide. In J. Waldenstrom, T. Larsson, &
         N. Ljungstedt (Eds.), <u>Suicide and attempted</u>
         <u>suicide</u> (pp. 30-44). Stockholm: Nordiska
         Bokhandlens Forlag.

* 3-009   Farberow, N. L. (1975). Cultural history of
          suicide. In N. L. Farberow (Ed.), Suicide in
          different cultures (pp. 1-15). Baltimore:
          University Park Press. (Reprinted from 3-008
          above.)

  3-010   Fedden, H. R. (1938). Suicide: A social and
          historical study. London: Peter Davies.
          (Reprinted, New York: B. Blom, 1972 and New
          York: Arno Press, 1980).

  3-011   Fitzpatrick, J. J. (1983). Suicidology and suicide
          prevention: Historical perspectives from the
          nursing literature. Journal of Psychosocial
          Nursing and Mental Health Services, 21, 20-28.

* 3-012   Gillon, R. (1969). Suicide and voluntary
          euthanasia: Historical perspective. In
          A. B. Downing (Ed.), Euthanasia and the right to
          death: The case for voluntary euthanasia
          (pp. 173-192). London: Peter Owen.

          The views and attitudes toward suicide of
          various historical people, places, times and
          religions are discussed.

  3-013   Grollman, E. A. (1971). Suicide: Prevention,
          intervention, postvention (pp. 17-29). Boston:
          Beacon Press, Chapter 2, "Views on suicide
          throughout history."

  3-014   Guernesy, R. S. (1963). Suicide: A history of the
          penal laws in reflection to it and their legal,
          social, moral, and religious aspects in ancient
          and modern times. New York: Strouse.
          (Originally published, 1883.)

  3-015   Lum, D. (1974). Responding to suicidal crisis:
          For church and community (pp. 23-36). Grand
          Rapids, MI: William B. Eerdmans, Chapter 2,
          "Surveying historical perspectives on suicide."

          Historical surveys of philosophical and
          religious aspects of suicide are presented.

  3-016   Morgan, H. G. (1979). Death wishes? The
          understanding and management of deliberate
          self-harm (pp. 3-7). New York: Wiley, Chapter
          1, "Historical review."

  3-017   Ringel, E. (1983). Suicide prevention: Retrospect
          and outlook (on the occassion of the ten-year
          anniversary of the German Society for Suicide
          Prevention). Crisis, 4, 3-15.

          Significant milestones in the history of

suicide prevention are noted as are future
needs and trends.

* 3-018   Rosen, G. (1975). History. In S. Perlin (Ed.), A
          handbook for the study of suicide (pp. 3-29).
          New York: Oxford University Press. (Reprinted
          from "History in the study of suicide."
          Psychological Medicine, 1971, 1(4), 267-285.)

          A historical presentation of suicide and views
          about suicide from ancient times up to, but
          not including, Durkheim.

  3-019   Topp, D. O. (1971). The stepping-stones to current
          knowledge on suicide. Medicine, Science and the
          Law, 11, 131-134.

* 3-020   Valente, M. (1984). History of suicide. In
          C. L. Hatton & S. M. Valente (Eds.), Suicide:
          Assessment and intervention (2nd ed.) (pp. 1-11;
          14-15). Norwalk, CT: Appleton-Century-Crofts.

  3-021   Vieth, I. (1969, August 11). Reflections on the
          medical history of suicide. Modern Medicine,
          pp. 116-121.

3.2 References Specific to Particular Times or Groups

  3-022   Bartel, R. (1959-60). Suicide in
          eighteenth-century England: The myth of a
          reputation. Huntington Library Quarterly, 23,
          148-158.

  3-023   Cavan, R. S. (1965). Suicide. New York: Russell
          & Russell. (Originally published, 1928.)

          Includes an overview of the views of suicide
          in ancient Europe and contemporary (1920's)
          Europe and the U.S. (pp. 12-55).

  3-024   Cohn, H. (1976). Suicide in Jewish legal and
          religious tradition. Mental Health and Society,
          3, 129-136.

  3-025   Crocker, L. G. (1952). The discussion of suicide
          in the eighteenth century. Journal of the
          History of Ideas, 13, 47-52.

  3-026   Gourevitch, D. (1969). Suicide among the sick in
          classical antiquity. Bulletin of the History of
          Medicine, 43, 501-518.

  3-027   Hankoff, L. D. (1979). A first century A.D. view
          of suicide: Flavius Josephus. In L. D. Hankoff
          & B. Einsider (Eds.), Suicide: Theory and
          clinical aspects (pp. 33-45). Littleton, MA:

PSG Publishing. (Reprinted, "The theme of
suicide in the works of Flavius Josephus." <u>Clio
Medica</u>, 1976, <u>11</u>(2), 15-24. Appears also,
"Flavius Josephus: First century A.D. view of
suicide." <u>New York State Journal of Medicine</u>,
1977, <u>77</u>, 1986-1992.)

3-028 Hankoff, L. D. (1979). Judaic origins of the
       suicide prohibition. In L. D. Hankoff &
       B. Einsidler (Eds.), <u>Suicide: Theory and
       clinical aspects</u> (pp. 3-20). Littleton, MA: PSG
       Publishing.

3-029 Hankoff, L. D. (1979). Suicide and the afterlife
       in ancient Egypt. In L. D. Hankoff &
       B. Einsidler (Eds.), <u>Suicide: Theory and
       clinical aspects</u> (pp. 21-31). Littleton, MA:
       PSG Publishing. (Reprinted, "Ancient Egyptian
       attitudes towards death and suicide." <u>The Pharos
       of Alpha Omega Honor Medical Society</u>, 1975,
       <u>38</u>(2), 60-64.)

3-030 Levine, M., & Kay, P. F. O. (1971, Fall). The
       Salvation Army's anti-suicide bureau,
       London-1905. <u>Bulletin of Suicidology</u>, No. 8,
       pp. 57-63.

3-031 MacDonald, M. (1977). The inner side of wisdom:
       Suicide in early modern England. <u>Psychological
       Medicine</u>, <u>7</u>(4), 565-582.

3-032 Speijer, N. (1948). Suicide in Jewish history.
       <u>Folia Psychiatrica Neerlandica</u>, <u>51</u>, 263-274.

See Shneidman (1971, reference 2-027) for a history of the
word "suicide."

See also Chapter 8, Sprott (1961, reference 8-096), and
Hoffman & Webb (1981, reference 8-134).

Theories of suicide are primarily intended to answer the question "Why?". While a great number of specific motivations or reasons for suicide could and have been suggested, theorists attempt to more generally explain the occurrence of suicide.

No single theory has been proposed and generally accepted as the explanation of suicidal behavior. Early theoretical attempts were primarily single-disciplined in nature, coming from either a sociological or psychological/psychoanalytic perspective. Freud (see Litman, references 4-059--4-061) suggested a death instinct and inwardly turned aggression as explanations of suicide. Durkheim (see reference 4-013), on the other hand, posited three major types of suicide and employed official statistics to provide evidence of their effects and the social forces which produces them. More recent theoretical approaches have stressed multi-disciplinary factors (i.e., some combination or interaction of psychological, social, and biological forces. See, e.g., Beall, 1965, reference 4-002).

Applying the strict use of the term "theory," sociological approaches have come closest to suggesting testable, specific postulates, axioms, etc. that portend to explain suicidal behavior (as usually measured by suicide rates). Psychological proposals are more properly "mini-theories" or specialized hypotheses which attempt to explain various components or single facets of suicidal behavior, but not the more general· phenomenon. It seems likely, however, that only a theory which encompasses and considers the variety of contributing factors to suicide will provide an understanding of suicidal behavior. Thus far, no such single theory exists. Present theoretical notions do however provide us with some insight into why people kill themselves.

4.1 General References on Suicide Theories

4-001   Alvarez, A. (1972). The savage god: A study of suicide (pp. 91-118). New York: Random House, "Theories."

4-002   Beall, L. (1965, March). The dynamics of suicide: A review of the literature, 1897-1965. Bulletin of Suicidology, No. 5, pp. 2-16.

Sociological, psychological, and social-psychological explanations of suicide are presented. It was concluded that interdisciplinary approaches were becoming more prominent.

4-003   Grollman, E. A. (1971). Suicide: Prevention, intervention, postvention (pp. 33-41). Boston: Beacon Press, Chapter 3, "The theorists."

A presentation of Durkheim's theory and several psychological explanations--those of Freud, Menninger, Adler, Jung, Hillman, Sullivan, and Horney.

4-004   Jackson, D. D. (1957). Theories of suicide. In E. S. Shneidman & N. L. Farberow (Eds.), Clues to suicide (pp. 11-21). New York: McGraw-Hill.

Psychoanalytic and nonpsychoanalytic theories are presented.

4-005   Krauss, H. H. (1976). Suicide--A psychosocial phenomenon. In B. B. Wolman (Ed.), Between survival and suicide (pp. 25-54). New York: Gardner.

The theories of Freud, Durkheim, Dollard, and Naroll are discussed, especially as they relate to interpersonal relations and suicide.

4-006   Leonard, C. V. (1967). Understanding and preventing suicide. Springfield, IL: Thomas.

Social, psychological, and psychosocial theories are discussed (pp. 305-312) as is a developmental theory (Chapter 7, pp. 313-328).

* 4-007   Lettieri, D. J. (1978). Theories of suicide. In D. J. Lettieri (Ed.), Drugs and suicide: When other coping strategies fail (pp. 13-30). Beverly Hill, CA: Sage Publications.

Brief coverage of many theories of suicide, including Jung, Adler, Sullivan, Freud, Kelly, Durkheim, and Henry and Short.

4-008 Lum, D. (1974). <u>Responding to suicidal crisis:</u>
<u>For church and community</u> (pp. 37-60). Grand
Rapids, MI: William B. Eerdmans, Chapter 3,
"Assessing theories of self-destruction and
suicide."

The sociological theories of Durkheim, Henry &
Short, Maris, Gibbs & Martin, and Porterfield
are discussed as well as the psychological
contributions to theory of Freud, Jung, Adler,
Sullivan, Horney, Menninger, Shneidman, and
Berne.

4-009 Peck, D. L. (1979). <u>Fatalistic suicide</u>
(esp. pp. 11-76). Palo Alto, CA: R & E Research
Associates, Chapter 2, "Theories of suicide,"
(pp. 11-46), Chapter 3, "Fatalism."

Peck presents psychological, sociological,
social-psychological theories and the Model of
Failure in Chapter 2 and in Chapter 3 he
advances fatalism as a contemporary theory of
suicidal behavior (this is tested and
discussed in later chapters, see references
4-044 and 4-045 below).

4-010a Rushing, W. A. (1968). Individual behavior and
suicide. In J. P. Gibbs (Ed.), <u>Suicide</u>
(pp. 96-121). New York: Harper & Row.

General theories of suicide--psychoanalytic,
interaction, symbolic interaction, field
theory, social integration, Durkheimian, and
Powell's--and of homicide and suicide are
summarized and evaluated.

4-010b Weisman, A., Feifel, H., Henley, C., Hiltner, S.,
Kalish, R. A., Kastenbaum, R., Nelson, Z., &
Tabachnick, N. D. (1973). Death and
self-destructive behaviors. In H. L. P. Resnik &
B. C. Hathorne (Eds.), <u>Suicide prevention in the</u>
<u>70's</u> (pp. 13-22). Washington, D.C.: USGPO, DHEW
Publication No. (HSM) 72-9054. SuDoc No. HE
20.2402:Sn3.

See reference 1-060 and its articles by Douglas, reference
1-060.01, Shneidman, reference 1-060.02, and Farberow,
reference 1-060.03 for discussions of theories of suicide.
See also Bohannan (1960, reference 5-424), Chapter 1,
"Theories of homicide and suicide," pp. 3-29.

4.2 <u>Sociological Theories/Explanations of Suicide</u>

4-011 Cresswell, P. (1972). Interpretations of
[Durkheim's] <u>Suicide</u>. <u>British Journal of</u>
<u>Sociology</u>, <u>23</u>, 133-145.

* 4-012 Douglas, J. D. (1967). The social meanings of
         suicide. Princeton, NJ: Princeton University
         Press.

              In addition to presenting Durkheim's theory of
              suicide (pp. 13-77), Post-Durkheimian theories
              (Gibbs & Martin, pp. 84-91; Powell,
              pp. 92-94; Ecological theories, pp. 95-108;
              Status change theories, pp. 109-123;
              Halbwach, pp. 124-131; Henry & Short,
              pp. 132-143; Gold, pp. 144-151), their
              weaknesses and contributions, Douglas focuses
              on the social meaning of suicide and its place
              in explaining suicidal behavior.

* 4-013 Durkheim, E. (1951). Suicide: A study in
         sociology (J. A. Spaulding & G. Simpson, Trans.;
         G. Simpson, Ed.). New York: Free Press.
         (Originally published, 1897.)

              The classic book putting forth and testing
              (using statistics) three types of suicide,
              altruistic, anomic, and egoistic (as well as a
              fourth type, fatalistic, in a footnote,
              p. 276). As seen below in Section 4.3, the
              theory continues to generate contemporary
              research and discussion.

  4-014 Gibbs, J. P. (1966). Suicide. In R. K. Merton &
         R. A. Nisbet (Eds.), Contemporary social problems
         (2nd ed.) (pp. 281-321, esp. pp. 308-321,
         "Particular theories on variation in suicide
         rates"). New York: Harcourt, Brace & World.

              Gibbs discusses various sociological theories
              of suicide, especially those of Durkheim,
              Henry and Short, and Gibbs and Martin.
              Detailed information on various demographic
              variables and suicide are also presented.

* 4-015 Gibbs, J. P., & Martin, W. T. (1964). Status
         integration and suicide. Eugene: University of
         Oregon Press. (Pages 14-31 are reprinted in
         A. Giddens (Ed.) (1971), The sociology of
         suicide: A selection of readings (pp. 67-86).
         London: Frank Cass & Co.)

              An elaboration of a portion of Durkheim's
              theory that has become recognized as a
              separate theory.

  4-016 Giddens, A. (1966). A typology of suicide.
         European Journal of Sociology, 7, 276-295.
         (Reprinted in A. Giddens (Ed.) (1971), The
         sociology of suicide: A selection of readings
         (pp. 97-120). London: Frank Cass & Co.)

Durkheim's theory and its applications are considered.

4-017   Ginsberg, R. B. (1980). Anomie and aspirations: A reinterpretation of Durkheim's theory. New York: Arno Press. (A reprint of Ginsberg's 1967 doctoral dissertation with additional prefacing comments and an appendix.)

4-018   Halbwachs, M. (1975). The causes of suicide. New York: Arno Press. (Originally published, 1930.)

* 4-019   Henry, A. F, & Short, J. F., Jr. (1954). Suicide and homicide: Some economic, sociological, and psychological aspects of aggression. New York: Free Press.

4-020   Henry, A. F., & Short, J. F., Jr. (1957). The sociology of suicide. In E. S. Shneidman & N. L. Farberow (Eds.), Clues to suicide (pp. 58-69). New York: McGraw-Hill. (A portion of this chapter is reprinted under the title "Suicide and external restraint," in A. Giddens (Ed.) (1971), The sociology of suicide: A selection of readings (pp. 58-66). London: Frank Cass and Co.)

4-021   Holland, R. F. (1970). Suicide as a social problem: Some reflections on Durkheim. Ratio, 12, 116-124.

4-022   Huff, T. E. (1975). Discovery and explanation in sociology: Durkheim on suicide. Philosophy of the Social Sciences, 5, 241-257.

4-023   Hynes, E. (1975). Suicide and homo-duplex: An interpretation of Durkheim's typology of suicide. Sociological Quarterly, 16, 87-104.

4-024   Johnson, B. D. (1965). Durkheim's one cause of suicide. American Sociological Review, 30, 875-886.

* 4-025   Lester, D. (1972). Why people kill themselves: A summary of research findings on suicidal behavior (pp. 75-114). Springfield, IL: Thomas, Chapter 10, "Sociological theories of suicide."

* 4-026   Lester, D. (1983). Why people kill themselves: A 1980's summary of research findings on suicidal behavior (2nd ed.) (pp. 31-34). Springfield, IL: Thomas, Chapter 5, "Sociological theories of suicide."

The 1972 edition (reference 4-025) presents

the various sociological theories of suicide
(Durkheim, Johnson, Powell, Ginsburg, Gibbs &
Martin, Henry & Short, Douglas) and research
related to them through the 1960's. The 1983
edition (reference 4-026) presents subsequent
studies conducted through the late 1970's on
the theories.

4-027   Lester, G., & Lester, D. (1971). Suicide: The
        gamble with death (pp. 116-126). Englewood
        Cliffs, NJ: Prentice-Hall, Chapter 15,
        "Sociological theories of suicide."

        A popularized version of the Lester (1972,
        reference 4-025) chapter.

4-028   Maris, R. W. (1969). Social forces in urban
        suicide. Homewood, IL: Dorsey Press.

        Durkheim's theory (pp. 20-44), its historical
        place and results (pp. 45-61), and the
        implications of Maris' research for Durkheim's
        theory (pp. 159-176) are given as is an
        attempt at a more systematic sociological
        theory of suicide (pp. 177-189).

4-029   Maris, R. W. (1981). Pathways to suicide: A
        survey of self-destructive behaviors. Baltimore:
        John Hopkins University Press.

        Following careful analyses and the comparing
        of 300 completed suicides with attempters and
        natural deaths, Maris posits a theory
        (esp. pp. 287-340).

4-030   Martin, W. T. (1968). Theories of variation in the
        suicide rate. In J. P. Gibbs (Ed.), Suicide
        (pp. 74-96). New York: Harper & Row.

        Martin gives and discusses the major
        sociological theories of suicide (Durkheim,
        Halbwach, Henry & Short, Gibbs & Martin).

4-031   Nolan, P. D. (1979). Role distance is suicide: A
        cumulative development in theory. Sociology and
        Social Research, 64, 99-104.

        A discussion of Durkheim's theory of suicide
        and how Goffman's "role distance" can be seen
        as an extension of it.

4-032   Pope, W. (1975). Concepts and explanatory
        structure in Durkheim's theory of suicide.
        British Journal of Sociology, 26, 417-434.

4-033   Pope, W. (1982). Durkheim's Suicide: A classic

analyzed. Chicago: University of Chicago Press.

4-034 Rootman, I. (1973). A cross-cultural note on
       Durkheim's theory of suicide. Life-Threatening
       Behavior, 3, 83-94.

* 4-035 Stack, S. (1982). Suicide: A decade review of the
         sociological literature. Deviant Behavior, ((4,
         41-66. (Abstract: PA, 1983, 70, No. 8230,
         p. 922)

         Similar to Lester (1983, reference 4-026)
         above, Stack reviews the sociological
         literature from the 1970's and highlights
         especially research findings as they relate to
         theories and explanations of suicide.

4-036 Taylor, S. (1982). Durkheim and the study of
       suicide. New York: St. Martin's Press.

       Durkheim's (pp. 3-21) and other sociological
       theories (pp. 22-40) are considered, and a
       social-psychological approach advanced
       (pp. 161-193).

4-037 Thompson, K. (1982). Emile Durkheim (pp. 109-121).
       London: Tavistock Publications.

       A book on Durkheim which includes a discussion
       of his book Suicide and the major theoretical
       points made therein.

4.3 Examples of Contemporary Research on Sociological Theory

4-038 Boor, M. (1979). Anomie and United States suicide
       rates, 1973-1976. Journal of Clinical
       Psychology, 35, 703-706.

4-039 Breault, K. D., & Barkey, K. (1982). A comparative
       analysis of Durkheim's theory of egoistic
       suicide. Sociological Quarterly, 23, 321-331.
       (Abstract: PA, 1983, 70, No. 1230, p. 144.)
       [Stack, S. (1983). A comparative analysis of
       Durkheim's theory of egoistic suicide: A
       comment. 24, 625-627. Breault, K. D., & Barkey,
       K. (1983). Reply to Stack: Durkheim scholarship
       and suicidology: Different ways of doing
       research in history of social thought, and
       different interpretations of Durkheim's Suicide.
       24, 629-632.]

4-040 Collette, J., Webb, S. D., & Smith, D. L. (1979).
       Suicide, alcoholism and types of social
       integration: Clarification of a theoretical
       legacy. Sociology and Social Work, 63, 699-721.

4-041   Danigelis, N., & Pope, W. (1979). Durkheim's
        theory of suicide as applied to the family: An
        empirical test. Social Forces, 57, 1081-1106.

4-042   Gibbs, J. P. (1982). Testing the theory of status
        integration and suicide rates. American
        Sociological Review, 47, 227-237.

4-043   Gibbs, J. P., & Martin, W. T. (1981). Still
        another look at status integration and suicide.
        Social Forces, 59, 815-823.

4-044   Peck, D. L. (1979). Fatalistic suicide
        (esp. pp. 77-111). Palo Alto, CA: R & E
        Research Associates, Chapter 4, "Research methods
        and procedures" (pp. 77-89), Chapter 5, "Results"
        (pp. 90-105), Chapter 6, "Summary and
        conclusions" (pp. 106-111).

4-045   Peck, D. L. (1980-81). Towards a theory of
        suicide: The case for modern fatatlism. Omega,
        11, 1-14.

        Peck argues that Durkheim's minor type of
        suicide--fatalistic--has more contemporary
        importance than Durkheim placed upon it.

4-046   Schalkwyk, J., Lazer, C., & Cumming, E. (1979).
        Another look at status integration and suicide.
        Social Forces, 57, 1063-1080.

4-047   Stack, S. (1979). Durkheim's theory of fatalistic
        suicide: A cross-national approach. Journal of
        Social Psychology, 107, 161-168.

4.4 Psychological & Psychoanalytic Theories/Explanations

4-048   Adler, A. (1958). Suicide. Journal of Individual
        Psychology, 14, 57-61. (Reprinted after
        translation and editing from Internationale
        Zeitschrift fur Individual Psychologie, 1937, 15,
        49-52. Reprinted in J. P. Gibbs (Ed.) (1968),
        Suicide (pp. 146-150). New York: Harper & Row.)

4-049   Ansbacher, H. L. (1969). Suicide as communication:
        Adler's concept and current applications.
        Journal of Individual Psychology, 25, 174-180.

4-050   Ansbacher, H. L. (1970). Suicide as communication:
        Adler's concept and current applications.
        Humanitas, 6, 5-11.

4-051   Farberow, N. L. (1961). Introduction and case
        history of Mr. A. S. In N. L. Farberow &
        E. S. Shneidman (Eds.), The cry for help
        (pp. 153-166). New York: McGraw-Hill.

Farberow presents a case followed by seven theoretical interpretations of the case from various psychological viewpoints.

4-051.01   Futterman, S. Suicide: Psychoanalytic point of view (pp. 167-180).

4-051.02   Hendin, H. Suicide: Psychoanalytic point of view (pp. 181-192).

4-051.03   Klopfer, B. Suicide: The Jungian point of view (pp. 193-203).

4-051.04   Ansbacher, H. L. Suicide: The Adlerian point of view (pp. 204-219).

4-051.05   Green, M. R. Suicide: The Sullivanian point of view (pp. 220-235).

4-051.06   De Rosis, L. E. Suicide: The Horney point of view (pp. 236-254).

4-051.07   Kelly, G. A. Suicide: The personal construct point of view (pp. 255-280).

4-052   Friedman, P. (Ed.) (1967). On suicide: With particular reference to suicide among young students. New York: International Universities Press.

A translation of 1910 discussions of the Vienna Psychoanalytic Society (prior to the secession of some members). Participants included Adler, Freud, Friedjung, Molitor, Oppenheim, Reitler, Sadger, and Stekel.

4-053   Hendin, H. (1963). The psychodynamics of suicide. Journal of Nervous and Mental Disease, 136, 236-244. (Reprinted in J. P. Gibbs (Ed.) (1968), Suicide (pp. 133-146). New York: Harper & Row.)

4-054   James, N. (1984). Psychology of suicide. In C. L. Hatton & S. M. Valente (Eds.), Suicide: Assessment and intervention (2nd ed.) (pp. 34-53). Norwalk, CT: Appleton-Century-Crofts.

4-055   Jeger, A. M. (1979). Behavior theories and their application. In L. D. Hankoff & B. Einsidler (Eds.), Suicide: Theory and clinical aspects (pp. 179-199). Littleton, MA: PSG Publishing.

4-056   Kilpatrick, E. (1948). A psychoanalytic understanding of suicide. American Journal of

Psychoanalysis, 8, 13-23. (Reprinted in
J. P. Gibbs (Ed.) (1968), Suicide (pp. 151-169).
New York: Harper & Row.)

4-057   Lester, D. (1972). Why people kill themselves: A
summary of research findings on suicidal behavior
(pp. 208-218). Springfield, IL: Thomas, Chapter
19, "Suicide as an act of aggression: The
psychoanalytic theory of suicide."

4-058   Lester, G., & Lester, D. (1971). Suicide: The
gamble with death (pp. 52-55). Englewood Cliffs,
NJ: Prentice-Hall, Chapter 7, "Suicide and
aggressiveness."

4-059   Litman, R. E. (1966). Sigmund Freud on suicide.
Psychoanalytic Forum, 2, 206-221.

* 4-060   Litman, R. E. (1967). Sigmund Freud on suicide.
In E. S. Shneidman (Ed.), Essays on
self-destruction (pp. 324-344). New York:
Science House. (Reprinted in E. S. Shneidman,
N. L. Farberow, & R. E. Litman (Eds.) (1970),
The psychology of suicide (pp. 565-586). New
York: Science House.)

4-061   Litman, R. E. (1968, July). Sigmund Freud on
suicide. Bulletin of Suicidology, pp. 11-23.

4-062   Litman, R. E., & Tabachnick, N. D. (1968).
Psychoanalytic theories of suicide. In
H. L. P. Resnik (Ed.), Suicidal behaviors:
Diagnosis and management (pp. 73-81). Boston:
Little, Brown.

4-063   Meissner, W. W. (1977). Psychoanalytic notes on
suicide. International Journal of Psychoanalytic
Psychotherapy, 6, 415-447.

* 4-064   Menninger, K. (1938). Man against himself. New
York: Harcourt, Brace & World.

4-065   Neimeyer, R. A. (1983). Toward a personal
construct conceptualization of depression and
suicide. Death Education, 7, 127-173.

4-066   Neuringer, C. (1974). Validation of the cognitive
aspect of Adler's theory of suicide. Journal of
Individual Psychology, 30, 59-64.

4-067   Shneidman, E. S. (1976). A psychological theory of
suicide. Psychiatric Annals, 6(11), 51, 53, 57,
60-62, 66. (Reprinted in Suicide and
Life-Threatening Behavior, 1981, 11(4), 221-231.)

4-068   Tabachnick, N. (1972). Theories of

self-destruction. <u>American Journal of
Psychoanalysis</u>, <u>32</u>, 53-61.

> Tabachnick presents psychological theories in
> three categories: those suggesting a death
> instinct, those centering on mental illness,
> and those speaking of adaptational failure.

4-069 Taylor, S. (1982). <u>Durkheim and the study of
suicide</u> (pp. 125-139). New York: St. Martin's
Press, Chapter 6, "Individualistic approaches to
suicide."

4.5 <u>Other Theories/Explanations of Suicide</u>

4-070 Atkinson, J. M. (1978). <u>Discovering suicide:
Studies in the social organization of sudden
death</u> (pp. 148-174). Pittsburgh, PA: University
of Pittsburgh Press, Chapter 7, "Common-sense
theorizing about suicide."

> Atkinson questions sociological theory on the
> basis that the data employed, usually official
> statistics, are flawed (see also Chapter 5),
> and suggests that "theorizing" to make sense
> of suicide deaths is common among coroners,
> medical examiners, etc.

4-071 Baechler, J. (1979). <u>Suicides</u> (B. Cooper, Trans.).
New York: Basic Books. (Originally published,
1975.) (Chapter 1, "A strategic theory,"
reprinted in <u>Suicide and Life-Threatening
Behavior</u>, 1980, <u>10</u>, 70-99, and in E. S. Shneidman
(Ed.) (1980), <u>Death: Current perspectives</u> (2nd
ed.) (pp. 491-519). Palo Alto, CA: Mayfield
Publishing.)

4-072 Blaker, K. P. (1972). Systems theory and
self-destructive behavior: A new theoretical
base. <u>Perspectives in Psychiatric Care</u>, <u>10</u>,
168-172.

4-073 deCatanzaro, D. (1980). Human suicide: A
biological perspective. <u>Behavioral and Brain
Sciences</u>, <u>3</u>, 265-290. (Article appears on
pp. 265-272, open peer commentary and the
author's response follow on pp. 272-290.)

> Pointing out the importance of biology in
> suicide, deCatanzaro suggests four heuristic
> models "to account for suicide in an
> evolutionary and sociobiological framework"
> (p. 265). After considering each model, he
> concludes that suicides come from a select
> subpopulation, those unlikely to promote their
> genes.

4-074   deCatanzaro, D. (1981).   Suicide and self-damaging
        behavior: A sociobiological perspective.   New
        York: Academic Press.

            Further elaboration and presentation of the
            arguments advanced in deCatanzaro (1980,
            reference 4-073), above.

4-075   Draper, E. (1976).   A developmental theory of
        suicide.   Comprehensive Psychiatry, 17, 63-80.

4-076   Farber, M. L. (1968).   Theory of suicide.   New
        York: Funk & Wagnalls.   (Reprinted 1977, New
        York: Arno Press.)

            Positing a general theory of suicide based on
            hope as the crucial element.

4-077   Goldney, R. D. (1980).   Attempted suicide: An
        ethological perspective.   Suicide and
        Life-Threatening Behavior, 10, 131-141.

4-078   Hamermesh, D. S., & Soss, N. M. (1974).   Economic
        theory of suicide.   Journal of Political Economy,
        82, 83-98.

4-079   Hendin, H. (1982).   Suicide in America (pp. 13-25).
        New York: Norton, Chapter 1, "A psychosocial
        perspective."

4-080   Kobler, A. L., & Stotland, E. (1964).   The end of
        hope: A social-clinical study of suicide.   New
        York: Free Press.

            The suggestion is made that the response of
            others to the individual's plea will determine
            whether one will commit suicide.

4-081   Krauss, H. H., & Krauss, B. J. (1968).
        Cross-cultural study of the
        thwarting-disorientation theory of suicide.
        Journal of Abnormal Psychology, 73, 353-357.

4-082   Nelson, F. L. (1980).   Social and hedonistic
        utility: A conceptual model of self-destructive
        behavior.   Crisis, 1, 125-133.

Chapter 5
DEMOGRAPHY AND EPIDEMIOLOGY OF SUICIDE:
STATISTICS AND RISK FACTORS

As can be seen from the length of this chapter, the greatest number of works in suicidology have been directed toward the determination of the factors associated with high risk of suicidal behavior and the extent of suicidal actions. This approach is directly traceable at least to Durkheim's 1897 work <u>Suicide</u> (reference 5-092) which put forth a theory of suicide and attempted to present evidence for that theory based on the suicide statistics of the time. The use of official statistics has been widespread in the suicide literature and has sparked great debate on the merits, usefulness, and detriments of such figures (see Section 5.2 especially). For other suicide-related behaviors, however, few if any statistics exist and available figures are based on estimates or empirically collected data (one such example is attempted suicide).

As stated in the introductory chapter, there are currently approximately 30,000 annual official suicides in the U.S., for a rate of 12-13 per 100,000 population. The highest risk groups among these suicides are most typically whites, males, the elderly, the widowed or divorced. Firearms are the most common method and their use is increasing among nearly all groups (see Section 5.10a). While suicide rates have increased dramatically in recent years for the young (making them an increasingly important target group for preventive measures and attention, see Section 5.6c) and decreased markedly for the old, the aged continue to have the highest rates of suicide (see Section 5.6f). Overall rates have increased for nonwhites as a whole, but the rates remain considerably lower than for whites (great variation exists between nonwhite groups, however, see Section 5.7). Discussions in the literature of lessening sex differences in suicide (see Section 5.5) have not been supported by post-1970 data. Female suicide rates are still considerably lower than those for males and remain at a ratio of approximately 3:1 (male to female suicides).

Suicide attempters have quite different characteristics

(see also Section 2.2). The young and females are the highest risk for non-fatal suicide attempts and drugs are the most common method.

While cultural differences are observed and often large, the basic relationships of the major demographic variables are found in most countries (see Section 5.9). Most of the literature presented here focuses on the U.S., England & Wales, and Australia because of the restriction made to include only articles written in English, but selected articles for other countries (written in English) have also been included (see Section 5.9c and the subject index).

Among the other high risk groups, aspects and factors that research has uncovered are: the socially isolated; those experiencing recent loss; those experiencing interpersonal conflict or problems, including marital or family discord; those lacking personal resources; the unemployed; those with mental disorders, especially depression, alcoholism, and schizophrenia; those who do not communicate well or at all with those around them; prisoners; physicians; police officers; those with physical illnesses. While Monday is consistently the highest day of the week for suicide, weather conditions seem to have little or no effect on suicidal behavior and the highest season is Spring.

The literature on the subjective experience of suicidal individuals indicates that among the feelings they have are: hopelessness, helplessness, haplessness, despair, pessimism, powerlessness, lack of (or out of) control, worthlessness, dysphoria (depression), and unhappiness. The suicidal typically have "tunnel vision," that is, they fail to see alternatives to their circumstances and ways of coping with them. However, those who contemplate suicide are also felt to experience ambivalence, i.e., the wish to die at the same time as the wish to live. The communications of intent of the suicidal are often interpreted as cries for help, appeals to help one escape from an existence perceived as unbearable and from which the person feels they cannot themselves escape.

5.1 Sources of Official U.S. Suicide Data

5-001   Diggory, J. C. (1976). United States suicide
        rates, 1933-1968: An analysis of some trends.
        In E. S. Shneidman (Ed.), Suicidology:
        Contemporary developments (pp. 30-69). New York:
        Grune & Stratton.

5-002   Grove, R. D., & Hetzel, A. M. (1968). Vital
        statistics rates in the United States 1940-1960.
        Washington, D.C.: United States Government
        Printing Office (USGPO).

5-003   Linder, F. E., & Grove, R. D. (1943). Vital
        statistics rates in the United States 1900-1940.
        Washington, D.C.: USGPO.

5-004   Massey, J. T. (1967). Suicide in the United
        States, 1950-1964. Vital and Health Statistics,
        Series 20, No. 5, Public Health Service
        Publication No. 1000.

5-005   McIntosh, J. L. (1980). A study of suicide among
        United States racial minorities based on official
        statistics: The influence of age, sex, and other
        variables (Doctoral dissertation, University of
        Notre Dame, 1980). Dissertation Abstracts
        International, 41, 1135B. (University Microfilms
        No. 8020965)

            This doctoral dissertation includes 144 pages
            of figures and tables which compile suicide
            data from many sources predominantly for the
            characteristics of age and race/ethnicity.

* 5-006   National Center for Health Statistics. Annual
        volumes of Vital Statistics of the United States,
        Parts I & II (for 1937-1949 data), Volume II (for
        1950-1959 data), Volume II--Mortality, Parts A &
        B (for 1960-1978 data currently). [Prior to
        1937, published data for 1900-1936 may be found
        in Mortality Statistics.] Washington, D.C.:
        USGPO.

5-007   National Center for Health Statistics. (1982,
        September 30). Advance report of final mortality
        statistics, 1979. Monthly Vital Statistics
        Report, 31(6, Supplement).

5-008   National Center for Health Statistics. (1982,
        December 20). Annual summary of births, deaths,
        marriages, and divorces: United States, 1981
        [provisional data]. Monthly Vital Statistics
        Report, 30(13).

5-009   National Center for Health Statistics. (1983,
        August 11). Advance report of final mortality
        statistics, 1980. Monthly Vital Statistics
        Report, 32(4, Supplement).

5-010   National Center for Health Statistics. (1983,
        October 5). Annual summary of births, deaths,
        marriages, and divorces: United States, 1982
        [provisional data]. Monthly Vital Statistics
        Report, 31(13).

5-011   National Office of Vital Statistics. (1956, August
        22). Death rates by age, race, and sex: United
        States, 1900-1953: Suicide. Vital Statistics

Special Reports, 43(30).

5-012   United States Bureau of the Census. Annual volumes
         of Statistical Abstract of the United States.
         Washington, D.C.: USGPO.

            Some suicide data may be found in the "Vital
            Statistics" chapter. The most current volume
            is for 1982-83 (103rd ed., published in 1982).
            The data presented are generally 3-4 years
            behind the year of the volume.

Other Countries:

5-013   United Nations. Annual volumes of Demographic
         Yearbook. New York: United Nations.

5-014   World Health Organization. Annual volumes of World
         health statistics annual. Geneva: WHO.

For other possible sources, see Lester et al. (1980,
reference 1-009), Chapter 7, "Suicide statistics."

The addresses of U.S. state vital statistics agencies are
available from the National Center for Health Statistics,
3700 East-West Highway, Hyattsville, Maryland 20782.

5.2 Discussions of Official Statistics as Sources of Data

5-015   Alderson, M. (1981). International mortality
         statistics. New York: Facts on File, Inc.

            While Alderson includes some suicide data, his
            main discussions center on the use, validity,
            and registration systems for mortality
            statistics in different countries.

5-016   Allen, N. (1984). Suicide statistics. In
         C. L. Hatton & S. M. Valente (Eds.), Suicide:
         Assessment and intervention (2nd
         ed.) (pp. 17-31). Norwalk, CT:
         Appleton-Century-Crofts.

5-017   Andress, V. R. (1977). Ethnic/racial
         misidentification in death: A problem which may
         distort suicide statistics. Forensic Science, 9,
         179-183.

5-018   Atkinson, J. M. (1968). On the sociology of
         suicide. Sociological Review, 16, 83-92.
         (Reprinted as "Suicide statistics" in A. Giddens
         (Ed.) (1971), The sociology of suicide: A
         selection of readings (pp. 87-96). London:
         Cass.)

5-019   Atkinson, J. M. (1978). Discovering suicide: Studies in the social organization of sudden death (pp. 33-67). Pittsburgh: University of Pittsburgh Press, Chapter 3, "Suicide research and data derived from official sources."

5-020   Atkinson, M. W., Kessel, N., & Dalgaard, J. B. (1975). The comparability of suicide rates. British Journal of Psychiatry, 127, 247-256.

5-021   Barraclough, B. M. (1970). The effect that coroners have on the suicide rate and the open verdict rate. In E. H. Hare & J. K. Wing (Eds.), Psychiatric epidemiology: Proceedings of the international symposium held at Aberdeen University, 22-5 July 1969 (pp. 361-365). London: Oxford University Press.

5-022   Barraclough, B. M. (1972). Are the Scottish and English suicide rates really different? British Journal of Psychiatry, 120, 267-273.

5-023   Barraclough, B. M. (1973). Differences between national suicide rates. British Journal of Psychiatry, 122, 95-96.

5-024   Barraclough, B. M. (1978). Reliability of violent death certification in one coroner's district. British Journal of Psychiatry, 132, 39-41.

5-025   Barraclough, B. M. (1978). The different incidence of suicide in Eire and in England and Wales. British Journal of Psychiatry, 132, 36-38.

5-026   Barraclough, B., Holding, T., & Fayers, P. (1976). Influences of coroners' officers and pathologists on suicide verdicts. British Journal of Psychiatry, 128, 471-474.

5-027   Brooke, E. M., & Atkinson, M. (1974). Ascertainment of deaths from suicide. In E. M. Brooke (Ed.), Suicide and attempted suicide (pp. 15-70). Geneva: World Health Organization, Public Health Papers No. 58.

5-028   Brown, J. H. (1975). Reporting of suicide: Canadian statistics. Suicide, 5, 21-28.

5-029   Brugha, T., & Walsh, D. (1978). Suicide past and present: The temporal constancy of under-reporting. British Journal of Psychiatry, 132, 177-179. (Abstract: PA, 1979, 61, No. 6198, p. 622)

5-030   Coombs, D., & Miller, H. (1975). The Scandinavian

suicide phenomenon: Fact or artifact? Another look. Psychological Reports, 37, 1075-1078.

5-031   Cresswell, P. (1974). Suicide: The stable rates argument. Journal of Biosocial Science, 6, 151-161.

5-032   Datel, W. E. (1979). The reliability of mortality count and suicide count in the United States Army. Military Medicine, 144, 509-512. [See also reference 5-034 below]

5-033   Douglas, J. D. (1967). The social meanings of suicide (pp. 163-231). Princeton, NJ: Princeton University Press, Chapter 12, "The nature and use of official statistics on suicide."

5-034   Editorial comment--The reliability of suicide statistics: A bomb-burst (1980). Suicide and Life-Threatening Behavior, 10, 67-69.

        Comments regarding Datel's (1979, reference 5-032 above) article on the reliability of mortality counts in the U.S. Army.

5-035   Farberow, N. L., MacKinnon, D. R., & Nelson, F. L. (1977). Suicide: Who's counting? Public Health Reports, 92, 223-232.

5-036   Gerdin, B. (1980). A case of disguised suicide. Forensic Science International, 16, 29-34.

5-037   Glasser, J. H. (1981). The quality and utility of death certificate data [Editorial]. American Journal of Public Health, 71, 231-233.

5-038   Gorwitz, K. (1975). Case registers. In S. Perlin (Ed.), A handbook for the study of suicide (pp. 213-226). New York: Oxford University Press.

        Gorwitz argues that because of suicide data inadequacies, the compilation of case registers is desireable. See also Boldt (1981, reference 5-070 below).

5-039   Gove, W. R., & Hughes, M. (1980). Reexamining the ecological fallacy: A study in which aggregate data are critical in investigating the pathological effects of living alone. Social Forces, 58, 1157-1177.

5-040   Hatton, C. L., Valente, S. M., & Rink, A. (1977). Variables in suicide statistics. In C. L. Valente, S. M. Valente, & A. Rink (Eds.), Suicide: Assessment and intervention

(pp. 133-143). New York:
Appleton-Century-Crofts.

5-041 Holding, T. A., & Barraclough, B. M. (1978).
Undetermined deaths: Suicide or accident?
British Journal of Psychiatry, 133, 542-549.
(Abstract: PA, 1980, 63, No. 12134, p. 1351)

* 5-042 Hopper, K., & Guttmacher, S. (1979). Rethinking
suicide: Notes toward a critical epidemiology.
International Journal of Health Services, 9,
417-438.

5-043 Jennings, C., & Barraclough, B. (1980). Legal and
administrative influences on the English suicide
rate since 1900. Psychological Medicine, 10,
407-418. (Abstract: PA, 1981, 66, No. 6036,
p. 635)

5-044 Kleinman, J. C. (1982). The continued vitality of
vital statistics [Editorial]. American Journal
of Public Health, 72, 125-127.

5-045 Kunitz, S. J., & Edland, J. F. (1973). The
epidemiology of autopsies in Monroe County, New
York. Journal of Forensic Sciences, 18, 370-379.

A study of the proportion of autopsies
performed over time reveals great changes and
likely affects on the classification of causes
of death (with suicide highlighted as one such
cause).

5-046 Liberakis, E. A., & Hoenig, J. (1978). Recording
of suicide in Newfoundland. Psychiatric Journal
of the University of Ottawa, 3, 254-259.
(Abstract: PA, 1980, 63, No. 12146,
pp. 1352-1353)

* 5-047 Linden, L. L., & Breed, W. (1976). The demographic
epidemiology of suicide. In E. S. Shneidman
(Ed.), Suicidology: Contemporary developments
(pp. 77-98). New York: Grune & Stratton.

5-048 Malla, A., & Hoenig, J. (1983). Differences in
suicide rates: An examination of
under-reporting. Canadian Journal of Psychiatry,
28, 291-293. (Abstract: PA, 1984, 71, No. 7035,
p. 744)

5-049 McCarthy, P. D., & Walsh, D. (1975). Suicide in
Dublin: I. The under-reporting of suicide and
the consequences for national statistics.
British Journal of Psychiatry, 126, 301-308.

5-050 McIntosh, J. L. (1983, November). Elderly suicide

data bases: Levels, availability, omissions.
Paper presented at the annual meeting of the
Gerontological Society of America, San Francisco.
[Copies available from the author]

* 5-051   Monk, M. (1975). Epidemiology. In S. Perlin
(Ed.), A handbook for the study of suicide
(pp. 185-211). New York: Oxford University
Press.

5-052   Moriyama, I. M., & Israel, R. A. (1968). Problems
in compilation of statistics on suicides in the
United States. In N. L. Farberow (Ed.),
Proceedings: Fourth international conference for
suicide prevention (pp. 16-21). Los Angeles:
Delmar.

5-053   Nelson, F. L., Farberow, N. L., & MacKinnon,
D. R. (1978). The certification of suicide in
eleven western states: An inquiry into the
validity of reported suicide rates. Suicide and
Life-Threatening Behavior, 8, 75-88.

5-054   Nuttall, E. A., Evenson, R. C., & Cho,
D. W. (1980). A comparison of suicide and
undetermined deaths in psychiatric patients.
Suicide and Life-Threatening Behavior 10,
167-174.

5-055   Ovenstone, I. M. K. (1973). A psychiatric approach
to the diagnosis of suicide and its effect upon
the Edinburgh statistics. British Journal of
Psychiatry, 123, 15-21.

5-056   Patel, N. S. (1973). Suicide, the coroner and the
declining suicide rate. Forensic Science, 2,
467-470.

5-057   Peck, D. L. (1983-84). "Official documentation" of
the black suicide experience. Omega, 14, 21-31.
(Abstract: PA, 1984, 71, No. 4224, p. 448)

5-058   Pokorny, A. D. (1973). The Scandinavian suicide
phenomenon--Myth or reality? Life-Threatening
Behavior, 3, 11-19.

5-059   Ross, O., & Kreitman, N. (1975). A further
investigation of differences in the suicide rates
of England and Wales and of Scotland. British
Journal of Psychiatry, 127, 575-582.

5-060   Sainsbury, P. (1973). Suicide: Opinions and
facts. Proceedings of the Royal Society of
Medicine, 66, 579-587.

5-061   Sainsbury, P., & Barraclough, B. (1968).

Differences between suicide rates. Nature, 220, 1252.

* 5-062 Sainsbury, P., & Jenkins, J. S. (1982). The accuracy of officially reported suicide statistics for purposes of epidemiological research. Journal of Epidemiology and Community Health, 36, 43-48.

5-063 Schwartz, A. J. (1980). Innaccuracy and uncertainty in estimates of college student suicide rates. Journal of the American College Health Association, 28, 201-204.

5-064 Suicide statistics: The problem of comparability (1975). WHO Chronicle, 29, 188-193.

5-065 Surtees, S. J. (1982). Suicide and accidental deaths at Beach Head. British Medical Journal, 2(284), 321-324.

The change in coroner greatly affected the number of deaths determined to be suicides.

5-066 Taylor, S. (1982). Durkheim and the study of suicide (pp. 43-64; 65-94). New York: St. Martin's Press, Part 2, "The social construction of official suicide rates," especially Chapters 3, "Some critiques of official suicide rates," and 4, "Proving suicide."

5-067 Walsh, B., Walsh, D., & Whelan, B. (1975). Suicide in Dublin: II. The influence of some social and medical factors on coroner's verdicts. British Journal of Psychiatry, 126, 309-312.

5-068 Warshauer, M. E., & Monk, M. (1978). Problems in suicide statistics for whites and blacks. American Journal of Public Health, 68, 383-388.

See also Gibbs (1968, reference 1-063), pp. 13-14, "The reliability of official statistics;" World Health Organization (1968, reference 1-047b), pp. 31-36 and 51-76; Atkinson (1971, reference 2-001a); Lester (1972, reference 1-041), Chapter 12, "The use of official statistics," pp. 140-148; Lester (1983, reference 1-042), Chapter 6, "The reliability of suicide rates," pp. 35-36.

5.3 Suicide Research: Official Statistics and Other Methods

5-069 Atkinson, J. M. (1978). Discovering suicide: Studies in the social organization of sudden death. Pittsburgh: University of Pittsburgh Press.

In addition to the chapter cited above in reference 5-019 on research and data, Atkinson discusses at great length other available methodologies and sources of data other than official statistics, most notably in Chapter 4, "Alternative sociological approaches to suicide research."

5-070   Boldt, M. (1981). A plan for improved research on suicidal behavior. Crisis, 2, 95-105.

* 5-071   Farberow, N. L. (1977). Research in suicide in 1971-1973: A review. In K. Achte, & J. Lonnqvist (Eds.), Suicide research: Proceedings of the seminars of suicide research in Yrjo Jahnsson Foundation 1974-1977 (pp. 23-47). Helsinki: Psychiatria Fennica (Psychiatria Fennica Supplementum 1976).

In addition to reviewing the suicide literature, Farberow suggests research needs as well.

* 5-072   Farberow, N. L., Breed, W., Bunney, W. E., Jr., Diggory, J. C., Lettieri, D. J., May, P., Murphy, G. E., & Sullivan, F. J.(1973). Research in suicide. In H. L. P. Resnik & B. C. Hathorne (Eds.), Suicide prevention in the 70s (pp. 45-80). Washington, D.C.: USGPO, DHEW Publication No. (HSM) 72-9054.

* 5-073   Lester, D. (1972). Why people kill themselves: A summary of research findings on suicidal behavior (pp. 5-12). Springfield, IL: Thomas, Chapter 1, "Methodological problems in suicide research."

  5-074   Lester, D. (1973). Basic research and suicide prevention [Letter]. American Journal of Psychiatry, 130, 1402-1403.

Lester notes that despite all the attention given to suicide prevention, there remains a great need for research to be done.

5-075   MacKinnon, D. R. (1977). Suicide research: Cautions and precautions in analysis. In K. Achte & J. Lonnqvist (Eds.), Suicide research: Proceedings of the seminars of suicide research by Yrjo Jahnsson Foundation 1974-1977 (pp. 49-57). Helsinki: Psychiatria Fennica (Psychiatria Fennica Supplementum 1976).

5-076   Murphy, G. E. (1983). Problems in studying suicide. Psychiatric Developments, 1, 339-350.

5-077   Neuringer, C. (1962). Methodological problems in

suicide research. _Journal of Consulting Psychology_, _26_, 273-278.

5-078   Neuringer, C., & Kolstoe, R. H. (1966). Suicide research and non-rejection of the null hypothesis. _Perceptual and Motor Skills_, _22_, 115-118.

5-079   Niemi, T. (1977). Can the epidemiology of suicide be considered epidemiological research? In K. Achte & J. Lonnqvist (Eds.), _Suicide research: Proceedings of the seminars of suicide research by Yrjo Jahnsson Foundation 1974-1977_ (pp. 79-81). Helsinki: Psychiatria Fennica (_Psychiatria Fennica_ Supplementum 1976).

5-080   Reynolds, D. K., & Farberow, N. L. (1973). Experiential research: An inside perspective on suicide and social systems. _Life-Threatening Behavior_, _3_, 261-269.

5-081   Reynolds, D. K., & Farberow, N. L. (1976). _Suicide: Inside and out_. Berkeley: University of California Press.

> This book describes the subjective experience ("experiential research") of being a suicidal patient in a psychiatric ward.

5-082   Selvin, H. C. (1958). Durkheim's _Suicide_ and problems of empirical research. _American Journal of Sociology_, _63_, 607-619.

5-083   Shershow, J. C. (1976). The sometimes science of suicidology [Editorial]. _New England Journal of Medicine_, _294_(6), 332-335.

> Shershow points to some problems in the prediction of suicidal behavior.

5-084   Simpson, G. (1950). Methodological problems in determining the aetiology of suicide. _American Sociological Review_, _15_, 658-663.

5-085   Whitehead, P. C., Johnson, F. G., & Ferrence, R. (1973). Measuring the incidence of self-injury: Some methodological and design considerations. _American Journal of Orthopsychiatry_, _43_, 142-148.

See also Wekstein (1979, reference 1-047a), pp. 38-42, "Statistics." Meer (1976, reference 5-444), Chapter 1, "Methodological problems in the study of suicide," pp. 3-17; Lester (1983, reference 1-042), Chapter 12, "Methodological issues: The problem of substitute subjects," pp. 81-82; Lester & Lester (1971, reference 1-043), Chapter 2,

"Problems in suicide research," pp. 9-16.

5.4 Overview Sources of Suicide Statistics/Risk Factors

5-086   Berman, A. L. (1975). The epidemiology of
        life-threatening events. Suicide, 5, 67-77.

5-087   Berman, A. L. (1975). Self-destructive behavior
        and suicide: Epidemiology and taxonomy. In
        A. R. Roberts (Ed.), Self-destructive behavior
        (pp. 5-20). Springfield, IL: Thomas.

5-088   Choron, J. (1972). Suicide. New York: Scribner.

5-089   deCatanzaro, D. (1981). Suicide and self-damaging
        behavior: A sociobiological perspective
        (pp. 13-23). New York: Academic Press, Chapter
        2, "The current incidence of suicide and
        self-injury."

5-090   Diekstra, R. F. W. (1982). Epidemiology of
        attempted suicide in the EEC. In J. Wilmotte,
        C. Mendlewicz, & J. Mendlewicz (Eds.), New trends
        in suicide prevention (pp. 1-16). New York:
        Karger (Bibliotheca Psychiatrica, No. 162).

5-091   Dublin, L. I. (1963). Suicide: A sociological and
        statistical study. New York: Ronald Press.

5-092   Durkheim, E. (1951). Suicide: A study in
        sociology (J. A. Spaulding & G. Simpson, Trans.;
        G. Simpson, Ed.). New York: Free Press.
        (Originally published, 1897.)

* 5-093 Frederick, C. J. (1978). Current trends in
        suicidal behavior in the United States. American
        Journal of Psychotherapy, 32, 172-200.

5-094   Gibbs, J. P. (1966). Suicide. In R. K. Merton &
        R. A. Nisbet (Eds.), Contemporary social problems
        (pp. 281-321). New York: Harcourt, Brace &
        World.

5-095   Hawton, K., & Catalan, J. (1982). Attempted
        suicide: A practical guide to its nature and
        management. New York: Oxford University Press.

5-096   Henry, A. F., & Short, J. F., Jr. (1954). Suicide
        and homicide: Some economic, sociological, and
        psychological aspects of aggression. New York:
        Free Press.

5-097   Holinger, P. C. (1980). Violent deaths as a
        leading cause of mortality: An epidemiological
        study of suicide, homicide, and accidents.
        American Journal of Psychiatry, 137, 472-476.

(Abstract: PA, 1980, 63, No. 12135, p. 1351)

* 5-098 Kramer, M., Pollack, E. S., Redick, R. W., & Locke,
         B. Z. (1972). Mental disorders/Suicide
         (pp. 173-227). Cambridge, MA: Harvard
         University Press, Chapter 7, "Suicide."
         (American Public Health Association, Vital and
         Health Statistics Monograph Series No. 12.)

  5-099 Kreitman, N. (1972). Some aspects of the
         epidemiology of suicide and "attempted suicide"
         (parasuicide). In J. Waldenstrom, T. Larsson, &
         N. Ljungstedt (Eds.), Suicide and attempted
         suicide (pp. 45-52). Stockholm: Nordiska
         Bokhandelns Forlag.

  5-100 Kreitman, N. (Ed.) (1977). Parasuicide
         (esp. pp. 12-40). New York: Wiley, Chapter 2,
         "The epidemiology of parasuicide."

  5-101 Kreitman, N. (1981). The epidemiology of suicide
         and parasuicide. Crisis, 2, 1-13.

  5-102 Labovitz, S. (1968). Variation in suicide rates.
         In J. P. Gibbs (Ed.), Suicide (pp. 57-73). New
         York: Harper & Row.

  5-103 Maris, R. W. (1969). Social forces in urban
         suicide. Homewood, IL: Dorsey.

         Maris analyzes detailed data for Chicago from
         1959-1963 for many variables and looks at
         their fit with Durkheim's theory of suicide.

  5-104 Maris, R. W. (1981). Pathways to suicide: A
         survey of self-destructive behaviors. Baltimore:
         John Hopkins University Press.

         A random sample of coroner's informants for
         suicides in Chicago from 1966-1968 are
         interviewed in order to collect data on a
         large number of factors and variables. The
         interviews were somewhat similar to
         "psychological autopsies" (see Section 9.8)
         and provide insight into the development of
         suicidal behavior over time.

  5-105 May, A. R. (1972). Suicide--A world health
         problem. In J. Waldenstrom, T. Larsson, &
         N. Ljungstedt (Eds.), Suicide and attempted
         suicide (pp. 15-25). Stockholm: Nordiska
         Bokhandelns Forlag.

* 5-106 Monk, M. (1975). Epidemiology. In S. Perlin
         (Ed.), A handbook for the study of suicide

(pp. 185-211). New York: Oxford University Press.

5-107   Morgan, H. G. (1979). Death wishes? The understanding and management of deliberate self-harm (pp. 8-21; 22-37; 87-98; 99-113). New York: Wiley, Chapters 2, "Suicide statistics," 3, "Correlates and causes of suicide," 8, "Incidence and methods" [non-fatal deliberate self-harm], 9, "Correlates" [non-fatal deliberate self-harm], respectively.

5-108   Ruzicka, L. T. (1976). Suicide, 1950-1971. World Health Statistics Report, 29(7), 396-413.

5-109   Sainsbury, P., Jenkins, J., & Levey, A. (1980). The social correlates of suicide in Europe. In R. D.T Farmer & S. R. Hirsch (Eds.), The suicide syndrome (pp. 38-53). London: Croom Helm.

5-110   Stengel, E. (1964). Suicide and attempted suicide (esp. pp. 17-32; 74-76). Baltimore: Penguin Books, Chapters 2, "The statistics" [suicide], and 8, "The statistics" [attempted suicide], respectively.

5-111   Victoroff, V. M. (1983). The suicidal patient: Recognition, intervention, management (pp. 9-22). Oradell, NJ: Medical Economics Books, Chapter 2, "Statistics and trends."

* 5-112   Weissman, M. M. (1974). The epidemiology of suicide attempts, 1960 to 1971. Archives of General Psychiatry, 30, 737-746.

* 5-113   Wexler, L., Weissman, M. M., & Kasl, S. V. (1978). Suicide attempts 1970-1975: Updating a United States study and comparisons with international trends. British Journal of Psychiatry, 132, 180-185.

See also Lester (1972, 1983, references 1-041 and 1-042); McCulloch & Philip (1972, reference 1-044), pp. 7-29; Shneidman & Farberow (1961, reference 2-048); Hopper & Guttmacher (1979, reference 5-042); and Linden & Breed (1976, reference 5-047).

5.5 Demographic Factors & Suicide: Sex

5.5a Bibliography

5-114   Miller, M. Female suicides [Non-annotated bibliography]. San Diego, CA: The Information Center. (Listed in the 1984 catalog.) Bibliography No. R-4.

5.5b Articles on Sex and Suicide

5-115   Beck, A. T., Lester, D., & Kovacs, M. (1973).
        Attempted suicide by males and females.
        Psychological Reports, 33, 965-966.

5-116   Bourque, L. B., Kraus, J. F., & Cosand,
        B. J. (1983). Attributes of suicide in females.
        Suicide and Life-Threatening Behavior, 13,
        123-138.

5-117   Burvill, P. W. (1972). Recent decreased ratio of
        male:female suicide rates: Analysis of rates in
        selected countries specific for age and sex.
        International Journal of Social Psychiatry, 18,
        137-139.

5-118   Clifton, A. K., & Lee, D. E. (1976).
        Self-destructive consequences of sex-role
        socialization. Suicide and Life-Threatening
        Behavior, 6, 11-22.

5-119   Cumming, E., Lazer, C., & Chisholm, L. (1975).
        Suicide as an index of role strain among employed
        and not employed married women in British
        Columbia. Canadian Review of Sociology and
        Anthropology, 12, 462-470.

5-120   Davis, F. B. (1968). Sex differences in suicide
        and attempted suicide. Diseases of the Nervous
        System, 29, 193-194.

5-121   Davis, R. A. (1981). Female labor force
        participation, status integration and suicide,
        1950-1969. Suicide and Life-Threatening
        Behavior, 11. 111-123. (Abstract: PA, 1982,
        67, No. 7963, p. 860)

5-122   Diggory, J. C., & Lester, D. (1976). Suicide rates
        of men and women: An instance of their
        independence. Omega, 7, 95-101.

5-123   French, L., & Bryce, F. O. (1978). Suicide and
        female aggression: A contemporary analysis of
        anomic suicide. Journal of Clinical Psychiatry,
        39, 761-765. (Abstract: PA, 1980, 63,
        No. 12127, p. 1350)

5-124   Goldney, R. D. (1981). Are young women who attempt
        suicide hysterical? British Journal of
        Psychiatry, 138, 141-146.

5-125   Goldney, R. D. (1981). Attempted suicide in young
        women: Correlate of lethality. British Journal
        of Psychiatry, 139, 382-390. (Abstract: PA,
        1982, 67, No. 12306, p. 1319)

5-126   Gove, W. R. (1972). Sex, marital status and
        suicide. Journal of Health and Social Behavior,
        13, 204-213.

5-127   Heshysius, L. (1980). Female self-injury and
        suicide attempts: Culturally reinforced
        techniques in human relations. Sex Roles, 6,
        843-855.

5-128   Hirsch, M. F. (1981). Women and violence
        (pp. 265-305; esp. pp. 290-300). New York: Van
        Nostrand Reinhold, Chapter 10, "To self-destruct:
        Alcoholism, drug addiction and suicide."

5-129   Johnson, K. K. (1979). Durkheim revisited: "Why
        do women kill themselves?" Suicide and
        Life-Threatening Behavior, 9, 145-153.
        (Abstract: PA, 1980, 64, No. 10598, p. 1140)

5-130   Kessler, R. C., & MacRae, J. A., Jr. (1983).
        Trends in the relationship between sex and
        attempted suicide. Journal of Health and Social
        Behavior, 24, 98-110. (Abstract: PA, 1984, 71,
        No. 7028, p. 743)

5-131   Kreitman, N., & Schreiber, M. (1979). Parasuicide
        in young Edinburgh women: 1968-75.
        Psychological Medicine, 9, 469-479. (Reprinted
        in R. D. T. Farmer & S. R. Hirsch (Eds.) (1980),
        The suicide syndrome (pp. 54-72). London: Croom
        Helm.)

5-132   Lester, D. (1969). Suicidal behavior in men and
        women. Mental Hygiene, 53, 340-345.

* 5-133 Lester, D. (1972). Why people kill themselves: A
        summary of research findings on suicidal behavior
        (pp. 36-46). Springfield, IL: Thomas, Chapter
        7, "Sexual differences in suicidal behavior."
        (Based on Lester, 1969, reference 5-132 above.)

5-134   Lester, D. (1973). Completed suicide and females
        in the labor force. Psychological Reports, 32,
        730.

        Lester presents results which are inconsistent
        with those of Newman et al., reference 5-140
        below.

* 5-135 Lester, D. (1979). Sex differences in suicidal
        behavior. In E. S. Gomberg & V. Franks (Eds.),
        Gender and disordered behavior: Sex differences
        in psychopathology (pp. 287-300). New York:
        Brunner/Mazel.

5-136   Linehan, M. M. (1971). Toward a theory of sex

differences in suicidal behavior. Crisis
Intervention, 3(4), 93-101. (Abstract: PA,
1972, 48, No. 7451, p. 808)

5-137   Linehan, M. M. (1973). Suicide and attempted
        suicide: Study of perceived sex differences.
        Perceptual and Motor Skills, 37, 31-34.

5-138   Maris, R. W. (1971). Deviance as therapy: The
        paradox of the self-destructive female. Journal
        of Health and Social Behavior, 12, 113-124.
        (Abstract: PA, 1972, 47, No. 9222, p. 1025)
        Hamblin, R. L., & Jacobsen, R. B. (1972).
        Suicide and pseudocide: A reanalysis of Maris'
        data. 13, 99-104. Alwin, D. F., & Eaton, W. W.,
        Jr. (1972). Additional comments on Maris' paper.
        13, 105. Maris' reply. 13, 106-109.

5-139   Neuringer, C. (1982). Suicidal behavior in women.
        Crisis, 3, 41-49. (Abstract: PA, 1983, 69,
        No. 5845, p. 637)

5-140   Newman, J. F., Wittemore, K. R., & Newman,
        H. G. (1973). Women in the labor force and
        suicide. Social Problems, 21, 220-230.
        (Abstract: PA, 1974, 52, No. 1222, p. 157)

5-141   Ornstein, M. D. (1983). The impact of marital
        status, age, and employment on female suicide in
        British Columbia. Canadian Review of Sociology
        and Anthropology, 20, 96-100.

5-142   Rosenthal, M. J. (1981). Sexual differences in the
        suicidal behavior of young people. In
        S. C. Feinstein, J. G. Looney,
        A. Z. Schwartzburg, & A. D. Sorosky (Eds.),
        Developmental and clinical studies (pp. 422-442).
        Chicago: University of Chicago Press (Adolescent
        Psychiatry, 9).

5-143   Suter, B. (1976). Suicide and women. In
        B. B. Wolman & H. H. Krauss (Eds.), Between
        survival and suicide (pp. 129-161). New York:
        Gardner Press.

5-144   Vigderhous, G., & Fishman, G. (1977).
        Socioeconomic determinants of female suicide
        rates: A cross-national comparison.
        International Review of Modern Sociology, 7,
        199-211.

5-145   Wilson, M. (1981). Suicidal behavior: Toward an
        explanation of differences in female and male
        rates. Suicide and Life-Threatening Behavior,
        11, 131-140.

See also Lester (1983, reference 1-042), Chapter 3, "Sex differences in suicide," pp. 14-19; Lester & Lester (1971, reference 1-043), Chapter 12, "Sex differences in suicidal behavior," pp. 88-93.

5.6 Demographic Factors and Suicide: Age

5.6a Bibliographies on Age Groups

5-146   American Association of Suicidology. Annotated bibliographies. Denver, CO: AAS. Available bibliographies include:

   5-146.01   Suicide and the elderly.

   5-146.02   Suicide and youth.

5-147   French, A. P. (1979). Annotated bibliography. In A. P. French & I. N. Berlin (Eds.), Depression in children and adolescents (pp. 218-290). New York: Human Sciences Press.

   A large number of research investigations on suicide in children and adolescents are included among these annotations.

5-148   Gallagher, D. (1981). Depression in the elderly: A selected bibliography (pp. 48-57). Los Angeles: Andrus Gerontology Center/University of Southern California, Technical Bibliographies on Aging Series III, Chapter 6, "Self-destructive behavior: Suicide."

5-149   McIntosh, J. L. (1981). Suicide among children, adolescents, and students: A comprehensive bibliography. Monticello, IL: Vance Bibliographies, Public Administration Series: Bibliography P-685. (107 pages)

5-150   McIntosh, J. L. (1981). Suicide among the elderly: A comprehensive bibliography. Monticello, IL: Vance Bibliographies, Public Administration Series: Bibliography P-686. [Includes references on "Age in general," pp. 6-10.] (37 pages)

5-151   Miller, M. Non-annotated bibliographies. San Diego: Suicide Information Center. The 1984 catalog lists:

   5-151.01   Childhood suicides. Bibliography R-5.

   5-151.02   Adolescent suicides. Bibliography R-6.

   5-151.03   Collegiate suicides. Bibliography R-7.

5-151.04 Geriatric suicides. Bibliography R-8.

5-152 National Clearinghouse for Mental Health
       Information (1981). Child and adolescent suicide
       (Literature Survey Series No. 2). Washington,
       D.C.: USGPO, DHHS Publication No. (ADM) 81-1135.
       SuDoc HE 20.8134.2 [Available only in microfiche]
       ERIC Document ED 218 558

       This annotated work presents 122 references
       from 1978-1980 and is 113 pages long.

5-153 Tedford, J. M., & Tedford, W. H. (1980, November).
       Youthful suicide: An annotated bibliography.
       Catalog of Selected Documents in Psychology, 10,
       p. 92, Manuscript No. 2155. (25 pages)

5-154 Wexler, P. (1979). Suicide or depression in
       childhood and adolescence. National Library of
       Medicine Literature Search No. 79-6.

       This bibliography includes 179 citations from
       January 1975-February 1979.

5.6b Age in General

5-155 Burvill, P. W. (1970). Age-sex variation in
       suicide in Western Australia. Medical Journal of
       Australia, 2(24), 1113-1116.

5-156 Goldney, R. D., & Katsikitis, M. (1983). Cohort
       analysis of suicide rates in Australia. Archives
       of General Psychiaty, 40, 71-74. (Abstract: PA,
       1983, 69, No. 10616, p. 1165)

5-157 Hellon, C. P., & Solomon, M. I. (1980). Suicide
       and age in Alberta, Canada, 1951 to 1977: The
       changing profile. Archives of General
       Psychiatry, 37, 505-510. (Abstract: PA, 1981,
       65, No. 13003, p. 1395)

5-158 Jarvis, G. K., Ferrence, R. G., Johnson, F. G., &
       Whitehead, P. C. (1976). Sex and age patterns in
       self-injury. Journal of Health and Social
       Behavior, 17, 145-154. (Abstract: EM, 1976,
       Sect. 20, 19, No. 2747, p. 499)

5-159 Kreitman, N. (1976). Age and parasuicide
       (attempted suicide). Psychological Medicine, 6,
       113-121. (Abstracts: PA, 1977, 57, No. 8456,
       p. 957; EM, 1977, Sect. 20, 20, No. 1418,
       p. 254)

5-160 Lester, D., & Beck, A. T. (1974). Age differences
       in patterns of attempted suicide. Omega, 5,
       317-322. (Abstract: EM, 1975, Sect. 20, 18,

No. 3168, p. 544)

5-161   Murphy, G. E., & Wetzel, R. D. (1980). Suicide
        risk by birth cohort in the United States, 1949
        to 1974. Archives of General Psychiatry, 37,
        519-523. (Abstract: PA, 1981, 65, No. 13014,
        p. 1396)

5-162   Seiden, R. H., & Freitas, R. P. (1980). Shifting
        patterns of deadly violence. Suicide and
        Life-Threatening Behavior, 10, 195-209.
        (Abstracts: PA, 1981, 66, No. 13048, p. 1359;
        CPA, 1981, 21, No. 1168, p. 270)

        The changing patterns of suicide by age are
        presented and discussed.

5-163   Solomon, M. I., & Hellon, C. P. (1980). Suicide
        and age in Alberta, Canada, 1951 to 1977: A
        cohort analysis. Archives of General Psychiatry,
        37, 511-513. (Abstract: PA, 1981, 65,
        No. 13024, p. 1397)

See also: Burvill (1972, reference 5-117 above); Darbonne
(1969, reference 9-169); Farberów & Shneidman (1957,
reference 9-173); McIntosh (1980, reference 5-005 above);
Ornstein (1983, reference 5-141 above); Ruzicka (1976,
reference 5-108 above).

5.6c Children & Adolescents

* 5-164 Berman, A. L., & Cohen-Sandler, R. (1982).
         Childhood and adolescent suicide research: A
         critique. Crisis, 3, 3-15. (Abstract: PA,
         1983, 69, No. 5808, p. 632)

5-165   Cantor, P. (1972). The adolescent attempter: Sex,
        sibling position, and family constellation.
        Life-Threatening Behavior, 2, 252-261.
        (Abstract: PA, 1973, 50, No. 11446,
        pp. 1256-1257)

5-166   Carlson, G. A. (1983). Depression and suicidal
        behavior in children and adolescents. In
        D. P. Cantwell & G. A. Carlson (Eds.), Affective
        disorders in childhood and adolescence: An
        update (pp. 335-352). Jamaica, NY: SP Medical &
        Scientific Books.

5-167   Carlson, G. A., & Cantwell, D. P. (1982). Suicidal
        behavior and depression in children and
        adolescents. Journal of the American Academy of
        Child Psychiatry, 21, 361-368.

5-168   Connell, P. H. (1971). Suicidal attempts in
        childhood and adolescence. In J. G. Howells

(Ed.), Modern perspectives in child psychiatry (pp. 403-427). New York: Brunner/Mazel.

5-169   Danto, B. L., & Kutscher, A. H. (Eds.) (1977). Suicide and bereavement. New York: MSS Information Corporation.

    5-169.01 Tallmer, M. Support work and self-destructive behavior: Childhood suicide. pp. 150-162.

    5-169.02 Schneider, L. Adolescents and suicide. pp. 163-175.

5-170   Davis, P. A. (1983). Suicidal adolescents. Springfield, IL: Thomas.

5-171   DenHouter, K. V. (1981). To silence one's self: A brief analysis of the literature on adolescent suicide. Child Welfare, 60, 2-10. (Abstract: CPA, 1981, 21, No. 1158, p. 268)

5-172   Emery, P. E. (1983). Adolescent depression and suicide. Adolescence, 18(70), 245-258. (Abstracts: PA, 1983, 70, No. 10468, p. 1172; CPA, 1983, 23, No. 1619, p. 345)

5-173   Evans, D. L. (1982). Explaining suicide among the young: An analytical review of the literature. Journal of Psychosocial Nursing and Mental Health Services, 20(8), 9-16.

5-174   Faigel, H. C. (1966). Suicide among young persons: A review of its incidence and causes, and methods for its prevention. Clinical Pediatrics, 5, 187-190.

* 5-175   Feinstein, S. C., Looney, J. G., Schwartzberg, A. Z., & Sorosky, A. D. (1981). Adolescent Psychiatry, 9: Developmental and clinical studies. Chicago: University of Chicago Press.

    This book/journal volume included a special section on adolescent suicide which included the following particularly relevant articles (as well as Rosenthal, reference 5-142 above):

    5-175.01 Doctors, S. The symptom of delicate self-cutting in adolescent females: A developmental view. pp. 443-460.

    5-175.02 Miller, D. Adolescent suicide: Etiology and treatment. pp. 327-342.

    5-175.03 Mintz, T. Clinical experience with suicidal adolescents. pp. 493-496.

5-175.04   Peck, M. L. The loner: An exploration
           of a suicidal subtype in adolescence.
           pp. 461-466.

5-175.05   Petzel, S. V., & Riddle, M. Adolescent
           suicide: Psychosocial and cognitive
           aspects. pp. 343-398.

5-175.06   Tabachnick, N. The interlocking
           psychologies of suicide and
           adolescence. pp. 399-410.

5-176   Finch, S. M., & Poznanski, E. O. (1971).
        Adolescent suicide. Springfield, IL: Thomas.

5-177   Fish, W. C., & Waldhart-Letzell, E. (1981).
        Suicide and children. Death Education, 5,
        215-222. (Abstract: PA, 1982, 67, No. 12305,
        p. 1319)

5-178   Frederick, C. J. (1977). Trends in mental health:
        Self-destructive behavior among younger age
        groups. Washington, D.C.: USGPO, DHEW
        Publication No. (ADM) 77-365. (Reprinted from
        Keynote, May 30, 1976, 4(3), 3-5.)

5-179   Garfinkel, B., & Golombek, H. (1977). Suicide and
        depression in children and adolescents. In
        P. Steinhauer & Q. Rae-Grant (Eds.),
        Psychological problems of the child and his
        family (pp. 151-164). Toronto: Macmillan of
        Canada.

5-180   Garfinkel, B. D., & Golombek, H. (1983). Suicidal
        behavior in adolescence. In H. Golombek &
        B. D. Garfinkel (Eds.), The adolescent and mood
        disturbance (pp. 189-217). New York:
        International Universities Press.

5-181   Glaser, K. (1978). The treatment of depressed and
        suicidal adolescents. American Journal of
        Psychotherapy, 32, 252-269. (Abstracts: PA,
        1979, 62, No. 3999, p. 409; ACP, 1979, 19,
        No. 288, p. 64)

5-182   Gould, R. (1975). Suicide problems in children and
        adolescents. In A. Esman (Ed.), Psychology of
        adolescence: Essential readings (pp. 285-301).
        New York: International Universities Press.

5-183   Haim, A. (1974). Adolescent suicide. New York:
        International Universities Press.
        (A. M. S. Smith, Trans.; Originally published,
        Paris: Payot, 1969.)

5-184   Hatton, C. L., & Valente, S. M. (Eds.) (1984).

Suicide: Assessment and intervention (2nd ed.).
Norwalk, CT: Appleton-Century-Crofts.

5-184.01 Kerfoot, M. Assessment of the young
          adolescent and the family.
          pp. 208-219.

5-184.02 Peck, M. Suicide in late adolescence and
          young adulthood. pp. 220-230.

5-184.03 Valente, S. M. Suicide in children.
          pp. 195-208.

5-185 Hatton, C. L., Valente, S. M., & Rink,
       A. (Eds) (1977). Suicide: Assessment and
       intervention. New York:
       Appleton-Century-Crofts.

       Included in this book are the following 2
       appropriate chapters:

5-185.01 Hatton, C. L., Valente, S. M., & Rink, A.
          Suicide in children. pp. 160-165.

5-185.02 Peck, M. Adolescent suicide.
          pp. 165-175.

5-186 Heillig, R. J. (1983). Adolescent suicidal
       behavior: A family systems model (Research in
       Clinical Psychology Series Volume No. 7). Ann
       Arbor, MI: UMI Research Press.

5-187 Herjanic, B., & Welner, Z. (1980). Adolescent
       suicide. In B. W. Camp (Ed.), Advances in
       behavioral pediatrics: A research annual, Volume
       1 (pp. 195-224). Greenwich, CT: JAI Press.

5-188 Holinger, P. C. (1977). Suicide in adolescence.
       American Journal of Psychiatry, 134, 1433-1434.
       (Abstracts: PA, 1978, 60, No. 9540, p. 1031;
       EM, 1979, Sect. 32, 39, No. 3093, pp. 544-545)

5-189 Holinger, P. C. (1978). Adolescent suicide: An
       epidemiological study of recent trends. American
       Journal of Psychiatry, 135, 754-756. (Abstract:
       PA, 1979, 62, No. 1273, p. 126)

5-190 Holinger, P. C. (1979). Violent deaths among the
       young: Recent trends in suicide, homicide, and
       accidents. American Journal of Psychiatry, 136,
       1144-1147. (Abstracts: PA, 1980, 63, No. 5657,
       p. 646; EM, 1980, Sect. 32, 41, No. 729,
       pp. 111-112)

5-191 Holinger, P. C., & Offer, D. (1981). Perspectives
       on suicide in adolescence. In R. G. Simmons

(Ed.), Research in community and mental health, Volume 2 (pp. 139-162). Greenwich, CT: JAI Press. (Abstract: PA, 1983, 69, No. 8096, pp. 887-888)

5-192 Holinger, P. C., & Offer, D. (1982). Prediction of adolescent suicide: A population study. American Journal of Psychiatry, 139, 302-307. (Abstract: PA, 1982, 67, No. 12308, p. 1319)

5-193 Husain, S. A., & Vandiver, T. (Eds.) (1983). Suicide in children and adolescents. Jamaica, NY: SP Medical & Scientific Books.

5-194 Jacobs, J. (1980). Adolescent suicide. New York: Irvington Publishers. (Originally published, 1971, New York: Wiley.)

5-195 Joffe, R. T., & Offord, D. R. (1983). Suicidal behaviour in childhood. Canadian Journal of Psychiatry, 28, 57-63. (Abstract: PA, 1983, 70, No. 10476, p. 1173)

5-196 King, M. (1971). Evaluation and treatment of suicide-prone youth. Mental Hygiene, 55, 344-350. Abstract: PA, 1972, 48, No. 11851, p. 1289)

5-197 Klagsbrun, F. (1976). Too young to die: Youth and suicide. Boston: Houghton Mifflin. (Reprinted, New York: Pocket Books, 1977.) [Popular press]

5-198 Madison, A. (1978). Suicide and young people. New York: Seabury Press. [Popular press]

5-199 Marfatia, J. C. (1975). Suicide in childhood and adolescence. Child Psychiatry Quarterly, 8(4), 13-16. (Abstract: PA, 1976, 55, No. 7352, p. 744)

5-200 Marks, P. A., & Haller, D. L. (1977). Now I lay me down for keeps: A study of adolescent suicide attempts. Journal of Clinical Psychology, 33, 390-400. (Abstracts: PA, 1978, 59, No. 3606, p. 394; EM, 1977, Sect. 32, 37, No. 1506, p. 275)

5-201 McAnarney, E. R. (1979). Adolescent and young adult suicide in the United States--A reflection of societal unrest? Adolescence, 14(56), 765-774. (Abstracts: PA, 1980, 63, No. 5665, p. 647; CPA, 1980, 20, No. 1797, p. 451)

5-202 McGuire, D. (1982). The problem of children's suicide: Ages 5-14. International Journal of Offender Therapy & Comparative Criminology, 26,

10-17. (Abstracts: PA, 1983, 69, No. 3683,
p. 398; CPA, 1982, 22, No. 1680, p. 354)

5-203   McIntire, M. S., & Angle, C. R. (Eds.) (1980).
Suicide attempts in children and youth. New
York: Harper & Row.

5-203.01   Angle, C. R. Recurrent adolescent
suicidal behavior. pp. 24-30.

5-203.02   Donaldson, J. Y., & Davis, J. A.
Evaluating the suicidal adolescent.
pp. 31-51.

5-203.03   Kenney, E. M., & Krajewski, K. J.
Hospital treatment of the adolescent
suicidal patient. pp. 70-86.

5-203.04   Long, W. A., Jr. Managing the suicidal
adolescent. pp. 64-69.

5-203.05   Lovejoy, F. H., Jr. Diagnosis and
treatment of acute overdose in
adolescents. pp. 52-63.

5-203.06   McIntire, M. S. The epidemiology and
taxonomy of suicide. pp. 1-23.

5-203.07   Moriarty, R. W. The poison center
perspective. pp. 87-91.

5-204   Parker, A. M., Jr. (1974). Suicide among young
adults. Hicksville, NY: Exposition Press.
[Popular press]

5-205   Paulson, M. J., Stone, D., & Sposto, R. (1978).
Suicide potential and behavior in children aged 4
to 12. Suicide and Life-Threatening Behavior, 8,
225-242. (Abstracts: ACP, 1979, 19, No. 1836,
p. 452; EM, 1980, Sect. 32, 41, No. 1945,
p. 307)

5-206   Petzel, S. V., & Cline, D. W. (1978). Adolescent
suicide: Epidemiological and biological aspects.
Adolescent psychiatry, 6, 239-266.

5-207   Pfeffer, C. R. (1981). Suicidal behavior of
children: A review with implications for
research and practice. American Journal of
Psychiatry, 138, 154-159. (Abstract: PA, 1981,
65, No. 8181, p. 866)

5-208   Pfeffer, C. R. (1982). Childhood and adolescent
suicidal behavior with an emphasis on girls. In
M. T. Notman & C. C. Nadelson (Eds.), Women in
context: Development and stresses, The woman

patient, Volume 3: Aggression, adaptation, and psychotherapy (pp. 115-130). New York: Plenum Press.

5-209   Rabkin, B. (1979). Growing up dead: A hard look at why adolescents commit suicide. Nashville, TN: Abingdon. [Popular press]

5-210   Rohn, R. D., Sarles, R. M., Kenny, T. J., Reynolds, B., & Heald, F. P. (1977). Adolescents who attempt suicide. Journal of Pediatrics, 90, 636-638. (Abstract: EM, 1977, Sect. 32, 37, No. 1119, p. 207)

5-211   Rosenkrantz, A. L. (1978). A note on adolescent suicide: Incidence, dynamics and some suggestions for treatment. Adolescence, 13(50), 209-214. (Abstract: PA, 1979, 62, No. 3863, pp. 395-396)

* 5-212   Seiden, R. H. (1969). Suicide among youth: A review of the literature, 1900-1967 (Supplement to the Bulletin of Suicidology). Washington, D.C.: USGPO, Public Health Service Publication No. 1971. (Excerpt reprinted as "Studies of adolescent suicidal behavior," in B. Q. Hafen & E. J. Faux (Eds.) (1972), Self-destructive behavior: A national crisis (pp. 153-191). Minneapolis: Burgess. Excerpt reprinted as "Studies of adolescent suicidal behavior: Etiology," in R. J. Morris (Ed.) (1974), Perspectives in abnormal behavior (pp. 117-143). New York: Pergamon Press.) (Abstract: PA, 1972, 47, No. 1213, p. 130)

* 5-213   Shaffer, D., & Fisher, P. (1981). The epidemiology of suicide in children and young adolescents. Journal of the American Academy of Child Psychiatry, 20, 545-565.

5-214   Stone, M. H. (1973). The parental factor in adolescent suicide. International Journal of Child Psychotherapy, 2, 163-201. (Abstract: PA, 1974, 52, No. 3340, p. 427)

5-215   Tishler, C. L. (1980). Intentional self-destructive behavior in children under age ten. Clinical Pediatrics, 19, 451-453.

5-216   Tishler, C. L., McKenry, P. C., & Morgan, K. C. (1981). Adolescent suicide attempts: Some significant factors. Suicide and Life-Threatening Behavior, 11, 86-92. (Abstracts: PA, 1982, 67, No. 7986, p. 862; CPA, 1981, 21, No. 2183, p. 497)

5-217 Toolan, J. M. (1978). Therapy of depressed and
       suicidal children. American Journal of
       Psychotherapy, 32, 243-251. (Abstracts: PA,
       1979, 62, No. 4015, p. 410; ACP, 1979, 19,
       No. 288, p. 64)

5-218 Toolan, J. M. (1981). Depression and suicide in
       children: An overview. American Journal of
       Psychotherapy, 35, 311-322. (Abstract: PA,
       1982, 67, No. 1602, p. 176)

5-219 Weiss, N. S. (1976). Recent trends in violent
       deaths among young adults in the United States.
       American Journal of Epidemiology, 103, 416-422.
       (Abstract: EM, 1977, Sect. 32, 35, No. 377,
       p. 67)

5-220 Wells, C. F., & Stuart, I. R. (Eds.) (1981).
       Self-destructive behavior in children and
       adolescents. New York: Van Nostrand Reinhold.

           Among the articles in this book are the
           following which are especially relevant here.

       5-220.01 Anderson, D. R. Diagnosis and prediction
                 of suicidal risk among adolescents.
                 pp. 45-59.

       5-220.02 McIntire, M. S., & Angle, C. R. The
                 taxonomy of suicide and self-poisoning:
                 A pediatric perspective. pp. 224-249.

       5-220.03 Pfeffer, C. R. The distinctive features
                 of children who threaten and attempt
                 suicide. pp. 106-120.

       5-220.04 Richman, J. Family treatment of suicidal
                 children and adolescents. pp. 274-290.

       5-220.05 Shaffer, D., & Fisher, P. Suicide in
                 children and young adolescents.
                 pp. 75-104.

See also: Pettifor et al. (1983, reference 6-135); Hersh
(1975, reference 7-088).

5.6d College Student Suicide

5-221 Bernard, J. L., & Bernard, M. L. (1982). Factors
       related to suicidal behavior among college
       students and the impact of institutional
       response. Journal of College Student Personnel,
       23, 409-413. (Abstract: PA, 1983, 69,
       No. 10600, p. 1163)

5-222 Hawton, K., Crowle, J., Simkin, S., & Bancroft,

J. (1978). Attempted suicide and suicide among Oxford University students. British Journal of Psychiatry, 132, 506-509. (Abstracts: PA, 1979, 62, No. 8806, p. 912; EM, 1979, Sect. 32, 39, No. 2325, p. 411)

5-223 Heinrichs, E. H. (1980). Suicide in the young: Demographic data of college-age students in a rural state. Journal of the American College Health Association, 28, 236-237.

5-224 Hendin, H. (1975a). Growing up dead: Student suicide. American Journal of Psychotherapy, 29, 327-338. (Abstracts: PA, 1976, 55, No. 975, p. 120; ACP, 1976, 16, No. 308, p. 95; ASW, 1976, 12(2), No. 442, p. 23)

5-225 Hendin, H. (1975b). Student suicide: Death as a life style. Journal of Nervous and Mental Diseases, 160, 204-219. (Abstract: EM, 1975, Sect. 32, 32, No. 3615, p. 619; ACP, 1976, 16, No. 307, p. 95)

5-226 Hendin, H. (1976). Growing up dead: Student suicide. In E. S. Shneidman (Ed.), Suicidology: Contemporary developments (pp. 322-333). New York: Grune & Stratton. (Adapted from Chapter 9 of Hendin's 1975 book, The age of sensation (pp. 223-258). New York: Norton.)

5-227 Hendrickson, S., & Cameron, C. A. (1975). Student suicide and college administrators: A perceptual gap. Journal of Higher Education, 46, 349-354. (Abstract: PA, 1975, 54, No. 8280, p. 1023)

5-228 Knight, J. A. (1968). Suicide among students. In H. L. P. Resnik (Ed.), Suicidal behaviors: Diagnosis and management (pp. 228-240). Boston: Little, Brown.

5-229 Knott, J. E. (1973). Campus suicide in America. Omega, 4, 65-71. (Abstracts: PA, 1974, 51, No. 9393, p. 1193; EM, 1974, Sect. 32, 29, No. 365, p. 62)

5-230 Kraft, D. P. (1980). Student suicides during a twenty-year period at a state university campus. Journal of the American College Health Association, 28, 258-262.

5-231 Patterson, J. E. (1975). Suicide Lethality Form: A guide to determining the potential lethality of university students' suicide threats (Doctoral dissertation, Kent State University, 1974). Dissertation Abstracts International, 35, 6465-6466A. (University Microfilms No. 75-7463)

5-232   Peck, D. L., & Bharadwaj, L. K. (1980). Personal stress and fatalism as factors in college suicide. Social Science, 55, 19-24.

5-233   Peck, M. L., & Schrut, A. (1971). Suicidal behavior among college students. HSMHA Health Reports, 86, 149-156.

5-234   Pepitone-Arreola-Rockwell, F., Rockwell, D., & Core, N. (1981). Fifty-two medical student suicides. American Journal of Psychiatry, 138, 198-201.

5-235   Schwartz, A. J., & Reifler, C. B. (1980). Suicide among American college and university students from 1970-71 through 1975-76. Journal of the American College Health Association, 28, 205-210.

5-236   Seiden, R. H. (1966). Campus tradegy: A study of student suicide. Journal of Abnormal Psychology, 71, 389-399. (Reprinted in G. D. Shean (Ed.) (1971), Studies in abnormal behavior (pp. 180-199). Chicago: Rand McNally. Reprinted in B. Kleinmuntz (Ed.) (1974), Readings in the essentials of abnormal psychology (pp. 214-222). New York: Harper & Row.)

5-237   Seiden, R. H. (1971). The problem of suicide on college campuses. Journal of School Health, 41, 243-248. (Abstract: ACP, 1972, 12, No. 1143, p. 348)

5-238   Sims, L., & Ball, M. J. (1973). Suicide among university students. Journal of the American College Health Association, 21, 336-338. (Abstract: PA, 1974, 52, No. 5663, p. 723)

5-239   Spalt, L. (1980). Suicide behavior and depression in university student psychiatric referrals. Psychiatric Quarterly, 52, 235-239.

5-240   Wolfe, R., & Cotler, S. (1973). Undergraduates who attempt suicide compared with normal and psychiatric controls. Omega, 4, 305-312. (Abstracts: PA, 1974, 52, No. 5675, p. 724; EM, 1975, Sect. 32, 31, No. 1039, p. 179)

See also Bernard & Bernard (1980, reference 8-009); Schwartz (1980, reference 5-063 above); Mishara et al. (1976, reference 5-823), Mishara (1982, reference 5-822), and Schotte & Clum (1982, reference 5-828).

5.6e Middle Aged

5-241   Boyd, J. H., & Weissman, M. M. (1981). The epidemiology of psychiatric disorders of middle

age: Depression, alcoholism, and suicide. In
J. G. Howells (Ed.), Modern perspectives in the
psychiatry of middle age (pp. 201-221;
esp. pp. 214-218). New York: Brunner/Mazel.

5-242   Burrows, G. D., & Dennerstein, L. (1981).
Depression and suicide in middle age. In
J. G. Howells (Ed.), Modern perspectives in the
psychiatry of middle age (pp. 222-250;
esp. pp. 241-245). New York: Brunner/Mazel.

5-243   Cath, S. H. (1980). Suicide in the middle years:
Some reflections on the annihilation of self. In
W. H. Norman & T. J. Scaramella (Eds.), Mid-life:
Developmental and clinical issues (pp. 53-72).
New York: Brunner/Mazel.

5-244   Lyons, M. J. (1982). Psychological concomitants of
the environment influencing suicidal behavior in
middle and later life (Doctoral dissertation,
University of Louisville, 1982). Dissertation
Abstracts International, 43, 1620B. (University
Microfilms No. DA8223898)

5-245   Sainsbury, P. (1962). Suicide in the middle and
later years. In H. T. Blumenthal (Ed.), Aging
around the world: Medical and clinical aspects
of aging (pp. 97-105). New York: Columbia
University Press.

5-246   Segal, B. E. (1969). Suicide and middle age.
Sociological Symposium, No. 3, pp. 131-141.
(Abstract: PA, 1972, 48, No. 3307, p. 368)

5.6f Elderly

5-247   Atchley, R. C. (1980). Aging and suicide:
Reflection of the quality of life? In
S. C. Haynes & M. Feinleib (Eds.), Second
conference on the epidemiology of aging
(pp. 141-161). Washington, D.C.: USGPO, NIH
Publication No. 80-969.

5-248   Batchelor, I. R. C., & Napier, M. B. (1953,
November 28). Attempted suicide in old age.
British Medical Journal, 2, 1186-1190.

5-249   Berdes, C. (1978). Social services for the aged
dying and bereaved in international perspective
(pp. 26-41). Washington, D.C.: International
Federation on Ageing, "Suicide and suicide
prevention."

5-250   Bock, E. W. (1972). Aging and suicide: The
significance of marital, kinship, and alternative
relations. Family Coordinator, 21, 71-79.

(Abstracts: PA, 1972, 48, No. 5237, p. 565;
ASW, 1972, 8, No. 799, p. 4; EM, 1972, Sect. 20,
15, No. 3074, p. 497)

5-251   Bock, E. W., & Webber, I. L. (1972). Social status
        and relational system of elderly suicides: A
        reexamination of the Henry-Short thesis.
        Life-Threatening Behavior, 2, 145-159.
        (Abstracts: PA, 1973, 50, No. 11437,
        pp. 1255-1256; ACP, 1973, 13, No. 1657, p. 462)
        Short, J. F., Jr. (1972). Comment on Bock &
        Webber's "Social status and relational system of
        elderly suicides," 2, 160-162.

5-252   Bock, E. W., & Webber, I. L. (1972). Suicide and
        the elderly: Isolating widowhood and mitigating
        alternatives. Journal of Marriage and the
        Family, 34, 24-31. (Abstracts: EM, 1972,
        Sect. 20, 15, No. 3077, p. 497; ASW, 1973, 9,
        No. 1, p. 3)

5-253   Breed, W., & Huffine, C. L. (1979). Sex
        differences in suicide among older white
        Americans: A role and developmental approach.
        In O. J. Kaplan (Ed.), Psychopathology of aging
        (pp. 289-309). New York: Academic Press.

5-254   Charatan, F. B. (1979). The aged. In
        L. D. Hankoff & B. Einsidler (Eds.), Suicide:
        Theory and clinical aspects (pp. 253-262).
        Littleton, MA: PSG Publishing.

5-255   Chynoweth, R. (1981). Suicide in the elderly.
        Crisis, 2, 106-116.

5-256   Farberow, N. L., & Moriwaki, S. Y. (1975).
        Self-destructive crises in the older person.
        Gerontologist, 15, 333-337.

5-257   Hendin, H. (1982). Suicide in America (pp. 59-82).
        New York: Norton, Chapter 3, "Suicide among
        older people."

5-258   Jarvis, G. K., & Boldt, M. (1980). Suicide in
        later years. Essence, 4(3), 145-158.

5-259   Marshall, J. R. (1978). Changes in aged white male
        suicide: 1948-1972. Journal of Gerontology, 33,
        763-768. (Abstracts: PA, 1980, 63, No. 3469,
        p. 397; EM, 1979, Sect. 20, 22, No. 541, p. 98)

5-260   McIntosh, J. L. (in press). Components of the
        decline in elderly suicide: Suicide among the
        young-old and old-old by race and sex. Death
        Education (to appear in a special issue on
        suicide).

5-261   McIntosh, J. L., Hubbard, R. W., & Santos,
         J. F. (1981). Suicide among the elderly: A
         review of issues with case studies. Journal of
         Gerontological Social Work, 4, 63-74. (Abstract:
         PA, 1983, 69, No. 1274, p. 138)

5-262   McIntosh, J. L., & Santos, J. F. (1981). Suicide
         among minority elderly: A preliminary
         investigation. Suicide and Life-Threatening
         Behavior, 11, 151-166. (Abstract: PA, 1982, 67,
         No. 10051, p. 1083)

5-263   Miller, M. (1978). Note: Toward a profile of the
         older white male suicide. Gerontologist, 18,
         80-82. (Abstracts: PA, 1979, 61, No. 8656,
         p. 868; EM, 1978, Sect. 20, 21, No. 3196,
         p. 590)

5-264   Miller, M. (1979). Suicide after sixty: The final
         alternative. New York: Springer.

5-265   Miller, M. (1979). A review of the research on
         geriatric suicide. Death Education, 3, 283-296.
         (Reprinted in Miller, 1979, reference 5-264
         above, pp. 95-105.)

5-266   O'Neal, P., Robins, E., & Schmidt, E. H. (1956). A
         psychiatric study of attempted suicide in persons
         over sixty years of age. Archives of Neurology
         and Psychiatry, 75, 275-284.

5-267   Payne, E. C. (1975). Depression and suicide. In
         J. G. Howells (Ed.), Modern perspectives in the
         psychiatry of old age (pp. 290-312). New York:
         Brunner/Mazel.

5-268   Pelizza, J. J. (1979). Suicide in the elderly:
         Can it be prevented? Long Term Care and Health
         Services Administration Quarterly, 3(2), 85-91.

5-269   Peretti, P. O., & Wilson, C. (1978-79).
         Contemplated suicide among voluntary and
         involuntary retirees. Omega, 9, 193-201.
         (Abstracts: PA, 1980, 63, No. 3473, p. 398; EM,
         1979, Sect. 20, 22, No. 1679, p. 296)

5-270a   Poldinger, W. J. (1981). Suicide and attempted
         suicide in the elderly. Crisis, 2, 117-121.

5-270b   Pollinger-Haas, A., & Hendin, H. (1983). Suicide
         among older people: Projections for the future.
         Suicide and Life-Threatening Behavior, 13,
         147-154.

5-271   Rachlis, D. (1970, Fall). Suicide and loss
         adjustment in the aging. Bulletin of

Suicidology, No. 7, pp. 23-26. (Abstracts: PA, 1972, 47, No. 7145, pp. 789-790; EM, 1972, Sect. 20, 15, No. 1186, pp. 194-195)

5-272   Resnik, H. L. P., & Cantor, J. M. (1970). Suicide and aging. *Journal of the American Geriatrics Society*, 18, 152-158. (Reprinted in V. M. Brantl & M. R. Brown (Eds.) (1973), *Readings in gerontology* (pp. 111-117). St. Louis: C. V. Mosby. Reprinted in S. Steury & M. L. Blank (Eds.) (1977), *Readings in psychotherapy with older people* (pp. 215-219). Washington, D.C.: USGPO.) (Abstracts: ACP, 1971, 11, No. 767, pp. 245-246; EM, 1970, Sect. 20, 13, No. 2808, p. 457)

5-273   Robins, L. N., West, P. A., & Murphy, G. E. (1977). The high rate of suicide in older white men: A study testing ten hypotheses. *Social Psychiatry*, 12, 1-20. (Abstracts: PA, 1977, 58, No. 3556, p. 370; ACP, 1977, 17, No. 1222, pp. 343-344; EM, 1977, Sect. 32, 36, No. 2327, p. 434)

5-274   Sainsbury, P. (1962). Suicide in later life. *Gerontologia Clinica*, 4, 161-170.

5-275   Sainsbury, P. (1963). Social and epidemiological aspects of suicide with special reference to the aged. In R. H. Williams, C. Tibbitts, & W. Donahue (Eds.), *Processes of aging: Social and psychological perspectives, Volume II* (pp. 153-175). New York: Atherton Press.

5-276   Seiden, R. H. (1981). Mellowing with age: Factors influencing the nonwhite suicide rate. *International Journal of Aging and Human Development*, 13, 265-284. (Abstracts: PA, 1982, 68, No. 1388, p. 155; SWRA, 1984, 20, No. 35, p. 32)

5-277   Sendbuehler, J. M., & Goldstein, S. (1977). Attempted suicide among the aged. *Journal of the American Geriatrics Society*, 25, 245-248. (Reprinted in M. Tallmer, D. J. Cherico, A. H. Kutscher, D. E. Sanders, & E. R. Prichard (Eds.) (1980), *Thanatological aspects of aging: Selected readings* (pp. 25-28). Brooklyn, NY: Highly Specialized Promotions.) (Abstract: EM, 1978, Sect. 20, 21, No. 1088, pp. 201-202)

5-278   Shulman, K. (1978). Suicide and parasuicide: A review. *Age and Ageing*, 7, 201-209. (Abstract: EM, 1979, Sect. 20, 22, No. 2980, p. 527)

5-279   Stenback, A. (1980). Depression and suicidal behavior in old age. In J. E. Birren &

R. B. Sloane (Eds.), Handbook of mental health and aging (pp. 616-652). Englewood Cliffs, NJ: Prentice-Hall. (Reprinted as "Suicidal behavior in old age" in K. W. Schaie & J. Geiwitz (Eds.) (1982), Readings in adult development and aging (pp. 369-384). Boston: Little, Brown.)

5-280   Stengel, E. (1965). Prevention of suicide in old age. Zeitschrift fur Praventivmedizin, 10, 474-481.

5-281   Walsh, D., & McCarthy, P. D. (1965). Suicide in Dublin's elderly. Acta Psychiatrica Scandinavica, 41, 227-235.

5-282   Weiss, J. M. A. (1968). Suicide in the aged. In H. L. P. Resnik (Ed.), Suicidal behaviors: Diagnosis and management (pp. 255-267). Boston: Little, Brown.

5-283   Wolff, K. (1970). Observations on depression and suicide in the geriatric patient. In K. Wolff (Ed.), Patterns of self-destruction: Depression and suicide (pp. 33-42). Springfield, IL: Thomas.

See also Holinger & Offer (1982, reference 5-192 above); Osgood (1982, reference 7-092); Ornstein (1983, reference 5-141); Darbonne (1969, reference 9-169); Farberow & Shneidman (1957, reference 9-173); McIntosh (1980, reference 5-005); Nelson & Farberow (1977, reference 2-082); Portwood (1978, reference 8-056); Sainsbury (1962, reference 5-245).

5.7 Suicide Among U.S. Racial/Ethnic Groups

5.7a Bibliographies

5-284   American Association of Suicidology. Suicide and minority groups. [Annotated bibliography]. Denver: AAS.

5-285   Hubbard, E. E., & Davis, L. G. (1975). Suicides in the black community: A preliminary survey. Monticello, IL: Council of Planning Librarians, Exchange Bibliography No. 887, available from Vance Bibliographies. (8 pages) [out of print]

5-286   McIntosh, J. L. (1981). Suicide among U.S. racial minorities: A comprehensive bibliography. Monticello, IL: Vance Bibliographies, Public Administration Series Bibliography No. P-684. (35 pages)

This bibliography includes references for Blacks, Native Americans, Asian-Americans (including separate sections for Chinese-, Japanese-, and Filipino-Americans) and Hispanics.

5-287   Miller, M. Non-annotated bibliographies. San Diego, CA: Center for Information on Suicide. The 1984 catalog includes:

5-287.01 Indian suicides. Bibliography No. R-1.

5-287.02 Black suicides. Bibliography No. R-2.

5-288   Peters, R. (1981). Suicidal behavior among Native Americans: An annotated bibliography. White Cloud Journal of American Indian/Alaska Native Mental Health, 2(3), 9-20. (Abstract: PA, 1982, 67, No. 12321, p. 1321)

5.7b References Considering Several Minorities

5-289   Green, J. (1977). Ethnic aspects of suicide statistics. In C. L. Hatton, S. M. Valente, & A. Rink (Eds.), Suicide: Assessment and intervention (pp. 138-143). New York: Appleton-Century-Crofts.

This article considers Los Angeles County, CA statistics for 1972-73 for white, black, Spanish Surname, and Oriental.

5-290   Kalish, R. A., & Reynolds, D. K. (1976). Death and ethnicity: A psychocultural study. Los Angeles: University of Southern California Press.

Among the questions about death that were asked were several regarding knowledge of and exposure to suicide. [See also Reynolds et al. (1975, reference 5-430.01).]

5-291   Lum, D. (1974). Responding to suicidal crisis: For church and community (esp. pp. 102-110). Grand Rapids, MI: Eerdmans.

Lum presents information for Black, Indian, and Japanese-American suicide.

5-292   McIntosh, J. L. (1980). A study of suicide among United States racial minorities based on official statistics: The influence of age, sex, and other variables (Doctoral dissertation, University of Notre Dame, 1980). Dissertation Abstracts International, 41, 1135B. (University Microfilms No. 8020965)

A study of official data for whites, blacks, Native Americans, Chinese-, Japanese-, and

Pilipino-Americans was conducted comparing 1976 figures compiled by the researcher with available data for 1959-61. A portion of these findings is presented in McIntosh & Santos (1981, reference 5-293 below).

5-293   McIntosh, J. L., & Santos, J. F. (1981). Suicide among minority elderly: A preliminary investigation. Suicide and Life-Threatening Behavior, 11, 151-166. (Abstract: PA, 1982, 67, No. 10051, p. 1083)

5-294   McIntosh, J. L., & Santos, J. F. (1982). Changing patterns in methods of suicide by race and sex. Suicide and Life-Threatening Behavior, 12, 221-233. (Abstracts: PA, 1983, 70, No. 12931, p. 1453; CPA, 1983, 23, No. 1252, pp. 264-265)

Official statistics for 1923-1978 were compiled for suicide methods by sex and race (white, black, Native American, Chinese-, and Japanese-Americans).

5-295   McIntosh, J. L., & Santos, J. F. (1984). Suicide counseling and intervention with racial/ethnic minorities. In C. L. Hatton & S. M. Valente (Eds.), Suicide: Assessment and intervention (2nd ed.) (pp. 175-194). Norwalk, CT: Appleton-Century-Crofts.

Information regarding counseling and intervention with suicidal minority members (blacks, Native Americans, Asian-Americans, Hispanics) is presented.

5-296   Seiden, R. H. (1974). Current developments in minority group suicidology. Journal of Black Health Perspectives, 1, 29-42.

5-297   Seiden, R. H. (1981). Mellowing with age: Factors influencing the nonwhite suicide rate. International Journal of Aging and Human Development, 13, 265-284. (Abstract: PA, 1982, 68, No. 1388, p. 155)

Seiden considers possible explanations for the low suicide rates observed among nonwhites in old age and the decline in rates with increasing age (see also McIntosh & Santos, 1981, reference 5-293 above for a similar consideration).

See also Santos et al. (1983, reference 5-360) below.

5.7c Blacks

5-298   Aldridge, D. F. (1980). Black female suicides: Is
        the excitement justified? In L. F. Rodgers-Rose
        (Ed.), The black woman (pp. 273-284). Beverly
        Hills, CA: Sage Publications.

5-299   Breed, W. (1970). The Negro and fatalistic
        suicide. Pacific Sociological Review, 13,
        156-162.

5-300   Bush, J. A. (Ed.) (1976). Suicide and blacks. Los
        Angeles: Charles Drew Postgraduate Medical
        School.

        Among the papers in this book are the
        following:

        5-300.01 Christian, E. An exploratory study into
                  suicides among urban blacks.
                  pp. 68-75.

        5-300.02 Douglas, F. Suicide in black adolescents
                  and children. pp. 51-61.

        5-300.03 Holmes, C. E. An underlying theory for
                  black suicides. pp. 77-80.

        5-300.04 Seiden, R. H. Current trends in minority
                  group suicidology. pp. 27-50.

5-301   Bush, J. A. (1976). Suicide and blacks: A
        conceptual framework. Suicide and
        Life-Threatening Behavior, 6, 216-222.

5-302   Bush, J. A. (1978). Similarities and differences
        in precipitating events between black and Anglo
        suicide attempts. Suicide and Life-Threatening
        Behavior, 8, 243-249. (Abstracts: ACP, 1979,
        19, No. 1833, pp. 243-249; EM, 1980, Sect. 32,
        41, No. 1939, p. 306)

5-303   Christian, E. R. (1977). Black suicide. In
        C. L. Hatton, S. M. Valente, & A. Rink (Eds.),
        Suicide: Assessment and intervention
        (pp. 143-159). New York:
        Appleton-Century-Crofts.

5-304   Davis, R. (1979). Black suicide in the seventies:
        Current trends. Suicide and Life-Threatening
        Behavior, 9, 131-140. (Abstracts: PA, 1980, 64,
        No. 10588, pp. 1138-1139; CPA, 1980, 20,
        No. 293, p. 73)

5-305   Davis, R. (1980). Suicide among young blacks:
        Trends and perspectives. Phylon, 41, 223-229.

5-306   Davis, R. (1980). Black suicide and relational
        system: Theoretical and empirical implications
        of communal and familial ties. Research in Race
        and Ethnic Relations, 2, 43-71.

5-307   Davis, R. (1981). Black suicide and support
        systems: An overview and some implications for
        mental health practitioners. Western Journal of
        Black Studies, 5, 219-223.

5-308   Davis, R. (1981). A demographic analysis of
        suicide. In L. E. Gury (Ed.), Black men
        (pp. 179-195). Beverly Hills, CA: Sage
        Publications.

5-309   Davis, R. (1983). Black suicide and social support
        systems: An overview and some implications for
        mental health practitioners. Phylon, 43,
        307-314.

5-310   Davis, R., & Short, J. F., Jr. (1978). Dimensions
        of black suicide: A theoretical model. Suicide
        and Life-Threatening Behavior, 8, 161-173.
        (Abstract: PA, 1980, 63, No. 7750, pp. 878-879)

5-311   Hamermesh, D. S. (1974). The economics of black
        suicide. Southern Economic Journal, 41, 188-199.

5-312   Hendin, H. (1969). Black suicide. Archives of
        General Psychiatry, 21, 407-422. (Abstracts:
        PA, 1970, 44, No. 8799, p. 923; ACP, 1971, 11,
        No. 753, p. 242)

5-313   Hendin, H. (1969). Black suicide. New York:
        Basic Books.

5-314   Howze, B. (1977). Suicide: Special references to
        black women. Journal of Non-White Concerns in
        Personnel & Guidance, 5(2), 65-72. (Abstract:
        PA, 1978, 59, No. 1274, p. 143)

5-315   Jedlicka, D., Shin, Y., & Lee, E. S. (1977).
        Suicide among blacks. Phylon, 38, 448-455.

5-316   Kiev, A., & Anumonye, A. (1976). Suicidal behavior
        in a black ghetto. International Journal of
        Mental Health, 5(2), 50-59.

5-317   Kirk, A. R. (1977). Suicide: A stress component
        in black males. Urban Health, 6(6), 38-40.

5-318   Kirk, A. R., & Zucker, R. A. (1979). Some
        sociopsychological factors in attempted suicide
        among urban black males. Suicide and
        Life-Threatening Behavior, 9, 76-86. (Abstracts:
        PA, 1980, 64, No. 8247, p. 896; ACP, 1979, 19,

No. 2800, p. 688)

5-319   Miles, D. E. (1979). The growth of suicide among
        black Americans. Crisis, 86, 430-433.

5-320   Poussaint, A. F. (1975). Black suicide. In
        R. A. Williams (Ed.), Textbook of black-related
        diseases (pp. 708-714). New York: McGraw-Hill.
        (Excerpt reprinted as "Rising suicide rates among
        blacks." Urban League Review, 1977, 3, 22-30.)

5-321   Seiden, R. H. (1970, August). We're driving young
        blacks to suicide. Psychology Today, pp. 24, 26,
        28.

5-322   Seiden, R. H. (1972). Why are suicides of young
        blacks increasing? HSMHA Health Reports, 87,
        3-8.

5-323   Steele, R. (1975, September/October). Suicide in
        the black community. Renaissance 2, Issue 2,
        pp. 4-6, 21-22.

5-324   Steele, R. (1977). Clinical comparison of black
        and white suicide attempters. Journal of
        Consulting and Clinical Psychology, 45, 982-986.
        (Abstract: PA, 1978, 60, No. 7665, p. 831) [See
        also: Bedrosian, R. C., & Beck, A. T. (1978).
        Premature conclusions regarding black and white
        suicide attempters: A reply to Steele. 46,
        1498-1499. And: Steele, R. (1978). Steele's
        reply to Bedrosian and Beck. 46, 1500-1501.]

5-325   Stein, M., Levy, M. T., & Glasberg, H. M. (1974).
        Separations in black and white suicide
        attempters. Archives of General Psychiatry, 31,
        815-821.

5-326   Stewart, J. B. (1980). The political economy of
        black male suicides. Journal of Black Studies,
        11, 249-261.

5-327   Swanson, W. C., & Breed, W. (1976). Black suicide
        in New Orleans. In E. S. Shneidman (Ed.),
        Suicidology: Contemporary developments
        (pp. 99-128). New York: Grune & Stratton.

5-328   Taylor, M. C. (1982). Black male-female suicide:
        A case study of occupation and rates of suicide
        by race and sex. Western Journal of Black
        Studies, 6, 124-130.

See also: Dennis & Kirk (1976, reference 6-292); Wenz
(1978-79, reference 6-164); Peck (1983-84, reference
5-057); Warshauer & Monk (1978, reference 5-068).

5.7d Native Americans (American Indians)

5-329 Bynum, J. (1972). Suicide and the American Indian:
       An analysis of recent trends. In H. M. Bahr,
       B. A. Chadwick, & R. C. Day (Eds.), Native
       Americans today: Sociological perspectives
       (pp. 367-377). New York: Harper & Row.

5-330 Foulks, E. F. (1980). Psychological continuities:
       From dissociative states to alcohol use and
       suicide in Arctic populations. Journal of
       Operational Psychiatry, 11, 156-161.

5-331 Frederick, C. J. (1975). Suicide, homicide, and
       alcoholism among American Indians: Guidelines
       for help. Washington, D.C.: USGPO, DHEW
       Publication No. (ADM) 76-42. (Formerly DHEW
       Publication No. (HSM) 73-9124, originally
       published, 1973.)

5-332 Handler, A. (1978). Mortality trends among
       American Indians 1955-1975. Washington, D.C.:
       Indian Health Service.

5-333 Havighurst, R. J. (1971). The extent and
       significance of suicide among American Indians
       today. Mental Hygiene, 55, 174-177. (Abstract:
       PA, 1972, 47, No. 1203, p. 129)

5-334 Hill, C. A., Jr., & Spector, M. I. (1971).
       Natality and mortality of American Indians
       compared with U. S. whites and nonwhites. HSMHA
       Health Reports, 86, 229-246.

5-335 Humphrey, J. A., & Kupferer, H. J. (1982).
       Homicide and suicide among the Cherokee and Lubee
       Indians of North Carolina. International Journal
       of Social Psychiatry, 28, 121-128.

5-336 Kost-Grant, B. L. (1983). Self-inflicted gunshot
       wounds among Alaska Natives. Public Health
       Reports, 98, 72-78.

5-337 May, P. A., & Dizmang, L. H. (1974). Suicide and
       the American Indian. Psychiatric Annals, 4,
       22-23; 27-28. (Abstract: PA, 1977, 57,
       No. 3588, p. 434)

* 5-338 McIntosh, J. L. (1983-84). Suicide among Native
         Americans: Further tribal data and
         considerations. Omega, 14, 215-229.

* 5-339 McIntosh, J. L., & Santos, J. F. (1980-81).
         Suicide among Native Americans: A compilation of
         findings. Omega, 11, 303-316. (Abstract: PA,
         1981, 66, No. 13039, p. 1358)

Combined, these two references (5-338 and
5-339) review in tabular form data found in
the numerous studies of specific tribes in the
U.S. In addition to this data review, the two
articles present the similarities of the
findings and the need to consider each tribal
group separately.

5-340   Pine, C. J. (1981). Suicide in American Indian and
        Alaska Native tradition. White Cloud Journal of
        American Indian/Alaska Native Mental Health,
        2(3), 3-8. (Abstracts: PA, 1982, 67, No. 12323,
        p. 1321; SWRA, 1984, 20, No. 202, p. 56)

5-341   Resnik, H. L. P., & Dizmang, L. H. (1971).
        Observations on suicidal behavior among American
        Indians. American Journal of Psychiatry, 127,
        882-887. (Reprinted in J. P. Carse &
        A. B. Dallery (Eds.) (1977), Death and society:
        A book of readings and sources (pp. 215-224).
        New York: Harcourt, Brace, Janovich.)

5-342   Santora, D., & Starkey, P. (1982, August).
        Research studies in American Indian suicides.
        Journal of Psychiatric Nursing and Mental Health
        Services, 20(8), 25-29.

5-343   Shore, J. H. (1975). American Indian suicide--Fact
        and fantasy. Psychiatry, 38, 86-91. (Abstracts:
        ACP, 1975, 15, No. 1792, p. 470; EM, 1975,
        Sect. 32, 32, No. 2835, p. 486)

5-344   Travis, R. (1983). Suicide in Northwest Alaska.
        White Cloud Journal of American Indian Mental
        Health, 3, 23-30. (Abstract: PA, 1984, 71,
        No. 9827, p. 1033)

5-345   Webb, J. P., & Willard, W. (1975). Six American
        Indian patterns of suicide. In N. L. Farberow
        (Ed.), Suicide in different cultures (pp. 17-33).
        Baltimore: University Park Press.

5-346   Willard, W. (1979). American Indians. In
        L. D. Hankoff & B. Einsidler (Eds.), Suicide:
        Theory and clinical aspects (pp. 299-307).
        Littleton, MA: PSG Publishing.

See also: Andress (1977, reference 5-017).

5.7e Asian-Americans

5-347   Bourne, P. G. (1973). Suicide among Chinese in San
        Francisco. American Journal of Public Health,
        63, 744-750.

5-348   Ibrahim, I. B., Carter, C., McLaughlin, D., &
        Rashad, M. N. (1977). Ethnicity and suicide in
        Hawaii. Social Biology, 24, 10-16. (Abstract:
        PA, 1979, 61, No. 13609, p. 1393)

5-349   Kalish, R. A. (1968, December). Suicide: An
        ethnic comparison in Hawaii. Bulletin of
        Suicidology, No. 4, pp. 37-43. (Abstract: PA,
        1970, 44, No. 21205, p. 2154)

5-350   Lum, D. (1972). Japanese suicides in Honolulu,
        1958-1969. Hawaii Medical Journal, 31, 19-23.

5-351   Yamamoto, J. (1976). Japanese-American suicides in
        Los Angeles. In J. Westermeyer (Ed.),
        Anthropology and mental health: Setting a new
        course (pp. 29-36). Paris: Mouton.

5.7f Hispanics

5-352   Andress, V. R., & Corey, D. M. (1976). The
        demographic distribution of suicide in Riverside
        County between 1965 and 1969. Loma Linda, CA:
        Department of Sociology and Anthropology,
        Occasional papers No. 3, Loma Linda University
        Press.

5-353   Hatcher, C., & Hatcher, D. (1975). Ethnic group
        suicide: An analysis of Mexican American and
        Anglo suicide rates for El Paso, Texas. Crisis
        Intervention, 6(1), 2-9. (Abstract: PA, 1980,
        63, No. 1177, p. 139)

5-354   Markides, K. S. (1981). Death-related attitudes
        and behavior among Mexican-Americans: A review.
        Suicide and Life-Threatening Behavior, 11, 75-85.

5-355   Monk, M., & Warshauer, M. E. (1974). Completed and
        attempted suicide in three ethnic groups.
        American Journal of Epidemiology, 100, 333-345.

5-356   Newton, F., Olmedo, E. L., & Padilla, A. M. (1982).
        Hispanic mental health research: A reference
        guide. Berkeley, CA: University of California
        Press.

            This compilation of over 2000 references
            includes only 14 references on Hispanic
            suicide, and not all of those are published
            papers.

5-357   Padilla, A. M., & Ruiz, R. A. (1976). Latino
        mental health: A review of the literature.
        Washington, D.C.: USGPO, DHEW Publication
        No. (ADM) 76-113. (Formerly DHEW Publication
        No. (HSM) 73-9143.)

5-358   Pokorny, A. D. (1968). Human violence: A
        comparison of homicide, aggravated assault,
        suicide, and attempted suicide. In J. P. Gibbs
        (Ed.), Suicide (pp. 227-246). New York: Harper
        & Row. (Reprinted from Journal of Criminal Law,
        Criminology and Police Science, 1965, 56,
        488-497.)

5-359   Sabin, J. E. (1975). Translating despair.
        American Journal of Psychiatry, 132, 197-199.

5-360   Santos, J. F., Hubbard, R. W., & McIntosh,
        J. L. (1983). Mental health and the minority
        elderly. In L. D. Breslau & M. R. Haug (Eds.),
        Depression and aging: Causes, care, and
        consequences (pp. 51-70; esp. pp. 59-60). New
        York: Springer.

5-361   Schneer, H. I., Perlstein, A., & Brozovsky,
        M. (1975). Hospitalized suicidal adolescents:
        Two generations. Journal of the American Academy
        of Child Psychiatry, 14, 268-280.

5-362   Trautman, E. C. (1961). Suicide attempts of Puerto
        Rican immigrants. Psychiatric Quarterly, 35,
        544-554.

5-363   Trautman, E. C. (1961). The suicidal fit: A
        psychobiologic study on Puerto Rican immigrants.
        Archives of General Psychiatry, 5, 76-83.

See also: Andress (1977, reference 5-017); Domino (1981,
reference 7-013); Green (1977, reference 5-289); Kalish &
Reynolds (1976, reference 5-290); Reynolds et al. (1975,
reference 5-430.01).

5.8 Marital Status & Family Circumstances

5.8a Bibliographic Source

5-364   International Bibliography of Research in Marriage
        and the Family. Ann Arbor, MI: Edwards
        Brothers. Volume 1: 1900-1964. Volume 2:
        1965-1972. Volume 3: 1973-1974. Subsequent
        volumes by pairs of years as was Volume 3. Under
        the header "Suicide" or "Suicide & the Family"
        090S.

5.8b Marital Status & Families

5-365   Bennett, M. (1979). Emotional responses of
        husbands to suicide attempts by their wives. In
        M. Cook & G. Wilson (Eds.), Love and attraction
        (pp. 205-208). Oxford, England: Pergamon Press.

5-366   Bonnar, J. W., & McGee, R. K. (1977). Suicidal

behavior as a form of communication in married couples. Suicide and Life-Threatening Behavior, 7, 7-16.

5-367   Cumming, E., & Lazer, C. (1981). Kinship structure and suicide: A theoretical link. Canadian Review of Sociology and Anthropology, 18, 271-282. (Abstract: CPA, 1981, 21, No. 2686, pp. 606-607)

5-368   Danigelis, N., & Pope, W. (1979). Durkheim's theory of suicide as applied to the family: An empirical test. Social Forces, 57, 1081-1106. (Abstract: CPA, 1980, 20, No. 297, p. 74)

5-369   Farber, M. L. (1977). Factors determining the incidence of suicide within families. Suicide and Life-Threatening Behavior, 7, 3-6.

5-370   Gibbs, J. P. (1969). Marital status and suicide in the United States: A special test of the status integration theory. American Journal of Sociology, 74, 521-533. Segal, B. E. (1979). Comment on Jack Gibbs' "Marital status and suicide" [and Gibbs' reply]. 75, 405-411.

5-371   Gove, W. R. (1972). Sex, marital status, and suicide. Journal of Health and Social Behavior, 13, 204-213.

5-372   Helsing, K. J., Comstock, G. W., & Szklo, M. (1982). Causes of death in a widowed population. American Journal of Epidemiology, 116, 524-532.

5-373   Herman, S. J. (1977). Women, divorce, and suicide. Journal of Divorce, 1, 107-117.

5-374   Jacobson, G. F., & Portuges, S. H. (1978). Relation of marital separation and divorce to suicide: A report. Suicide and Life-Threatening Behavior, 8, 217-224. (Abstract: CPA, 1979, 19, No. 1835, p. 452)

5-375   Koskenvuo, M., Sarna, S., Kaprio, J., & Lonnqvist, J. (1979). Cause-specific mortality by marital status and social class in Finland during 1969-1971. Social Science and Medicine (Medical Psychology & Medical Sociology), 13A, 691-697.

5-376   Kozak, C. M., & Gibbs, J. O. (1979). Dependent children and suicide of married parents. Suicide and Life-Threatening Behavior, 9, 67-75. (Abstracts: PA, 1980, 64, No. 8248, p. 896; CPA, 1979, 19, No. 2804, pp. 688-689)

5-377   Leviton, D. (1973). The significance of sexuality
        as a deterrent to suicide among the aged. Omega,
        4, 163-174.

5-378   MacMahon, B., & Pugh, T. F. (1965). Suicide in the
        widowed. American Journal of Epidemiology, 81,
        23-31.

5-379   Miller, M. (1979). Cooperation of some wives in
        their husbands' suicides. Psychological Reports,
        44, 39-42. (Reprinted in Miller, M. (1979).
        Suicide after sixty: The final alternative
        (pp. 76-81). New York: Springer.)

5-380   Pfeffer, C. R. (1981). The family system of
        suicidal children. American Journal of
        Psychotherapy, 35, 330-341. (Abstract: PA,
        1982, 67, No. 1451, p. 160)

5-381   Rao, A. V. (1974). Marriage, parenthood, sex and
        suicidal behaviour. Indian Journal of
        Psychiatry, 16, 92-94.

5-382   Rico-Velasco, J., & Mynko, L. (1973). Suicide and
        marital status: A changing relationship?
        Journal of Marriage and the Family, 35, 239-244.
        Heer, D., & MacKinnon, D. (1974). Suicide and
        marital status: A rejoinder to Rico-Velasco and
        Mynko. 36, 6-10.

5-383   Schrut, A., & Michels, T. (1974). Suicidal
        divorced and discarded women. Journal of the
        American Academy of Psychoanalysis, 2, 329-348.

5-384   Simon, W., & Lumry, G. K. (1970). Suicide of the
        spouse as a divorce substitute. Diseases of the
        Nervous System, 31, 608-612.

5-385   Stack, S. (1980). The effects of marital
        dissolution on suicide. Journal of Marriage and
        the Family, 42, 83-91. (Abstract: PA, 1981, 65,
        No. 7878, p. 833)

5-386   Stack, S. (1981). Divorce and suicide: A time
        series analysis, 1933-1970. Journal of Family
        Issues, 2, 77-90.

5-387   Stroebe, M. S., & Stroebe, W. (1983). Who suffers
        more? Sex differences in health risks of the
        widowed. Psychological Bulletin, 93, 279-301
        (esp. pp. 293-294).

5-388   Veevers, J. E. (1973). Parenthood and suicide: An
        examination of a neglected variable. Social
        Science and Medicine, 7, 135-144.

5-389   Wenz, F. V. (1977). Marital status, anomie, and
        forms of social isolation: A case of high
        suicide rate among the widowed in an urban
        sub-area. Diseases of the Nervous System, 38,
        891-895. (Abstract: PA, 1979, 61, No. 3872,
        p. 389)

5-390   Wenz, F. V. (1979). Family constellation factors,
        depression, and parent suicide potential.
        American Journal of Orthopsychiatry, 49, 164-167.

See also Section 5.11b on bereavement. See also Gibbs &
Martin (1964, reference 4-015), Chapter 8, "Suicide and
marital status," pp. 86-103; Bock (1972, reference 5-250);
Bock & Webber (1972, 1972, references 5-251 & 5-252); Demi
(1978, 1978, references 9-024 and 9-025); Cain & Fast
(1966, reference 9-009.06); Goldberg & Mudd (1968,
reference 9-031); Nayha (1983, reference 5-513).

5.8c Other Family Issues

5-391   Dorpat, T. L., Jackson, J. K., & Ripley,
        H. S. (1965). Broken homes and attempted and
        completed suicide. Archives of General
        Psychiatry, 12, 213-216. (Reprinted in
        J. P. Gibbs (Ed.) (1968), Suicide (pp. 170-176).
        New York: Harper & Row.)

5-392   Jacobs, J., & Teicher, J. D. (1967). Broken homes
        and social isolation in attempted suicides of
        adolescents. International Journal of Social
        Psychiatry, 13, 139-149. (Reprinted in Jacobs,
        J. (1982). The moral justification of suicide
        (pp. 112-126). Springfield, IL: Thomas.)

5-393   Murphy, G. E., & Wetzel, R. D. (1982). Family
        history of suicidal behavior among suicide
        attempters. Journal of Nervous and Mental
        Diseases, 170, 86-90. (Abstract: CPA, 1982, 22,
        No. 723, pp. 144-145)

5-394   Trout, D. L. (1980). The role of social isolation
        in suicide. Suicide and Life-Threatening
        Behavior, 10, 10-23.

See also: Gove & Hughes (1980, reference 5-039) for a
discussion of social isolation and suicide; World Health
Organization (1968, reference 1-047b, presents a table of
research investigations on broken homes and suicide on
pp. 57-58.

5.8d Homosexuals & Suicide

5-395   Bell, A. P., & Weinberg, M. S. (1978).
        Homosexualities: A study of diversity among men
        and women. New York: Simon & Schuster.

5-396   Enright, M. F., & Parsons, B. V. (1976). Training
        crisis intervention specialists and peer group
        counselors as therapeutic agents in the gay
        community. Community Mental Health Journal, 12,
        383-391.

5-397   Fitzgerald, T. K. (1981). Suicide prevention and
        gay self-help groups in Sweden and Finland.
        Crisis, 2, 58-94.

5-398   Harry, J. (1983). Parasuicide, gender, and gender
        deviance. Journal of Health and Social Behavior,
        24, 350-361.

5-399   Hendin, H. (1982). Suicide in America
        (pp. 107-123). New York: Norton, Chapter 5,
        "Suicide and homosexuality."

5-400   Oberstone, A. K., & Sukoneck, H. (1976).
        Psychological adjustment and life style of single
        lesbians and single heterosexual women.
        Psychology of Women Quarterly, 1, 172-188.

5-401   Rofes, E. E. (1983). I thought people like that
        killed themselves: Lesbians, gay men and
        suicide. Eugene, OR: Grey Fox Press.

5-402   Tabachnick, N. (1970, May). Sex and suicide.
        Medical Aspects of Human Sexuality, 4(5), 48-63.

5.9 Culture & Suicide

5.9a Bibliographic Source

5-403   Favazza, A. R., & Faheem, A. D. (1982). Themes in
        cultural psychiatry: An annotated bibliography,
        1975-1980. Columbia: University of Missouri
        Press.

        This collection includes a large number of
        articles on suicide in various cultures.

5.9b Culture in General

5-404   De Vos, G. A. (1968). Suicide in cross-cultural
        perspective. In H. L. P. Resnik (Ed.), Suicidal
        behaviors: Diagnosis and management
        (pp. 105-134). Boston: Little, Brown.

5-405   Ellner, M. (1977). Research of international
        suicide. International Journal of Social
        Psychiatry, 23, 187-194.

5-406   Leigh, D. (1973). The transcultural aspects of
        suicide. Transactions of the Medical Society of
        London, 89, 121-123.

5-407   Lester, D. (1971a). The incidence of suicide and
        fear of the dead in nonliterate societies.
        Journal of Cross-Cultural Psychology, 2, 207-208.

5-408   Lester, D. (1971b). Suicide and mutilation
        behaviors in nonliterate societies.
        Psychological Reports, 28, 801-802.

5-409   Lester, D. (1973). Suicide, homicide, and
        age-dependency ratios. International Journal of
        Aging and Human Development, 4, 127-132.

5-410   Lester, D. (1974). A cross-national study of
        homicide and suicide. Behavioral Science
        Research, 9, 307-318.

5-411   Lester, D. (1977). The prediction of suicide and
        homicide rates cross-nationally by means of
        stepwise multiple regression. Behavioral Science
        Research, 12, 61-69.

5-412   Lester, D. (1982). The distribution of sex and age
        among completed suicides: A cross-national
        study. International Journal of Social
        Psychiatry, 28, 256-260.

5-413   Lynn, R. (1971). Personality and national
        character (pp. 6-15; 48-56). New York:
        Pergamon Press, Chapters 2, "Suicide and
        alcoholism," and 5, "Suicide, calorie intake and
        alcoholism."

        Lynn explains suicide levels, alcoholism
        levels and other factors within particular
        countries on the basis of their national or
        cultural anxiety levels.

5-414   Nanda, S. (1982). Death from a cross-cultural
        perspective. In B. A. Backer, N. Hannon, &
        Russell, N. A. (Eds.), Death and dying:
        Individuals and institutions (pp. 273-297,
        esp. pp. 285-288, "Suicide"). New York: Wiley.

5-415   Palmer, S. (1965). Murder and suicide in forty
        non-literate societies. Journal of Criminal Law,
        Criminology and Police Science, 56, 320-324.
        (Reprinted in J. Gibbs (Ed.) (1968), Suicide
        (pp. 246-254). New York: Harper & Row.)

5-416   Palmer, S. (1971). Characteristics of suicide in
        54 nonliterate societies. Life-Threatening
        Behavior, 1, 178-183.

5-417   Smith, D. H., & Hackathorn, L. (1982). Some social
        and psychological factors related to suicide in
        primitive societies: A cross-cultural

comparative study. Suicide and Life-Threatening Behavior, 12, 195-211. (Abstract: PA, 1983, 70, No. 12944, p. 1455)

5-418   Snyder, B. J. (1977). A note on the importance of cultural factors in suicide studies. Suicide and Life-Threatening Behavior, 7, 230-235.

5-419   Stack, S. (1980). Effects of age composition on suicide in traditional and industrial societies. Journal of Social Psychology, 111, 143-144.

* 5-420   Tousignant, M., & Mishara, B. L. (1981). Suicide and culture: A review of the literature (1969-1980). Transcultural Psychiatric Research Review, 18, 5-32.

5-421   Tseng, W.-S., & McDermott, J. F., Jr. (1981). Culture, mind and therapy: An introduction to cultural psychiatry (pp. 88-108). New York: Brunner/Mazel, Chapter 7, "Suicide."

5-422   Vigderhous, G. (1975). Suicide and homicide as causes of death and their relationship to life expectancy: A cross-cultural comparison. Social Biology, 22, 338-343.

See also: Krauss & Krauss (1968, reference 4-081); Lester (1972, reference 1-041), Chapter 8, "Cultural differences in suicidal behavior," pp. 47-56; Ruzicka (1976, reference 5-108); Sainsbury et al. (1980, reference 5-109); World Health Organization (1968, reference 1-047b).

5.9c Selected Articles on Other Countries

5-423   Aponte, R. (1980). Epidemiological aspects of suicide in Latin America. Crisis, 1, 35-41.

5-424   Bohannon, P. (Ed.) (1960). African homicide and suicide. Princeton, NJ: Princeton University Press.

5-425   Bolander, A.-M. (1972). Nordic suicide statistics. In J. Waldenstrom, T. Larsson, & N. Ljungstedt (Eds.), Suicide and attempted suicide (pp. 57-88). Stockholm: Nordiska Bokhandelns Forlag. [statistics for Denmark, Finland, Norway, Sweden]

5-426   Burvill, P. W. (1980). Changing patterns of suicide in Australia, 1910-1977. Acta Psychiatrica Scandinavica, 62, 258-268. (Abstract: PA, 1981, 66, No. 8193, p. 856)

5-427   Choron, J. (1968, December). Concerning suicide in Soviet Russia. Bulletin of Suicidology, No. 4,

pp. 31-36.

5-428   Dorsch, M. M., & Roder, D. M. (1983).   A comparison
        of Australian suicide rates in 1969-73 and
        1976-80. Australian & New Zealand Journal of
        Psychiatry, 17, 254-258.

5-429   Farber, M. L. (1979).   Suicide in France: Some
        hypotheses. Suicide and Life-Threatening
        Behavior, 9, 154-162.

* 5-430 Farberow, N. L. (Ed.) (1975).   Suicide in different
        cultures. Baltimore: University Park Press.

        In addition to references 3-009 and 5-345, the
        following articles on various cultures are
        included.

        5-430.01 Reynolds, D. K., Kalish, R., & Farberow,
                  N. L. A cross-ethnic study of suicide
                  attitudes and expectations in the
                  United States. pp. 35-50.

        5-430.02 Yampey, N. Suicide in Buenos Aires:
                  Social and cultural influences.
                  pp. 51-75.

        5-430.03 Retterstol, N. Suicide in Norway.
                  pp. 77-94.

        5-430.04 Achte, K. A., & Lonnqvist, J. Suicide in
                  Finnish culture. pp. 95-113.

        5-430.05 Rudestam, K. E. Suicide in Sweden and
                  the United States. pp. 115-133.

        5-430.06 Atkinson, M. Some cultural aspects of
                  suicide in Britain. pp. 135-158.

        5-430.07 Speijer, N. The attitude of Dutch
                  society toward the phenomenon of
                  suicide. pp. 159-164.

        5-430.08 Noomen, P. Suicide in the Netherlands.
                  pp. 165-177.

        5-430.09 Farber, M. L. Psychological variables in
                  Italian suicide. pp. 179-184.

        5-430.10 Farberow, N. L., & Simon, M. D. Suicide
                  in Los Angeles and Vienna.
                  pp. 185-203. (Reprinted from Public
                  Health Reports, 1969, 84, 389-403.)

        5-430.11 Schipkowensky, N., Milenkov, K., &
                  Bogdanova, A. Self-destruction in

Bulgarian folk songs. pp. 205-213.

5-430.12   Headley, L. Jewish suicide in Israel.
           pp. 215-230.

5-430.13   Rao, A. V. Suicide in India.
           pp. 231-238.

5-430.14   Rin, H. Suicide in Taiwan. pp. 239-254.

5-430.15   Iga, M., & Tatai, K. Characteristics of
           suicides and attitudes toward suicide
           in Japan. pp. 255-280.

5-431   Foulks, E. F. (1980). Psychological continuities:
        From dissociative states to alcohol use and
        suicide in Arctic populations. Journal of
        Operational Psychiatry, 11, 156-161.

5-432   Fuse, T. (1980a). Some characteristics of suicide
        in Japan. Psychiatric Journal of the University
        of Ottawa, 5, 89-94. (Abstract: PA, 1981, 66,
        No. 1514, p. 162)

5-433   Fuse, T. (1980b). Suicide and culture in Japan: A
        study of seppuku as an institutionalized form of
        suicide. Social Psychiatry, 15, 57-63.
        (Abstract: PA, 1981, 66, No. 1515, p. 162)

5-434   Giddens, A. (1971). The sociology of suicide: A
        selection of readings. London: Cass.

5-434.01   Leighton, A. H., & Hughes, C. C. Notes
           on Eskimo patterns of suicide.
           pp. 158-169. (Reprinted from
           Southwestern Journal of Anthropology,
           1955, 11, 327-338.)

5-434.02   La Fontaine, J. Suicide among the Gisu.
           pp. 170-184. (Reprinted from Bohannan,
           1960, reference 5-424 above).

5-434.03   Jeffreys, M. D. W. Samsonic suicides:
           Or suicides of revenge among Africans.
           pp. 185-196. (Reprinted from African
           Studies, 1952, 11, 118-122.)

5-434.04   Firth, R. Suicide and risk-taking in
           Tikopia society. pp. 197-222.
           (Reprinted from Psychiatry, 1961, 24,
           1-17.)

5-434.05   Iga, M., & Ohara, K. Suicide attempts of
           Japanese youth and Durkheim's concept
           of anomie. pp. 223-239. (Reprinted
           from Human Organization, 1967, 26,

59-68.)

5-435 Hendin, H. (1964). Suicide and Scandinavia. New
       York: Grune & Stratton.

       Hendin considers child rearing practices of
       Sweden, Norway, and Denmark as possible
       explanations for the differences in suicide
       levels in those countries.

5-436 Hendin, H. (1978). Suicide: The psychosocial
       dimension. Suicide and Life-Threatening
       Behavior, 8, 99-117.

5-437 Iga, M. (1978). Regional differences in Japanese
       suicide and its change. In T. L. Smith &
       M. S. Das (Eds.), Sociocultural change since 1950
       (pp. 69-93). New Delhi: Vikas Publishing.

5-438 Iga, M. (1981). Suicide of Japanese youth.
       Suicide and Life-Threatening Behavior, 11, 17-30.

5-439 Ishii, K. (1981). Adolescent self-destructive
       behavior and crisis intervention in Japan.
       Suicide and Life-Threatening Behavior, 11, 51-61.

5-440 Jennings, C., & Barraclough, B. (1980). Legal and
       administrative influences on the English suicide
       rate since 1900. Psychological Medicine, 10,
       407-418.

5-441 Kruijt, C. S. (1977). The suicide rate in the
       Western world since World War II. Netherlands
       Journal of Sociology, 13, 55-64. [Germany,
       France, Netherlands, Belgium, Great Britain &
       Wales]

5-442 Lindelius, R. (1979). Trends in suicide in Sweden
       1749-1975. Acta Psychiatrica Scandinavica, 60,
       295-310.

5-443a Low, A. A., Farmer, R. D., Jones, D. R., & Rohde,
       J. R. (1981). Suicide in England and Wales: An
       analysis of 100 years, 1876-1975. Psychological
       Medicine, 11, 359-368.

5-443b McClure, G. M. G. (1984). Trends in suicide rate
       for England and Wales 1975-80. British Journal
       of Psychiatry, 144, 119-126.

5-444 Meer, F. (1976). Race and suicide in South Africa.
       London: Routledge & Kegan Paul.

5-445 Okasha, A., & Lotaif, F. (1979). Attempted
       suicide: An Egyptian investigation. Acta
       Psychiatrica Scandinavica, 60, 69-75.

5-446   Paerregaard, G. (1980). Suicide in Denmark: A
        statistical review for the past 150 years.
        Suicide and Life-Threatening Behavior, 10,
        150-156.

5-447   Retterstol, N. (1972). Suicide in Norway. In
        J. Waldenstrom, T. Larsson, & N. Ljungstedt
        (Eds.), Suicide and attempted suicide
        (pp. 89-97). Stockholm: Nordiska Bokhandelns
        Forlag.

5-448   Rudestam, K. E. (1972). Demographic factors in
        suicide in Sweden and the United States.
        International Journal of Social Psychiatry, 18,
        79-90.

5-449   Shichor, D., & Bergman, S. (1979). Patterns of
        suicide among the elderly in Israel.
        Gerontologist, 19, 487-495.

5-450   Walsh, D. (1978). The recent increase in reported
        suicide in Ireland. Irish Medical Journal, 71,
        613-616.

A large number of the articles cited in this reference guide
consider suicide in other cultures. One need only look at
titles of the articles and journals to determine the
likelihood that non-U.S. suicide is being considered. Among
the works to consider are: Brown (1975, reference 5-028);
Diekstra (1982, reference 5-090);   Farmer & Rohde (1980,
reference 5-463);   Goldney & Katsikitis (1983, reference
5-156);   Solomon & Hellon (1980, reference 5-163);   Weiss &
Perry (1975, reference 7-051);   Wexler et al. (1978,
reference 5-113).

5.10 Other Factors and Suicide

5.10a Methods of Suicide

5-451   Boor, M. (1981). Methods of suicide and
        implications for suicide prevention. Journal of
        Clinical Psychology, 37, 70-75.

5-452   Bostic, R. A. (1973). Self-immolation: A survey
        of the last decade. Life-Threatening Behavior,
        3, 66-74.

5-453   Boyd, J. H. (1983). The increasing rate of suicide
        by firearms. New England Journal of Medicine,
        308, 872-874. (Abstract: PA, 1984, 71,
        No. 7007, p. 741) Hudgens, R. W. (1983).
        Preventing suicide [Editorial re: suicide
        methods and Boyd's article]. 308, 897-898.
        (Abstract: PA, 1984, 71, No. 7024, p. 743)

5-454   Brown, J. H. (1979). Suicide in Britain: More

attempts, fewer deaths, lessons for public
policy. _Archives of General Psychiatry_, _36_,
1119-1124. (Abstract: _PA_, 1980, _64_, No. 12840,
p. 1378)

5-455   Browning, C. H. (1974). Suicide, firearms, and
public health. _American Journal of Public
Health_, _64_, 313-317.

5-456   Browning, C. H. (1974). Epidemiology of suicide:
Firearms. _Comprehensive Psychiatry_, _15_, 549-553.

5-457   Card, J. J. (1974). Lethality of suicidal methods
and suicide risk: Two distinct concepts. _Omega_,
_5_, 37-45. Pallis, D. J., & Barraclough,
B. M. (1977-78). Seriousness of suicide attempt
and future risk of suicide: A comment on Card's
paper. _8_, 141-149.

5-458   Crosby, K., Rhee, J.-O., & Holland, J. (1977).
Suicide by fire: A contemporary method of
political protest. _International Journal of
Social Psychiatry_, _23_, 60-69.

5-459   Danto, B. L. (1971). Firearms and their role in
homicide and suicide. _Life-Threatening Behavior_,
_1_, 10-17.

5-460   Danto, B. L. (1972). Firearm suicide in the home
setting. _Omega_, _3_, 111-119.

5-461   Danto, B. L. (1982). Gun control to prevent
homicide and suicide. In B. L. Danto, J. Bruhns,
& A. H. Kutscher (Eds.), _The human side of
homicide_ (pp. 209-221). New York: Columbia
University Press.

5-462   Farmer, R. D. T. (1979). Suicide by different
methods. _Postgraduate Medical Journal_, _55_,
775-779.

5-463   Farmer, R., & Rohde, J. (1980). Effect of
availability and acceptability of lethal
instuments on suicide mortality: An analysis of
some international data. _Acta Psychiatrica
Scandinavica_, _62_, 436-446. (Abstract: _PA_, 1981,
_66_, No. 13026, p. 1357)

5-464   Fox, K., & Weissman, M. (1975). Suicide attempts
and drugs: Contradiction between method and
intent. _Social Psychiatry_, _10_, 31-38.

5-465   Hendin, H. (1982). _Suicide in America_
(pp. 143-159). New York: Norton, Chapter 7,
"Method and motive."

5-466 Kreitman, N. (1976). The coal gas story: United
       Kingdom suicide rates, 1960-71. British Journal
       of Preventative and Social Medicine, 30, 86-93.

5-467 Lester, D. (1970a). Factors affecting choice of
       method of suicide. Journal of Clinical
       Psychology, 26, 437.

5-468 Lester, D. (1970b). Personality correlates [MMPI]
       associated with choice of method of committing
       suicide. Personality, 1, 261-264.

5-469 Lester, D. (1971). Choice of method for suicide
       and personality. Omega, 2, 76-80.

5-470 Lester, D. (1979). Preference for method of
       suicide and attitudes toward death in normal
       people. Psychological Reports, 45, 638.

5-471 Lester, D., Beck, A. T., & Bruno, S. (1976).
       Correlates of choice of method for suicide.
       Psychology, 13, 70-73.

5-472 Lester, D., & Murrell, M. E. (1980). The influence
       of gun control laws on suicidal behavior.
       American Journal of Psychiatry, 137, 121-122.

5-473 Lester, D., & Murrell, M. E. (1982). The
       preventive effect of strict gun control laws on
       suicide and homicide. Suicide and
       Life-Threatening Behavior, 12, 131-140.
       (Abstract: PA, 1983, 69, No. 12936, p. 1429)

5-474 Markush, R. E., & Bartolucci, A. A. (1984).
       Firearms and suicide in the United States.
       American Journal of Public Health, 74, 123-127.

5-475 Marks, A. (1977). Sex differences and their effect
       upon cultural evaluations of methods of
       self-destruction. Omega, 8, 65-70.

5-476 Marks, A., & Abernathy, T. (1974). Toward a
       sociocultural perspective on means of
       self-destruction. Life-Threatening Behavior, 4,
       3-17.

5-477 Marks, A., & Stokes, C. S. (1976). Socialization,
       firearms, and suicide. Social Problems, 23,
       622-629.

5-478 McIntosh, J. L., & Santos, J. F. (1982). Changing
       patterns in methods of suicide by race and sex.
       Suicide and Life-Threatening Behavior, 12,
       221-233. (Abstract: PA, 1983, 70, No. 12931,
       p. 1453)

5-479   McIntosh, J. L., & Santos, J. F. (in press).
        Methods of suicide by age: Sex and race
        differences among the young and old.
        International Journal of Aging and Human
        Development.

5-480   Medoff, M. H., & Magaddino, J. P. (1983). Suicides
        and firearm control laws. Evaluation Review, 7,
        357-372. (Abstract: PA, 1984, 71, No. 7036,
        p. 744)

5-481   Oliver, R. G. (1972). Rise and fall of suicide
        rates in Australia: Relation to sedative
        availability. Medical Journal of Australia, 2,
        1208-1209.

5-482   Oliver, R. G., & Hetzel, B. S. (1972). Rise and
        fall of suicide rates in Australia: Relation to
        sedative availability. Medical Journal of
        Australia, 2, 919-923.

5-483   Proudfoot, A. T., & Park, J. (1978, January 14).
        Changing pattern of drugs used for
        self-poisoning. British Medical Journal,
        1(6105), 90-93.

5-484   Robertson, J. (1977). The epidemiology of
        self-poisoning. Public Health Reports, 91,
        75-82.

5-485   Seiden, R. H., & Spence, M. (1983-84). A tale of
        two bridges: Comparative suicide incidence on
        the Golden Gate and San Francisco-Oakland Bay
        bridges. Omega, 14, 201-209. (Reprinted from
        Crisis, 1982, 3, 32-40.)

5-486   Sims, M. (1974). Sex and age differences in
        suicide rates in a Canadian province: With
        particular reference to suicides by means of
        poison. Life-Threatening Behavior, 4, 139-159.

5-487   Taylor, M. C., & Wicks, J. W. (1980). The choice
        of weapons: A study of methods of suicide by
        sex, race, and region. Suicide and
        Life-Threatening Behavior, 10, 142-149.
        (Abstract: PA, 1981, 66, No. 3858, p. 407)

5-488   Watanbe, T., Kobayashi, Y., & Hata, S. (1973).
        Harakiri and suicide by sharp instruments in
        Japan. Forensic Science, 2, 191-199.

5-489   Weissman, M. M. (1975). Wrist cutting:
        Relationship between clinical observations and
        epidemiological findings. Archives of General
        Psychiatry, 32, 1166-1171.

* 5-490   Westermeyer, J. (1984).   Firearms, legislation, and
          suicide prevention [Editorial].   American Journal
          of Public Health, 74, 108.

          A succinct statement of the pro and con
          arguments regarding firearm legislation and
          suicide is presented.

See also: Lester (1983, reference 1-042), Chapter 15, "The
method chosen for suicide," pp. 91-97;   Burvill et
al. (1973, reference 5-544, and 1983, reference 5-547).

5.10b Temporal Factors & Suicide

5-491   Barraclough, B. M. (1976).   Time of day chosen for
        suicide.   Psychological Medicine, 6, 303-305.

5-492   Barraclough, B. M., & Shepherd, D. M. (1976).
        Birthday blues: The association of birthday with
        self-inflicted death in the elderly.   Acta
        Psychiatrica Scandinavica, 54, 146-149.
        (Abstract: PA, 1977, 57, No. 6046, p. 704)

5-493   Barraclough, B. M., & White, S. J. (1978a).
        Monthly variation of suicide and undetermined
        death compared.   British Journal of Psychiatry,
        132, 275-278.

5-494   Barraclough, B. M., & White, S. J. (1978b).
        Monthly variation of suicidal, accidental and
        undetermined poisoning death.   British Journal of
        Psychiatry, 132, 279-282.

5-495   Bazas, T., Jemos, J., Stefanis, K., & Trichopoulos,
        D. (1979).   Incidence and seasonal variation of
        suicide mortality in Greece.   Comprehensive
        Psychiatry, 20, 15-20.

5-496   Beck, A. T., & Lester, D. (1973).   Attempted
        suicide and month of birth.   Psychological
        Reports, 33, 506.

5-497   Bollen, K. A. (1983).   Temporal variations in
        mortality: A comparison of U. S. suicides and
        motor vehicle fatalities, 1972-1976.   Demography,
        20, 45-59.

5-498   Bunch, J., & Barraclough, B. (1971).   The influence
        of parental death anniversaries upon suicide
        dates.   British Journal of Psychiatry, 118,
        621-626.

5-499   de Maio, D., Carandente, F., & Riva, C. (1982).
        Evaluation of circadian, circaseptan and
        circannual periodicity of attempted suicides.
        Chronobiologia, 9, 185-193.   (Abstract: PA,

1983, <u>69</u>, No. 3661, p. 396)

5-500 Eastwood, M. R., & Peacocke, J. (1976). Seasonal patterns of suicide, depression and electroconvulsive therapy. <u>British Journal of Psychiatry</u>, <u>129</u>, 472-475.

* 5-501 Kevan, S. M. (1980). Perspectives on season of suicide: A review. <u>Social Science & Medicine</u>, <u>14D</u>, 369-378.

5-502 Kunz, P. R. (1978). Relationship between suicide and month of birth. <u>Psychological Reports</u>, <u>42</u>, 794.

5-503 Lester, D. (1971). Seasonal variation in suicidal deaths. <u>British Journal of Psychiatry</u>, <u>118</u>, 627-628.

5-504 Lester, D. (1973). Seasonal variation in suicide rates. <u>Lancet</u>, <u>1</u>, 611-612.

5-505 Lester, D. (1979). Temporal variation in suicide and homicide. <u>American Journal of Epidemiology</u>, <u>109</u>, 517-520.

5-506 Lester, D., & Beck, A. T. (1974). Suicide in the spring: A test of Durkheim's explanation. <u>Psychological Reports</u>, <u>35</u>, 893-894.

5-507 Lester, D., & Beck, A. T. (1975). Suicide and national holidays. <u>Psychological Reports</u>, <u>36</u>, 52.

5-508 Lester, D., Reeve, C. L., & Prieve, K. (1970). Completed suicide and month of birth. <u>Psychological Reports</u>, <u>27</u>, 210.

5-509 Lyster, W. R. (1973). Seasonal variation in suicide rates. <u>Lancet</u>, <u>1</u>, 725.

5-510 MacMahon, K. (1983). Short-term temporal cycles in the frequency of suicide, United States, 1972-1978. <u>American Journal of Epidemiology</u>, <u>117</u>, 744-750.

5-511 Meares, R., Mendelsohn, F. A. O., & Milgrom-Friedman, J. (1981). A sex difference in the seasonal variation of suicide rate: A single cycle for men, two cycles for women. <u>British Journal of Psychiatry</u>, <u>138</u>, 321-325.

5-512 Nayha, S. (1982). Autumn incidence of suicides re-examined: Data from Finland by sex, age and occupation. <u>British Journal of Psychiatry</u>, <u>141</u>, 512-517. (Abstract: <u>PA</u>, 1983, <u>70</u>, No. 1259,

p. 147)

5-513   Nayha, S. (1983). The bi-seasonal incidence of
        some suicides: Experience from Finland by
        marital status, 1961-1976. Acta Psychiatrica
        Scandinavica, 67, 32-42. (Abstract: PA, 1983,
        70, No. 10490, p. 1175)

5-514   Parker, G., & Walter, S. (1982). Seasonal
        variation in depressive disorders and suicidal
        deaths in New South Wales. British Journal of
        Psychiatry, 140, 626-632.

5-515   Phillips, D. P., & Liu, J. (1980). The frequency
        of suicides around major public holidays: Some
        surprising findings. Suicide and
        Life-Threatening Behavior, 10, 41-50.

5-516   Reid, P., Smith, H., & Greene, S. (1980). Seasonal
        variation in Irish suicidal deaths.
        Psychological Reports, 46, 306.

5-517   Rogot, E., Fabsitz, R., & Feinleib, M. (1976).
        Daily variation in USA mortality. American
        Journal of Epidemiology, 103, 198-211.

5-518   Sanborn, D. E., III, Casey, T. M., & Niswander,
        G. D. (1970). Suicide: Seasonal patterns and
        related variables. Diseases of the Nervous
        System, 31, 702-704.

5-519   Sanborn, D. E., III, & Sanborn, C. J. (1974).
        Suicide and months of birth. Psychological
        Reports, 34, 950.

5-520   Sanborn, D. E., III, & Sanborn, C. J. (1978). Sex,
        season and suicide. Psychological Reports, 42,
        1332.

5-521   Spiers, P. S. (1972). Seasonal variation in
        suicide rates. Lancet, 2, 428-429.

5-522   Vollen, K. H., & Watson, C. G. (1975). Suicide in
        relation to time of day and day of week.
        American Journal of Nursing, 75, 263.

5-523   Warren, C. W., Smith, J. C., & Tyler, C. W. (1983).
        Seasonal variation in suicide and homicide: A
        question of consistency. Journal of Biosocial
        Science, 15, 349-356.

5-524   Wenz, F. V. (1977). Seasonal suicide attempts and
        forms of loneliness. Psychological Reports, 40,
        807-810.

5-525   Wenz, F. V. (1977). Effects of seasons and

sociological variables on suicidal behavior.
Public Health Reports, 92, 233-239.

5-526 Zung, W. W. K., & Green, R. L. (1974). Seasonal
       variation of suicide and depression. Archives of
       General Psychiatry, 30, 89-91.

See also: Lester (1972, reference 1-041), Chapter 13,
"Temporal factors in suicidal behavior," pp. 149-153;
Lester (1983, reference 1-042), Chapter 8, "Temporal factors
in suicidal behavior," pp. 58-62; Lester & Lester (1972,
reference 1-043), Chapter 18, "Time, season, weather, and
suicide."

5.10c Meteorological Conditions & Suicide

5-527 Anderson, A. C. (1982). Environmental factors and
       aggressive behavior. Journal of Clinical
       Psychiatry, 43, 280-283. (Abstract: PA, 1983,
       69, No. 3647, p. 394)

5-528 De Voge, S. D., & Mikawa, J. K. (1977). Moon
       phases and crisis calls: A spurious
       relationship. Psychological Reports, 40,
       387-390.

5-529 Dixon, K. W., & Shulman, M. D. (1983). A
       statistical investigation into the relationship
       between meteorological parameters and suicide.
       International Journal of Biometeorology, 27,
       93-105.

5-530 Garth, J. M., & Lester, D. (1978). Moon and
       suicide. Psychological Reports, 43, 678.

5-531 Jones, P. K., & Jones, S. L. (1977). Lunar
       association with suicide. Suicide and
       Life-Threatening Behavior, 7, 31-39.

5-532 Ossenkopp, K. P., & Ossenkopp, M. D. (1978).
       Self-inflicted injuries and the lunar cycle: A
       preliminary report. Journal of Interdisciplinary
       Cycle Research, 4, 337-348.

5-533 Perry, F. S. (1981). Environmental power-frequency
       magnetic fields and suicide. Health Physics, 41,
       267-277. Comments: Smith, C. W. (1982). 43,
       439-441. Other comments: 1983, 44, 697-700.

* 5-534 Pokorny, A. D. (1968). Myths about suicide. In
         H. L. P. Resnik (Ed.), Suicidal behaviors:
         Diagnosis and management (pp. 57-72,
         esp. pp. 66-71). Boston: Little, Brown.

         Pokorny has been a major researcher in the
         area of weather and suicidal behavior. He

reviews the literature to the mid-1960s on
pages 66-71 and concludes that there is not
relationship between any weather or
atmospheric condition and suicidal behavior.

5-535   Reichmanis, M., Perry, F. S., Marino, A. A., &
        Becker, R. O. (1979). Relation between suicide
        and the electromagnetic field of overhead power
        lines. Physiological Chemistry & Physics, 11,
        395-403.

5-536   Taylor, L. J., & Diespecker, D. D. (1972). Moon
        phases and suicide attempts in Australia.
        Psychological Reports, 31, 110-120.

For other reviews of the literature, See: Lester (1972,
reference 1-041), Chapter 14, "Meteorlogical correlates of
suicidal behavior," pp. 154-158; Lester (1983, reference
1-042), Chapter 10, "Meteorological correlates of suicidal
behavior," pp. 70-71; Lester & Lester (1971, reference
1-043), Chapter 18, "Time, season, weather, and suicide",
pp. 144-148.

5.10d Geographic/Regional Differences & Migration

5-537   Alley, J. C. (1982). Life-threatening indicators
        among Indochinese refugees. Suicide and
        Life-Threatening Behavior, 12, 46-51.

5-538   Barton, S. N., Coombs, D. W., & Murkherjer,
        D. (1980). Urban-rural suicide differentials in
        Minnesota 1967-1973. Minnesota Medicine, 63,
        415-418.

5-539   Boor, M. (1981). Relationship of 1977 state
        suicide rates to population increases and
        immigration. Psychological Reports, 49, 856-858.

5-540   Burke, A. W. (1976). Attempted suicide among Asian
        immigrants in Birmingham. British Journal of
        Psychiatry, 128, 528-533.

5-541   Burke, A. W. (1976). Socio-cultural determinants
        of attempted suicide among West Indians in
        Birmingham: Ethnic origin and immigrant status.
        British Journal of Psychiatry, 129, 261-266.

5-542   Burke, A. W. (1978). Attempted suicide among
        Commonwealth immigrants in Birmingham.
        International Journal of Social Psychiatry, 24,
        7-11.

5-543   Burvill, P. W., Armstrong, B. K., & Carlson,
        D. J. (1983). Attempted suicide and immigration
        in Perth, Western Australia, 1969-1978. Acta
        Psychiatrica Scandinavica, 68, 89-99.

5-544   Burvill, P. W., McCall, M. G., Reid, T. A., &
        Stenhouse, N. S. (1973). Methods of suicide of
        English and Welsh immigrants in Australia.
        British Journal of Psychiatry, 123, 285-294.

5-545   Burvill, P. W., McCall, M. G., Stenhouse, N. S., &
        Reid, T. A. (1973). Deaths from suicide, motor
        vehicle accidents and all forms of violent deaths
        among migrants in Australia, 1962-66. Acta
        Psychiatrica Scandinavica, 49, 28-50.

5-546   Burvill, P. W., McCall, M. G., Stenhouse, N. S., &
        Woodings, T. L. (1982). The relationship between
        suicide, undetermined deaths and accidental
        deaths in Australian born and migrants in
        Australia. Australia & New Zealand Journal of
        Psychiatry, 16, 179-184. (Abstract: PA, 1983,
        69, No. 12903, p. 1425)

5-547   Burvill, P. W., McCall, M. G., Woodings, T. L., &
        Stenhouse, N. S. (1983). Comparison of suicide
        rates and methods in English, Scots, and Irish
        migrants in Australia. Social Science &
        Medicine, 17, 705-708. (Abstract: PA, 1984, 71,
        No. 7009, p. 741)

5-548   Burvill, P. W., Woodings, T. L., Stenhouse, N. S.,
        & McCall, M. G. (1982). Suicide during 1961-70
        migrants in Australia. Psychological Medicine,
        12, 295-308.

5-549   Coombs, D. W., Barton, S. N., & Moore, R. (1977).
        Urban-rural suicide differentials in Alabama
        1967-1973. Alabama Journal of Medical Science,
        14, 306-315.

5-550   Dorpat, T. L., & Ripley, H. S. (1981). The social
        geography of urban suicide behavior. Crisis, 2,
        14-19.

5-551   Frederick, C. J. (1982). Violent behavior in rural
        areas. In P. A. Keller & J. D. Murray (Eds.),
        Handbook of rural community mental health
        (pp. 74-84; esp. pp. 78-82). New York: Human
        Sciences Press.

5-552   French, L. A., & Wailes, S. N. (1980). Regional
        comparisons of suicidal aggression. Corrective
        and Social Psychiatry and Journal of Behavior
        Technology, Methods and Therapy, 26, 180-192.
        (Abstract: PA, 1981, 66, No. 8199, p. 856)

5-553   Gelfand, M. (1976). Suicide and attempted suicide
        in the urban and rural African in Rhodesia.
        Central Africa Medican Journal, 22, 203-205.

5-554   Koller, K. M., & Cotgrove, R. C. (1976). Social
        geography of suicidal behaviour in Hobart.
        Australia & New Zealand Journal of Psychiatry,
        10, 237-242.

5-555   Krupinski, J. (1979). Urbanization and mental
        health: Psychiatric morbidity, suicide and
        violence in the State of Victoria. Australia &
        New Zealand Journal of Psychiatry, 13, 139-145.

5-556   Lester, D. (1970). Completed suicide and latitude.
        Psychological Reports, 27, 818.

5-557   Lester, D. (1971). Completed suicide and
        longitude. Psychological Reports, 28, 662.

5-558   Lester, D. (1972). Migration and suicide. Medical
        Journal of Australia, 1, 941-942.

5-559   Lester, D. (1980). Variation of suicide and
        homicide by latitude and longitude. Perceptual &
        Motor Skills, 51, 1346.

5-560   Miller, M. (1980). The geography of suicide.
        Psychological Reports, 47, 699-702.

5-561   Morgan, H. G. (1980). Social correlates of
        non-fatal deliberate self-harm. In
        R. D. T. Farmer & S. R. Hirsch (Eds.), The
        suicide syndrome (pp. 90-102). London: Croom
        Helm.

5-562   Morgan, H. G., Pocock, H., & Pottle, S. (1975).
        The urban distribution of non-fatal deliberate
        self-harm. British Journal of Psychiatry, 126,
        319-328.

5-563   Morris, J. B., Kovacs, M., Beck, A. T., & Wolfe,
        A. (1974). Notes toward an epidemiology of urban
        suicide. Comprehensive Psychiatry, 15, 537-547.

5-564   Renwick, M. Y., Olsen, G. G., & Tyrrell,
        M. S. (1982). Suicide in rural New South Wales:
        Comparison with metropolitan experience. Medical
        Journal of Australia, 1, 377-380.

5-565   Stack, S. (1980). The effects of interstate
        migration on suicide. International Journal of
        Social Psychiatry, 26, 17-26.

5-566   Stack, S. (1981). Comparative analysis of
        immigration and suicide. Psychological Reports,
        49, 509-510.

5-567   Whitlock, F. A. (1971). Migration and suicide.
        Medical Journal of Australia, 2, 840-848.

See also: Niskanen et al. (1975, reference 6-423); Lester
(1983, reference 1-042), Chapter 9, "Studies of regional
suicide rates," pp. 63-69.

5.10e Religiosity and Religious Affiliation

5-568   Bainbridge, W. S., & Stark, R. (1981). Suicide,
         homicide, and religion: Durkheim reassessed.
         Annual Review of the Social Sciences of Religion,
         5, 33-56.

5-569   Bankston, W. B., Allen, H. D., & Cunningham,
         D. S. (1983). Religion and suicide: A research
         note on sociology's "one law." Social Forces,
         62, 521-528.

5-570   Beck, R. W., & Morris, J. B. (1974). Moral
         attitudes and suicidal behavior. Psychological
         Reports, 34, 697-698.

5-571   Beit-Hallahmi, B. (1975). Religion and suicidal
         behavior. Psychological Reports, 37, 1303-1306.

5-572   Best, J. B., & Kirk, W. G. (1982). Religiosity and
         self-destruction. Psychological Record, 32,
         35-39. (Abstract: PA, 1982, 68, No. 8148,
         p. 899)

5-573   Comstock, G. W., & Partridge, K. B. (1972). Church
         attendance and health. Journal of Chronic
         Diseases, 25, 665-672.

5-574   Danto, B. L., & Danto, J. M. (1983). Jewish and
         non-Jewish suicide in Oakland County, Michigan.
         Crisis, 4, 33-60. (Abstract: PA, 1984, 71,
         No. 9772, p. 1027)

5-575   Goss, M. E. W., & Reed, J. I. (1971). Suicide and
         religion: A study of white adults in New York
         City, 1963-1967. Life-Threatening Behavior, 1,
         163-177.

5-576   Hoelter, J. W. (1979). Religiosity, fear of death
         and suicide acceptability. Suicide and
         Life-Threatening Behavior, 9, 163-172.

5-577   Jasperse, C. W. G. (1976). Self-destruction and
         religion. Mental Health and Society, 3, 154-168.

5-578   Kranitz, L., Abrahams, J., Spiegel, D., &
         Keith-Spiegel, P. (1968). Religious beliefs of
         suicidal patients. Psychological Reports, 22,
         936.

5-579   Miller, L. (1976). Some data on suicide and

attempted suicide of the Jewish population in Israel. Mental Health and Society, 3, 178-181.

5-580   Morphew, J. A. (1968). Religion and attempted suicide. International Journal of Social Psychiatry, 14, 193-200.

5-581   Neal, C. D. (1981). Religion and self-poisoning. International Journal of Social Psychiatry, 27, 257-260.

5-582   Nelson, F. L. (1977). Religiosity and self-destructive crises in the institutionalized elderly. Suicide and Life-Threatening Behavior, 7, 67-74.

5-583   Pope, W., & Danigelis, N. (1981). Sociology's "one law." Social Forces, 60, 495-516.

Using cross-national longitudinal data, these authors find no evidence that Catholics have lower suicide rates than Protestants.

5-584   Stack, S. (1980). Religion and suicide: A reanalysis. Social Psychiatry, 15, 65-70.

5-585   Stack, S. (1981). Suicide and religion: A comparative analysis. Sociological Focus, 14, 207-220.

5-586   Stack, S. (1983). A comparative analysis of suicide and religiosity. Journal of Social Psychology, 119, 285-286. (Abstracts: PA, 1984, 71, No. 1657, p. 179; CPA, 1983, 23, No. 1751, p. 371)

5-587   Stack, S. (1983). The effect of the decline in instutionalized religion on suicide, 1954-1978. Journal for the Scientific Study of Religion, 22, 239-252.

5-588   Stack, S. (1983). The effect of religious commitment on suicide: A cross-national analysis. Journal of Health and Social Behavior, 24, 362-374.

5-589   Stark, R., Doyle, D. P., & Rushing, J. L. (1983). Beyond Durkheim: Religion and suicide. Journal for the Scientific Study of Religion, 22, 120-131.

5-590   Templer, D. I., & Veleber, D. M. (1980). Suicide rate and religion within the United States. Psychological Reports, 47, 898. (Abstract: PA, 1981, 66, No. 13054, p. 1360)

5-591   Unkovic, C., Adler, R., & Brown, W. (1981).
        Religion and college suicides: A dynamic
        relationship? Free Inquiry in Creative
        Sociology, 9(1), 39-42.

5-592   Whalley, E. A. (1964). Religion and suicide.
        Review of Religious Research, 5, 91-110.

5-593   Whitt, H. P., Gordon, C. C., & Hofley,
        J. R. (1972). Religion, economic development and
        lethal aggression. American Sociological Review,
        37, 193-201.

See also: Breault & Barkey (1982, 1983) and Stark (1983),
reference 4-039; See especially Sections 8.4 and 10.1. See
also Headley (1975, reference 5-430.12). See also Maris
(1981, reference 5-104), Chapter 9, "The religious factor:
Religion, culture, and concepts of death in suicide",
pp. 236-263.

5.11 Other Risk Factors

5.11a Personality and Suicide

5-594   Bhagat, M. (1976). The spouses of attempted
        suicides: A personality study. British Journal
        of Psychiatry, 128, 44-46.

5-595   Cantor, J. M. (1970). The search for the suicidal
        personality. In K. Wolff (Ed.), Patterns of
        self-destruction: Depression and suicide
        (pp. 56-66). Springfield, IL: Thomas.

5-596   Cantor, P. C. (1976). Personality characteristics
        found among youthful female suicide attempters.
        Journal of Abnormal Psychology, 85, 324-329.

5-597   Conte, H. R., & Plutchik, R. (1974). Personality
        and background characteristics of suicidal mental
        patients. Journal of Psychiatric Research, 10,
        181-188.

5-598   Eastwood, M. R., Henderson, A. S., & Montgomery,
        F. M. (1972). Personality and parasuicide:
        Methodological problems. Medical Journal of
        Australia, 1, 170-175.

5-599   Geller, A. M., & Atkins, A. (1978). Cognitive and
        personality factors in suicidal behaviors.
        Journal of Consulting and Clinical Psychology,
        46, 860-868. (Abstract: PA, 1979, 62, No. 6251,
        p. 649)

5-600   Irfani, S. (1978). Personality correlates of
        suicidal tendency among Iranian and Turkish
        students. Journal of Psychology, 99, 151-153.

5-601   Kinsinger, J. R. (1973). Women who threaten
        suicide: Evidence for an identifiable
        personality type. Omega, 4, 73-84. (Abstract:
        PA, 1974, 51, No. 9391, p. 1192)

5-602   Mehryar, A. H., Hekmat, H., & Khajavi, F. (1977).
        Some personality correlates of contemplated
        suicide. Psychological Reports, 40, 1291-1294.

5-603   Pallis, D. J., & Birtchnell, J. (1976).
        Personality and suicidal history in psychiatric
        patients. Journal of Clinical Psychology, 32,
        246-253.

5-604   Pallis, D. J., & Birtchnell, J. (1977).
        Seriousness of suicide attempt in relation to
        personality. British Journal of Psychiatry, 130,
        253-259.

5-605   Schwartz, D. A. (1979). The suicidal character.
        Psychiatric Quarterly, 51, 64-70.

5-606   Tucker, S. J., & Cantor, P. C. (1975). Personality
        and status profiles of peer counselors and
        suicide attempters. Journal of Counseling
        Psychology, 22, 423-430. (Abstract: PA, 1975,
        54, No. 12398, p. 1543)

*See also: Lester (1972, reference 1-041), Chapter 23,
"Personality correlates of suicidal inclincations,"
pp. 259-300; Lester (1983, reference 1-042), Chapter 22,
"The personality of suicidal people," pp. 147; Lester &
Lester (1971, reference 1-043), Chapter 6, "Personality
difference and suicide," pp. 41-51.

See also: Section 6.3 on assessment, especially reference
on scales, e.g., MMPI, Rorschach, etc.

5.11b Bereavement, Parental Loss, and Loss in General

Bibliographic Source:

5-607   Mace, G. S., Akins, F. R., & Akins, D. L. (1981).
        The bereaved child: Analysis, education and
        treatment: An abstracted bibliography. New
        York: Plenum.

Articles:

5-608   Adam, K. S., Bouckoms, A., & Streiner, C. (1982).
        Parental loss and family stability in attempted
        suicide. Archives or General Psychiatry, 39,
        1081-1085.

5-609   Birtchnell, J. (1970). The relationship between
        attempted suicide and parent death. British

Journal of Psychiatry, 116, 307-313.

5-610   Bunch, J. (1972).   Recent bereavement in relation
         to suicide.   Journal of Psychosomatic Research,
         16, 361-366.

5-611   Bunch, J., & Barraclough, B. (1971).   The influence
         of parental death anniversaries upon suicide
         deaths.   British Journal of Psychiatry, 118,
         621-626.

5-612   Bunch, J., Barraclough, B., Nelson, B., &
         Sainsbury, P. (1971).   Early parental bereavement
         and suicide.   Social Psychiatry, 6, 200-202.

5-613   Bunch, J., Barraclough, B., Nelson, B., &
         Sainsbury, P. (1971).   Suicide following
         bereavement of parents.   Social Psychiatry, 6,
         193-199.

5-614   Clayton, P. J. (1982).   Bereavement.   In
         E. S. Paykel (Ed.), Handbook of affective
         disorders (pp. 403-415, esp. p. 410, "Suicide").
         New York: Guilford.

5-615   Crook, T., & Raskin, A. (1973).   Association of
         childhood parental loss with attempted suicide
         and depression.   Journal of Consulting and
         Clinical Psychology, 43, 277.

5-616   Danto, B. L. (1974).   Drug ingestion and suicide
         during anticipatory grief.   In B. Shoenberg,
         A. C. Carr, A. H. Kutscher, D. Peretz, &
         I. K. Goldberg (Eds.), Anticipatory grief
         (pp. 311-314).   New York: Columbia University
         Press.

5-617   Danto, B. L., & Kutscher, A. H. (Eds.) (1977).
         Suicide and bereavement.   New York: MSS
         Information Corporation.

5-618   Dorpat, T. L. (1973).   Suicide, loss, and mourning.
         Life-Threatening Behavior, 3, 213-224.
         (Reprinted in Danto & Kutscher, 1977, reference
         5-617 above, pp. 21-31.)

5-619   Goldney, R. D. (1981).   Parental loss and reported
         childhood stress in young women who attempt
         suicide.   Acta Psychiatrica Scandinavica, 64,
         34-47.

5-620   Humphrey, J. A. (1977).   Suicidal loss: A
         comparison of suicide victims, homicide offenders
         and non-violent individuals.   Diseases of the
         Nervous System, 38, 157-160.

5-621 Lester, D., & Beck, A. T. (1976). Early loss as a
       possible "sensitizer" to later loss in attempted
       suicides. Psychological Reports, 39, 121-122.

5-622 Murphy, G. E., Armstrong, J. W., Hermele, S. L.,
       Fischer, J. R., & Clendenin, W. W. (1979).
       Suicide and alcoholism: Interpersonal loss
       confirmed as a predictor. Archives of General
       Psychiatry, 36, 65-69.

5-623 Taylor, D. A. (1983-84). Views of death from
       sufferers of early loss. Omega, 14, 77-82.

See also references on suicide survivors, Chapter 9; See
also: Adam (1973), Adam et al. (1973, 1982), references
5-805--5-807, respectively.

5.11c Life Stress, Circumstances, Events

5-624 Cochrane, R., & Robertson, A. (1975). Stress in
       the lives of parasuicides. Social Psychiatry,
       10, 161-171.

5-625 Cohen-Sandler, R., Berman, A. L., & King,
       R. A. (1982). Life stress and symptomatology:
       Determinants of suicidal behavior in children.
       Journal of the American Academy of Child
       Psychiatry, 21, 178-186. (Abstract: PA, 1983,
       69, No. 5671, p. 617)

5-626 Farmer, R. D. T., & Hirsch, S. R. (1980). The
       suicide syndrome. London: Croom-Helm. Includes
       the following articles:

       5-626.01 Paykel, E. S. Recent life events and
                 attempted suicide. pp. 105-115.

       5-626.02 Katschnig, H. Measuring life stress: A
                 comparison of two methods.
                 pp. 116-123.

       5-626.03 O'Brien, S. E. M., & Farmer, R. D. T.
                 The role of life events in the
                 aetiology of episodes. pp. 124-130.

5-627 Hagnell, O., & Rorsman, B. (1980). Suicide in the
       Lundby study: A controlled prospective
       investigation of stressful life events.
       Neuropsychobiology, 6, 319-332.

5-628 Humphrey, J. A., French, L., Niswander, G. D., &
       Casey, T. M. (1974). The process of suicide:
       The sequence of disruptive events in the lives of
       suicide victims. Diseases of the Nervous System,
       35, 275-277.

5-629 Humphrey, J. A., Puccio, D., Niswander, G. D., & Casey, T. M. (1972). An analysis of the sequence of selected events in the lives of a suicidal population: A preliminary report. Journal of Nervous & Mental Disease, 154, 137-140.

5-630 Isherwood, J., Adam, K. S., & Hornblow, A. R. (1982). Life event stress, psychosocial factors, suicide attempt and auto-accident proclivity. Journal of Psychosomatic Research, 26, 371-383. (Abstract: PA, 1983, 69, No. 5828, p. 635)

5-631 Isherwood, J., Adam, K. S., & Hornblow, A. R. (1982). Readjustment, expectedness, mastery and outcome dimensions of life stress suicide attempt and auto-accident. Journal of Human Stress, 8, 11-18. (Abstract: PA, 1983, 69, No. 1265, p. 137)

5-632 Luscomb, R. L., Clum, G. A., & Patsiokas, A. T. (1980). Mediating factors in the relationship between life stress and suicide attempting. Journal of Nervous and Mental Disease, 168, 644-650. (Abstract: CPA, 1981, 21, No. 690, pp. 160-161)

5-633 Papa, L. L. (1980). Responses to life events as predictors of suicidal behavior. Nursing Research, 29, 362-369.

5-634 Paykel, E. S. (1976). Life stress, depression and attempted suicide. Journal of Human Stress, 2, 3-12.

5-635 Paykel, E. S. (1979). Life stress. In L. D. Hankoff & B. Einsidler (Eds.), Suicide: Theory and clinical aspects (pp. 225-234.). Littleton, MA: PSG Publishing.

5-636 Paykel, E. S., Prusoff, B. A., & Myers, J. K. (1975). Suicide attempts and recent life events: A controlled comparison. Archives of General Psychiatry, 32, 327-333.

5-637 Ripley, H. S., & Dorpat, T. L. (1981). Life change and suicidal behavior. Psychiatric Annals, 11, 219-226.

5-638 Slater, J., & Depue, R. A. (1981). The contribution of environmental events and social supports to serious suicide attempts in primary depressive disorder. Journal of Abnormal Psychology, 90, 275-285. (Abstract: PA, 1981, 66, No. 8116, p. 848)

5.11d <u>Mental Disorders & Suicidal Behavior</u>

Bibliographies:

5-639   American Association of Suicidology. <u>Suicide and</u>
         <u>alcoholism</u> [Annotated bibliography]. Denver, CO:
         AAS.

5-640   Miller, M. Non-annotated bibliographies. San
         Diego, CA: The Information Center. 1984 catalog
         includes:

         5-640.01 <u>Alcoholism and suicide</u>. Bibliography
                   R-11.

         5-640.02 <u>Drug abuse and suicide</u>. Bibliography
                   R-29.

         5-640.03 <u>Schizophrenia and suicide</u>. Bibliography
                   R-38.

         5-640.04 <u>Mental Illness/Suicide</u>. Bibliography
                   R-43.

         5-640.05 <u>Depression and suicide</u>. Bibliography
                   R-44.

Articles:

5-641   Achte, K., & Lonnqvist, J. (Eds.) (1979).
         <u>Psychopathology of direct and indirect</u>
         <u>self-destruction</u>. Helsinki: Psychiatria Fennica
         (<u>Psychiatria Fennica</u> Supplementum 1978).

            This book includes a section on
            "Psychopathology of direct self-destruction,"
            pp. 43-80, which includes 7 articles on
            various aspects.

5-642   Barraclough, B., & Pallis, D. (1975). Depression
         followed by suicide: A comparison of depressed
         suicides with living depressives. <u>Psychological</u>
         <u>Medicine</u>, <u>5</u>, 55-61.

5-643   Beskow, J. (1979). Suicide in mental disorder in
         Swedish men. <u>Acta Psychiatrica Scandinavica</u>,
         Supplement 277, pp. 1-138.

5-644   Copas, J. B., & Robin, A. (1982). Suicide in
         psychiatric in-patients. <u>British Journal of</u>
         <u>Psychiatry</u>, <u>141</u>, 503-511. (Abstract: <u>PA</u>, 1983,
         <u>70</u>, No. 1783, p. 205)

5-645   Corey, D. M., & Andress, V. R. (1977). Alcohol
         consumption and suicidal behavior. <u>Psychological</u>
         <u>Reports</u>, <u>40</u>, 506.

5-646 Evenson, R. C., Wood, J. B., Nuttall, E. A., & Cho, D. W. (1982). Suicide rates among public mental health patients. Acta Psychiatrica Scandinavica, 66, 254-264.

5-647 Flynn, P., & MacMahon, R. C. (1983). Indicators of depression and suicide ideation among drug abusers. Psychological Reports, 52, 784-786. (Abstract: PA, 1984, 71, No. 5616, p. 589)

5-648 Garvey, M. J., & Spoden, F. (1980). Suicide attempts in antisocial personality disorder. Comprehensive Psychiatry, 21, 146-149.

5-649 Goodwin, D. W. (1973). Alcohol in suicide and homicide. Quarterly Journal of Studies on Alcohol, 34, 144-156.

5-650 Harris, R., Linn, M. W., & Hunter, K. I. (1979). Suicide attempts among drug abusers. Suicide and Life-Threatening Behavior, 9, 25-32.

5-651 Hogan, T. P., & Awad, A. G. (1983). Pharmacotherapy and suicide risk in schizophrenia. Canadian Journal of Psychiatry, 28, 277-281. (Abstract: PA, 1984, 71, No. 7433, p. 784)

5-652 Johnson, G. F., & Hunt, G. (1979). Suicidal behavior in bipolar manic-depressive patients and their families. Comprehensive Psychiatry, 20, 159-164.

5-653 Khuri, R., & Akiskal, H. S. (1983). Suicide prevention: The necessity of treating contributory psychiatric disorders. Psychiatric Clinics of North America, 6, 193-207.

5-654 Leonard, C. V. (1974). Depression and suicidality. Journal of Consulting and Clinical Psychology, 42, 98-104.

5-655 Lester, D. (1971). Relationship of mental disorder to suicidal behavior: Review of recent issues. New York State Journal of Medicine, 71, 1503-1505.

5-656 Lettieri, D. J. (Ed.) (1978). Drugs and suicide: When other coping strategies fail. Beverly Hills, CA: Sage.

5-656.01 Saxon, S., Aldrich, S. Y., & Kuncel, E. E. Suicide and drug abuse. pp. 167-191.

5-656.02 Cuskey, W. R. Self-destruction: Suicide

and drugs. pp. 193-222.

5-657   Levitt, E. E., Lubin, B., & Brooks, J. M. (1983).
Depression: Concepts, controversies, and some
new facts (2nd ed.) (pp. 51-56, "Depression and
suicidal behavior"). Hillsdale, NJ: Lawrence
Erlbaum.

* 5-658   Miles, C. P. (1977). Conditions predisposing to
suicide: A review. Journal of Nervous and
Mental Disease, 164, 231-246.

5-659   Motto, J. A. (1979). The psychopathology of
suicide: A clinical model approach. American
Journal of Psychiatry, 136, 516-520.

5-660   Motto, J. A. (1980). Suicide risk factors in
alcohol abuse. Suicide and Life-Threatening
Behavior, 10, 230-238.

5-661   Motto, J. A. (1980). Suicide risk factors in drug
abuse. Crisis, 1, 8-15.

5-662   Noriek, K. (1975). Attempted suicide and suicide
in functional psychoses. Acta Psychiatrica
Scandinavica, 52, 81-106.

5-663   Pohlmeier, H. (1980). Suicide as a psychodynamic
problem in depression. Crisis, 1, 27-34.

5-664   Pokorny, A. D. (1977). Suicide in depression. In
W. E. Fann, I. Karacan, A. D. Pokorny, &
R. L. Williams (Eds.), Phenomenology and
treatment of depression (pp. 197-216). New York:
Spectrum Publications.

5-665   Pokorny, A. D. (1983). Prediction of suicide in
psychiatric patients. Archives of General
Psychiatry, 40, 249-257.

5-666   Rabiner, C. J., Wegner, J. T., & Kane,
J. M. (1982). Suicide in a psychiatric
population. Psychiatric Hospital, 13, 55-59.
(Abstract: PA, 1983, 69, No. 10636, p. 1168)

5-667   Rorsman, B., Hagnell, O., & Lanke, J. (1982).
Violent death and mental disorders in the Lundby
study: Accidents and suicides in a total
population during a 25-year period.
Neuropsychobiology, 8, 233-240.

5-668   Roy, A. (1982). Risk factors for suicide in
psychiatric patients. Archives of General
Psychiatry, 39, 1089-1095.

5-669   Roy, A. (1982). Suicide in chronic schizophrenia.

British Journal of Psychiatry, 141, 171-177.

5-670   Roy, A. (1983). Suicide in depressives.
         Comprehensive Psychiatry, 24, 487-491.

5-671   Sainsbury, P. (1982). Suicide: Epidemiology and
         relationship to depression. In J. K. Wing (Ed.),
         Handbook of psychiatry, Volume 3, Psychoses of
         uncertain aetiology (pp. 134-140). Cambridge,
         MA: Cambridge University Press.

5-672   Sainsbury, P. (1982). Depression and suicide
         prevention. In J. Wilmotte, C. Mendlewicz, &
         J. Mendlewicz (Eds.), New trends in suicide
         prevention (pp. 17-32). New York: Karger.
         (Bibliotheca Psychiatrica No. 162.)

5-673   Saxon, S., Kuncel, E., & Aldrich, S. (1978). Drug
         abuse and suicide. American Journal of Drug and
         Alcohol Abuse, 5, 485-495.

5-674   Saxon, S., Kuncel, E., & Kaufman, E. (1980).
         Self-destructive behavior patterns in male and
         female drug abusers. American Journal of Drug
         and Alcohol Abuse, 7, 19-29.

5-675   Solomon, J., & Arnon, D. (1979). Alcohol and other
         substance abusers. In L. D. Hankoff &
         B. Einsidler (Eds.), Suicide: Theory and
         clinical aspects (pp. 263-278). Littleton, MA:
         PSG Publishing.

5-676   Stallone, F., Dunner, D. L., Ahearn, J., & Fieve,
         R. R. (1980). Statistical predictions of suicide
         in depressives. Comprehensive Psychiatry, 21,
         381-387.

5-677   Tsuang, M. T. (1978). Suicide in schizophrenics,
         manics, depressives, and surgical controls: A
         comparison with general population suicide
         mortality. Archives of General Psychiatry, 35,
         153-155. (Abstract: PA, 1979, 61, No. 1130,
         p. 126)

5-678   Tsuang, M. T. (1983). Risk of suicide in the
         relatives of schizophrenics, manics, depressives,
         and controls. Journal of Clinical Psychiatry,
         44, 396-400.

5-679   Virkkunen, M. (1974). Suicides in schizophrenia
         and paranoid psychoses. Acta Psychiatrica
         Scandinavica, Supplement 250, pp. 1-305.

5-680   Ward, N. G., & Schuckit, M. A. (1980). Factors
         associated with suicidal behavior in polydrug
         abusers. Journal of Clinical Psychiatry, 41,

379-385.

See also: Hendin (1982, reference 5-399), Chapter 6,
"Suicide and alcoholism," pp. 124-140; Lester (1972,
reference 1-041), Chapter 17, "Mental disorder and suicide,"
pp. 193-202 and Chapter 25, "The effect of drugs on suicidal
behavior," pp. 308-313; Lester (1983, reference 1-042),
Chapter 18, "Mental disorder and suicide," pp. 106-121;
Lester & Lester (1971, reference 1-043), Chapter 17,
"Suicide and mental illness," pp. 135-143; Wekstein (1979,
reference 1-047a), Chapter 5, "Clinical syndromes,"
pp. 75-93; World Health Organization (1968, reference
1-047b), pp. 59-67.

5.11e Physical Illness & Conditions

Bibliographies:

5-681   American Association of Suicidology. Suicide and
         cancer, euthanasia [Annotated bibliography].
         Denver, CO: AAS.

5-682   Miller, M. Non-annotated bibliographies. San
         Diego, CA: The Information Center, 1984 catalog
         includes:

         5-682.01 Menstruation/Suicide. Bibliography R-33.

         5-682.02 Pregnancy and suicide. Bibliography
                   R-34.

Articles:

5-683   Abram, H. S., Moore, G. L., & Westervelt, F. B.,
         Jr. (1971). Suicidal behavior in chronic
         dialysis patients. American Journal of
         Psychiatry, 127, 1199-1204. [Letters and Reply:
         1971, 128, 495-497.]

5-684   Bryan, D. P., & Herjanic, B. (1980). Depression
         and suicide among adolescents and young adults
         with selective handicapping conditions.
         Exceptional Education Quarterly, 1(2), 57-65.
         (Abstract: PA, 1982, 67, No. 7805, p. 844)

5-685   Birtchnell, J., & Floyd, S. (1974). Attempted
         suicide and the menstrual cycle--A negative
         conclusion. Journal of Psychosomatic Research,
         18, 361-369.

5-686   Birtchnell, J., & Floyd, S. (1975). Further
         menstrual characteristics of suicide attemptors.
         Journal of Psychosomatic Research, 19, 81-85.

5-687   Danto, B. L. (1981). Suicide among cancer
         patients. In S. E. Wallace & A. Eser (Eds.),

Suicide and euthanasia: The rights of personhood
(pp. 26-36). Knoxville: University of Tennessee
Press.

5-688   DiBianco, J. T. (1979). The hemodialysis patient.
In L. D. Hankoff & B. Einsidler (Eds.), Suicide:
Theory and clinical aspects (pp. 291-297).
Littleton, MA: PSG Publishing.

5-689   Dorpat, T. L., Anderson, W. F., & Ripley,
H. S. (1968). The relationship of physical
illness to suicide. In H. L. P. Resnik (Ed.),
Suicide: Diagnosis and management (pp. 209-219).
Boston: Little, Brown.

5-690   Dubovsky, S. L. (1978). Averting suicide in
terminally ill patients. Psychosomatics, 19,
113-115.

5-691   Fawcett, J. (1972). Suicidal depression and
physical illness. Journal of the American
Medical Association, 219, 1303-1306.

5-692   Flanagan, T. A., & Murphy, G. E. (1978). Body
donation and suicide: Is there a relationship?
Archives of General Psychiatry, 28, 732-734.

5-693   Forman, B. F. (1979). Cancer and suicide. General
Hospital Psychiatry, 1(2), 108-114.

5-694   Fox, B. H., Stanek, E. J., III, Boyd, S. C., &
Flannery, J. T. (1982). Suicide rates among
cancer patients in Connecticut. Journal of
Chronic Diseases, 35, 89-100.

5-695   Goodwin, J., & Harris, D. (1979). Suicide in
pregnancy: The Hedda Gabler syndrome. Suicide
and Life-Threatening Behavior, 9, 105-115.

5-696   Gruner, O. P., Naas, R., Gjone, E., Flatmark, A., &
Fretheim, B. (1978). Mental disorders in
ulcerative colitis: Suicide, divorce, psychosis,
hospitalization for mental disease, alcoholism,
and consumption of psychotropic drugs in 178
patients subjected to colectomy. Disease of the
Colon & Rectum, 21, 37-39.

5-697   Haenel, T., Brunner, F., & Battegay, R. (1980).
Renal dialysis and suicide: Occurrence in
Switzerland and in Europe. Comprehensive
Psychiatry, 21, 140-145.

5-698   Hawton, K., Fagg, J., & Marsack, P. (1980).
Association between epilepsy and attempted
suicide. Journal of Neurology, Neurosurgery &
Psychiatry, 43, 168-170.

5-699   Holding, T. A., & Minkoff, K. (1973). Parasuicide
        and the menstrual cycle. Journal of
        Psychosomatic Research, 17, 365-368.

5-700   Jeffreys, D. B., & Volans, G. N. (1983). Self
        poisoning in diabetic patients. Human
        Toxicology, 2, 345-348.

5-701   Josefowitz, N., Gurvey, M., Dobson, R., & Weichel,
        C. (1983). Recognizing and helping the suicidal
        patient in chiropractic practice. Journal of
        Manipulative and Physiological Therapeutics,
        6(2), 71-75.

5-702   Krugman, M. E., Shneidman, E., Ward, P. H., &
        Davis, J. (1977). Suicide in the head and neck
        cancer patient. In B. L. Danto & A. H. Kutscher
        (Eds.), Suicide and bereavement (pp. 144-149).
        New York: MSS Information Corporation.

5-703   Levitan, H. (1983). Suicidal trends in patients
        with asthma and hypertension: A chart study.
        Psychotherapy and Psychosomatics, 39, 165-170.
        (Abstract: PA, 1984, 71, No. 7182, p. 760)

5-704   Louhivuori, K. A., & Hakama, M. (1979). Risk of
        suicide among cancer patients. American Journal
        of Epidemiology, 109, 59-65.

5-705   Mackay, A. (1979). Self-poisoning--A complication
        of epilepsy. British Journal of Psychiatry, 134,
        277-282.

5-706   Marshall, J. R., Burnett, W., & Brasure, J. (1983).
        On precipitating factors: Cancer as a cause of
        suicide. Suicide and Life-Threatening Behavior,
        13, 15-27.

* 5-707 Matthews, W. S., & Barabas, G. (1981). Suicide and
        epilespy: A review of the literature.
        Psychosomatics, 22, 515-524.

5-708   Minaire, P., Price, M., Almagro, P., Ravichandran,
        G., Silver, J. R., Nuseibeh, I., & Burr,
        R. G. (1982). Life expectancy following spinal
        cord injury. Paraplegia, 20, 277-279.

5-709   Missel, J. L. (1978). Suicide risk in the medical
        rehabilitation setting. Archives of Physical
        Medicine & Rehabilitation, 59, 371-376.

5-710   Neale, R. (1976). Attempted suicide in labour.
        British Medical Journal, 1, 321-322.

5-711   Pallis, D. J., & Holding, T. A. (1976). The
        menstrual cycle and suicidal intent. Journal of

Biosocial Science, 8, 27-33.

5-712   Resnik, H. L. P. (1971). Abortion and suicidal
        behaviors: Observations on the concept of
        "endangering the mental health of the mother."
        Mental Hygiene, 55, 10-20.

5-713   Sanborn, D. E., III, & Seibert, D. J. (1976).
        Cancerophobic suicides and history of cancer.
        Psychological Reports, 38, 602.

5-714   Schwartz, M. L., & Pierron, M. (1972). Suicide and
        fatal accidents in multiple sclerosis. Omega, 3,
        291-293.

5-715   Viskum, K. (1975). Ulcer, attempted suicide and
        suicide. Acta Psychiatrica Scandinavica, 51,
        221-227.

5-716   Weinberg, S. (1970). Suicidal intent in
        adolescence: A hypothesis about the role of
        physical illness. Journal of Pediatrics, 77,
        579-586.

5-717   Weisman, A. D. (1976). Coping behavior and suicide
        in cancer. In J. W. Cullen, B. H. Fox, &
        R. N. Isom (Eds.), Cancer: The behavioral
        dimensions (pp. 331-341). New York: Raven.

* 5-718 Wetzel, R. D., & McClure, J. N., Jr. (1972).
        Suicide and the menstrual cycle: A review.
        Comprehensive Psychiatry, 13, 369-374.
        (Abstract: PA, 1973, 50, No. 9320, p. 990)

5-719   Whitlock, F. (1978). Suicide, cancer and
        depression. British Journal of Psychiatry, 132,
        269-274.

See also: Goldstein & Reznikoff (1971, reference 5-847);
Lester (1983, reference 1-042), Chapter 19, "Suicide and
medical illness, pp. 122-125; Maris (1981, reference
4-029), Chapter 7, "The physical context of suicide:
Alcohol, drug use, and physical illness," pp. 170-204.

See also: Section 5.15, Biological Factors and Suicide.

5.11f Homicide & Suicide

Relationship Between Homicide & Suicide:

5-720   Franke, R. H., Thomas, E. W., & Queenen,
        A. J. (1977). Suicide and homicide: Common
        sources and consistent relationships. Social
        Psychiatry, 12, 149-156.

5-721   Holinger, P. C., & Klemen, E. H. (1982). Violent

death in the United States, 1900-1975:
Relationship between suicide, homicide, and
accidental deaths. Social Science and Medicine,
16, 1929-1938. (Abstract: PA, 1983, 70,
No. 3607, p. 409)

5-722   Lester, D. (1977). The relationship between
suicide and homicide. Corrective and Social
Psychiatry and Journal of Behavior Technology,
Methods and Therapy, 23(3), 83-84.

5-723   Lester, D. (1978). Internal conflict and personal
violence: A cross-national study of suicide and
homicide. International Journal of Group
Tensions, 8(3-4), 68-70. (Abstract: PA, 1981,
66, No. 8205, p. 857)

5-724   Lester, D. (1982). Conformity, suicide and
homicide. Behavior Science Research, 17, 24-30.
(Abstract: PA, 1984, 71, No. 1629, p. 176)

5-725   Levi, K. (1982). Homicide and suicide: Structure
and process. Deviant Behavior, 3, 91-115.

5-726   Palmer, S., & Humphrey, J. A. (1977). Suicide and
homicide: A test of a role theory of
self-destructive behavior. Omega, 8, 45-58.

5-727   Wilbanks, W. (1982). Fatal accidents, suicide and
homicide: Are they related? Victimology, 7,
213-217.

See also: Braucht et al. (1980, reference 2-053); Henry &
Short (1954, 4-019); Lester & Lester (1971, reference
1-043), Chapter 8, "Suicide and homicide," pp. 56-64.

Homicide Followed by Suicide:

5-728a Allen, N. H. (1983). Homicide followed by suicide:
Los Angeles, 1970-1979. Suicide and
Life-Threatening Behavior, 13, 155-165.

5-728b Berman, A. L. (1979). Dyadic death:
Murder-suicide. Suicide and Life-Threatening
Behavior, 9, 15-24.

5-729   Coid, J. (1983). The epidemiology of abnormal
homicide and murder followed by suicide.
Psychological Medicine, 13, 855-860.

5-730   Goldney, R. D. (1977). Family murder followed by
suicide. Forensic Science, 9, 219-228.

5-731   Palmer, S., & Humphrey, J. A. (1980).
Offender-victim relationships in criminal
homicide followed by offender's suicide, North

Carolina, 1972-1977. Suicide and
Life-Threatening Behavior, 10, 106-118.

5-732   Selkin, J. (1976).   Rescue fantasies in
homicide-suicide. Suicide and Life-Threatening
Behavior, 6, 79-85.

5-733   West, D. J. (1967). Murder followed by suicide.
Cambridge, MA: Harvard University Press.

See also: Rosenbaum (1983, reference 5-775); Phillips
(1980, reference 5-924).

5.11g Economic & Employment Conditions

5-734a Ahlburg, D. A., & Schapiro, M. O. (1984).
Socioeconomic ramifications of changing cohort
size: An analysis of U.S. postwar suicide rates
by age and sex. Demography, 21, 97-108.

* 5-734b Bedeian, A. G. (1982).   Suicide and occupation: A
review. Journal of Vocational Behavior, 21,
206-223.   (Abstract: PA, 1983, 69, No. 8074,
p. 885)

5-735   Boor, M. (1980).   Relationships between
unemployment rates and suicide rates in eight
countries, 1962-1976. Psychological Reports, 47,
1095-1101. (Abstract: PA, 1981, 66, No. 13020,
pp. 1356-1357)

5-736   Boor, M. (1982).   Relationship of anomie to
perceived changes in financial status, 1973-1980.
Journal of Clinical Psychology, 38, 891-892.

5-737   Brodsky, C. M. (1977).   Suicide attributed to work.
Suicide and Life-Threatening Behavior, 7,
216-229.

5-738   Karcher, C. J., & Linden, L. L. (1982).   Is work
conducive to self-destruction? Suicide and
Life-Threatening Behavior, 12, 151-175.
(Abstract: ACP, 1982, 22, No. 2720, pp. 580-581)

5-739   Labovitz, S., & Hagedorn, R. (1971).   An analysis
of suicide rate among occupational categories.
Sociological Inquiry, 41, 67-72.

5-740   Lester, D. (1970).   Suicide and unemployment: A
reexamination. Archives of Environmental Heatlh,
20, 277-278.

5-741   Marks, A. (1980).   Socioeconomic status and suicide
in the state of Washington: 1950-1971.
Psychological Reports, 46, 924-926.

5-742   Olsen, J., & Lajer, M. (1979). Violent death and
         unemployment in two trade unions in Denmark.
         Social Psychiatry, 14, 139-145. (Abstract: PA,
         1981, 65, No. 6483, p. 680)

5-743   Pierce, A. (1967). The economic cycle and the
         social suicide rate. American Sociological
         Review, 32, 457-462. (Reprinted in A. Giddens
         (Ed.), The sociology of suicide: A selection of
         readings (pp. 271-279). London: Cass.)

5-744   Reinhart, G. R., & Linden, L. L. (1982). Suicide
         by industry and occupation: A structural change
         approach. Suicide and Life-Threatening Behavior,
         12, 34-45.

5-745   Rushing, W. A. (1968). Occupation, status, and
         suicide: An occupational study. Sociological
         Quarterly, 9, 493-503.

5-746   Sanborn, D. E., III, Sanborn, C. J., & Cimbolic,
         P. (1974). Occupation and suicide. Diseases of
         the Nervous System, 35, 7-12.

5-747   Schapiro, M. O., & Ahlburg, D. A. (1982-83).
         Suicide: The ultimate cost of unemployment.
         Journal of Post-Keynesian Economics, 5, 276-280.

5-748   Shepherd, D. M., & Barraclough, B. M. (1980). Work
         and suicide: An empirical investigation.
         British Journal of Psychiatry, 136, 469-478.

5-749   Simon, J. L. (1968). Effect of income on the
         suicide rate: A paradox resolved. American
         Journal of Sociology, 74, 302-303. Barnes,
         C. B. (1975). The partial effect of income on
         suicide is always negative [Comment]. 80,
         1454-1460. Simon's reply, 1460-1462.

5-750a   Stack, S. (1980). Occupational status and suicide:
         A relationship reexamined [A research note].
         Aggressive Behavior, 6, 233-234. (Abstract: PA,
         1981, 66, No. 13050, p. 1359)

5-750b   Stack, S. (1982). The effect of strikes on
         suicide: A cross-national analysis.
         Sociological Focus, 15, 135-146.

5-751   Stack, S., & Haas, A. (1984). The effect of
         unemployment duration on national suicide rates:
         A time series analysis, 1948-1982. Sociological
         Focus, 17, 17-29.

5-752   Vigderhous, G., & Fishman, G. (1978). The impact
         of unemployment and familial integration on
         changing suicide rates in the U.S.A., 1920-1969.

Social Psychiatry, 13, 239-248.

5-753   Wenz, F. V. (1978). Economic status, family
        anomie, and adolescent suicide. Journal of
        Psychology, 98, 45-47.

5-754   Wenz, F. V. (1979). Self-injury behavior, economic
        status and the family anomie syndrome among
        adolescents. Adolescence, 14(54), 387-398.

See also: Cumming et al. (1975, reference 5-119); Davis
(1981, reference 5-121); Hammermesh & Soss (1974, reference
4-078); Henry & Short (1954, reference 4-019); Lester
(1973, reference 5-134); Newman et al. (1973, reference
5-140); Ornstein (1983, reference 5-141); Peretti & Wilson
(1978-79, reference 5-269); Taylor (1982, reference 5-328);
Vigderhous & Fishman (1977, reference 5-144); Lunden (1977,
reference 5-794).

For a consideration of physician suicide, see Section 10.3.

5.11h Jails, Prisons and Suicide

Bibliography:

5-755   Miller, M. Prison suicides [Non-annotated
        bibliography]. San Diego, CA: The Information
        Center. (Listed in the 1984 catalog.)
        Bibliography R-23.

Articles:

5-756   Albanese, J. S. (1983). Preventing inmate
        suicides: A case study. Federal Probation,
        46(2), 65-72.

5-757   Burtch, B. E. (1979). Prisoner suicides
        reconsidered. International Journal of Law and
        Psychiatry, 2, 307-413.

* 5-758 Danto, B. L. (1973). Jail house blues: Studies of
        suicidal behavior in jail and prison. Orchard
        Lake, MI: Epic Publications. [20 articles on
        jail and prison suicide]

5-759   Flaherty, M. G. (1980, August). An assessment of
        the national incidence of juvenile suicide in
        adult jails, lockups, and juvenile detention
        centers. Washington, D.C.: USGPO, prepared by
        Community Research Forum, University of Illinois
        at Urbana-Champaign for the Office of Juvenile
        Justice and Delinquency Prevention of the United
        States Department of Justice.

5-760   Flaherty, M. G. (1983). The national incidence of
        juvenile suicide in adult jails and juvenile

detention centers. Suicide and Life-Threatening
Behavior, 13, 85-94.

* 5-761 Gaston, A. W. (1979). Prisoners. In L. D. Hankoff
& B. Einsidler (Eds.), Suicide: Theory and
clinical aspects (pp. 335-342). Littleton, MA:
PSG Publishing.

5-762 Hankoff, L. D. (1980). Prisoner suicide.
International Journal of Offender Therapy and
Comparative Criminology, 24, 162-166.

5-763 Haviland, L. S., & Larew, B. L. (1980). Dying in
jail: The phenomenon of adolescent suicide in
correctional facilities. Children and Youth
Services Review, 2, 331-342.

5-764 Johnson, R. (1978). Youth in crisis: Dimensions
of self-destructive conduct among adolescent
prisoners. Adolescence, 13(51), 461-482.

5-765 Niemi, T. (1978). The time-space distances of
suicides committed in the lock-up in Finland in
1963-1967. Israel Annals of Psychiatry, 16,
39-45.

5-766 Payson, H. E. (1975). Suicide among males in
prison--Why not? Bulletin of the American
Academy of Psychiatry and the Law, 3(3), 152-161.

5-767 Topp, D. (1979). Suicide in prison. British
Journal of Psychiatry, 134, 24-27.

5-768 Tuskan, J. J., Jr., & Thase, M. E. (1983).
Suicides in jails and prisons. Journal of
Psychosocial Nursing and Mental Health Services,
21, 29-33.

See also Section 10.2 for law enforcement officers.

5.12 Additional Aspects and Factors

5.12a Suicide Pacts

Bibliography:

5-769 Miller, M. Suicide pacts [Non-annotated
bibliography]. San Diego, CA: The Information
Center, Bibliography R-37 (listed in the 1984
catalog).

Articles:

5-770 Hemphill, E., & Thornley, F. L. (1969). Suicide
pacts. South African Medical Journal, 43,
1335-1338.

5-771   Mehta, D., Mathew, P., & Mehta, S. (1978).   Suicide
        pact in a depressed elderly couple: Case report.
        Journal of the American Geriatrics Society, 26,
        136-138.

5-772   Noyes, R., Frye, S. J., & Hartford, C. E. (1977).
        Conjugal suicide pact.   Journal of Nervous and
        Mental Disease, 165, 72-75.

5-773   Ohara, K., & Reynolds, D. (1970).   Love-pact
        suicides.   Omega, 1, 159-166.

* 5-774   Rosen, B. K. (1981).   Suicide pacts: A review.
        Psychological Medicine, 11, 525-533.

5-775   Rosenbaum, M. (1983).   Crime and punishment--The
        suicide pact.   Archives of General Psychiatry,
        40, 979-982.

5-776   Sathyavathi, K. (1975).   Usual and unusual suicide
        pacts in Bangalore.   Indian Journal of Social
        Work, 36, 173-180.

5.12b Mass Suicides & Jonestown, Guyana

5-777   Calhoun, L. G., Selby, J. W., & Moira, J. (1980).
        Mass suicide: A note on popular conceptions of
        suicidal behavior.   Journal of Community
        Psychology, 8, 366-369.   (Abstract: PA, 1981,
        66, No. 8194, p. 856)

5-778   Curran, W. J. (1979).   Law-medicine notes: The
        Guyana mass suicides: Medicolegal re-evaluation.
        New England Journal of Medicine, 300, 1321.
        Siegler, R. (1979).   Medical complicity in the
        Guyana tradegy [Letter].   301, 559.   Glaser,
        F. B. (1979).   Doctor's role not 'pivotal' in
        Jonestown [Letter].   301, 1401.

5-779   Dwyer, P. M. (1979).   An inquiry into the
        psychological dimensions of cult suicide.
        Suicide and Life-Threatening Behavior, 9,
        120-127.

5-780   Eckert, W. G. (1980).   Catastrophes et morts
        collectives.   Recent American experiences in mass
        deaths.   American Journal of Forensic Medicine
        and Pathology, 1, 77-79.

5-781   Hall, J. R. (1979).   Apocalypse at Jonestown.
        Society, 16(6), 52-61.

5-782   Lasaga, J. I. (1980).   Death in Jonestown:
        Techniques of political control by a paranoid
        leader.   Suicide and Life-Threatening Behavior,
        10, 210-213.

5-783   Seiden, R. H. (1979). Reverend Jones on suicide.
        Suicide and Life-Threatening Behavior, 9,
        116-119. [A transcript of a Jim Jones speech at
        an anti-suicide rally in 1977]

5-784   Spencer, J. D. (1983). George Armstrong Custer and
        the Battle of the Little Big Horn: Homicide or
        mass suicide? Journal of Forensic Science, 28,
        756-761.

5-785   Spero, M. H. (1978). Samson and Masada:
        Altruistic suicides reconsidered. Psychoanalytic
        Review, 65, 631-639.

5-786   Stack, S. (1983). The effect of the Jonestown
        suicides on American suicide rates. Journal of
        Social Psychology, 119, 145-146. (Abstract: PA,
        1983, 70, No. 8231, p. 922)

5-787   Zee, H. J. (1980). The Guyana incident: Some
        psychoanalytic considerations. Bulletin of the
        Menninger Clinic, 44, 345-363.

5.12c Global Factors Affecting Suicidal Behaviors

5-788   Andress, V. R., & Corey, D. M. (1976). Regional
        suicide rates as a function of national political
        change. Psychological Reports, 39, 955-958.

5-789   Biller, O. A. (1977). Suicide related to the
        assassination of President John F. Kennedy.
        Suicide and Life-Threatening Behavior, 7, 40-44.

5-790   Bjarnason, O. (1982). Association between changes
        in psychiatric services and increases in suicide
        rates. Archiv fur Psychiatrie und
        Nervenkrankheiten, 232, 15-23.

5-791   Boor, M. (1981). Effects of United States
        presidential elections on suicide and other
        causes of death. American Sociological Review,
        46, 616-618.

5-792   Boor, M. (1982). Reduction in deaths by suicide,
        accidents, and homicide prior to United States
        presidential elections. Journal of Social
        Psychology, 118, 135-136. (Abstract: PA, 1983,
        69, No. 12900, p. 1425)

5-793   Lester, D. (1973). National homicide and suicide
        rates as a function of political stability.
        Psychological Reports, 33, 298.

* 5-794 Lunden, W. A. (1977). The suicide cycle: Suicides
        in war, peace and depressions in twenty Western
        and Eastern nations. Montezuma, IA: Sutherland

Printing Company.

5-795   Marshall, J. R. (1981). Political integration and
         the effect of war on suicide: United States,
         1933-76. Social Forces, 59, 771-785.

5-796   O'Malley, P. (1975). Suicide and war: A case
         study and theoretical appraisal. British Journal
         of Criminology, 15, 348-359.

5-797   Robertson, A., & Cochrane, R. (1976). Attempted
         suicide and cultural change: An empirical
         investigation. Human Relations, 29, 863-883.

5-798   Rojcewicz, S. J., Jr. (1971). War and suicide.
         Life-Threatening Behavior, 1, 46-54.

5-799   Wasserman, I. M. (1983). Political business
         cycles, presidental elections, and suicide and
         mortality patterns. American Sociological
         Review, 48, 711-720.

See also: Henry & Short (1954, reference 4-019); Weightman
(1983, reference 1-098).

5.12d Other Factors

5-800   Lingens, E. (1972). Suicide in extreme situations.
         In J. Waldenstrom, T. Larsson, & N. Ljungstedt
         (Eds.), Suicide and attempted suicide
         (pp. 114-121). Stockholm: Nordiska Bokhandelns
         Forlag. [ghettos, concentration camps]

5-801   Lester, D. (1973). Suicide in released prisoners
         of war. Journal of the American Medical
         Association, 225, 747.

5-802   Roberts, J., & Hawton, K. (1980). Child abuse and
         attempted suicide. British Journal of
         Psychiatry, 137, 319-323.

5-803   Roden, R. G. (1982). Suicide and holocaust
         survivors. Israel Journal of Psychiatry and
         Related Sciences, 19, 129-135.

5-804   Shneidman, E. S. (1971). Perturbation and
         lethality as precursors of suicide in a gifted
         group. Life-Threatening Behavior, 1, 23-45.
         (Reprinted in E. S.Shneidman (Ed.) (1976),
         Suicidology: Contemporary developments
         (pp. 341-368). New York: Grune & Stratton, as
         "Suicide among the gifted." Reprinted in
         E. S. Shneidman (Ed.) (1976), Death: Current
         perspectives (2nd ed.) (pp. 446-466) (3rd ed.,
         1984, pp. 321-341). Palo Alto, CA: Mayfield, as
         "Suicide among the gifted." Reprinted in Suicide

and Life-Threatening Behavior, 11(4), 1981, 254-281, as "Suicide among the gifted." Reprinted with some omissions in L. D.Hankoff & B. Einsidler (Eds.) (1979), Suicide: Theory and clinical aspects (pp. 309-322). Littleton, MA: PSG Publishing, as "The gifted.")

5.13 Suicide Ideation & Past Exposure to Suicide

5-805   Adam, K. S. (1973). Childhood parental loss, suicidal ideation, and suicidal behavior. In E. J. Anthony & C. Koupernik (Eds.), The child in his family: The impact of disease and death, Volume 2 (pp. 275-297). New York: Wiley.

5-806   Adam, K. S., Lohrenz, J. G., & Harper, D. (1973). Suicidal ideation and parental loss: A preliminary report. Canadian Psychiatric Association Journal, 18, 95-100.

5-807   Adam, K. S., Lohrenz, J. G., Harper, D., & Streiner, D. (1982). Early parental loss and suicidal ideation in university students. Canadian Journal of Psychiatry, 27, 275-281.

5-808   Bagley, C. (1975). Suicidal behavior and suicidal ideation in adolescents: A problem for counselors in education. British Journal of Guidance and Counseling, 3, 190-208. (Abstract: PA, 1976, 55, No. 7332, p. 742)

5-809   Bell, R. A., Lin, E., Ice, J., & Bell, R. J. (1978). Drinking patterns and suicidal ideation and behavior in a general population. Currents in Alcoholism, 5, 317-332.

5-810   Cantor, P. (1976). Frequency of suicidal thought and self-destructive behavior among females. Suicide and Life-Threatening Behavior, 6, 92-100.

5-811   Craig, L. E., & Senter, R. J. (1972). Student thoughts about suicide. Psychological Record, 22, 355-358. (Abstracts: PA, 1973, 49, No. 2598, p. 286; ACP, 1973, 13, No. 742, p. 191)

5-812   Flinn, D. E., & Leonard, C. V. (1972). Prevalence of suicidal ideation and behavior among basic trainees and college students. Military Medicine, 137, 317-320.

5-813   Friedrich, W., Reams, R., & Jacobs, Jane (1982). Depression and suicidal ideation in early adolescents. Journal of Youth and Adolescence, 11, 403-408. (Abstract: PA, 1983, 70, No. 12793, p. 1437)

5-814   Goldberg, E. L. (1981). Depression and suicide
        ideation in the young adult. American Journal of
        Psychiatry, 138, 35-40.

5-815   Hallstrom, T. (1977). Life-weariness, suicidal
        thoughts and suicidal attempts among women in
        Gothenburg, Sweden. Acta Psychiatrica
        Scandinavica, 56, 15-20.

5-816   Humphrey, J. A., Niswander, D., & Casey,
        T. M. (1971). A comparison of suicidal thinkers
        and attempters: Interim findings. Diseases of
        the Nervous System, 32, 825-830.

5-817   Leonard, C. V., & Flinn, D. E. (1972). Suicidal
        ideation and behavior in youthful nonpsychiatric
        populations. Journal of Consulting and Clinical
        Psychology, 38, 366-371. (Abstract: PA, 1972,
        48, No. 11852, p. 1289)

5-818   Lester, D., & Beck, A. T. (1977). Suicidal wishes
        and depression in suicidal ideators: A
        comparison with attempted suicides. Journal of
        Clinical Psychology, 33, 92-94.

5-819   Linehan, M. M., & Laffaw, J. A. (1982). Suicidal
        behaviors among clients at an outpatient
        psychology clinic versus the general population.
        Suicide and Life-Threatening Behavior, 12,
        234-239.

5-820   Melges, F. T., & Weisz, A. E. (1971). The personal
        future and suicidal ideation. Journal of Nervous
        and Mental Disease, 153, 244-250.

5-821   Mintz, R. S. (1970, Fall). Prevalence of persons
        in the city of Los Angeles who have attempted
        suicide: A pilot study. Bulletin of
        Suicidology, No. 7, pp. 9-16.

5-822   Mishara, B. L. (1982). College students'
        experiences with suicide and reactions to
        suicidal verbalizations: A model for prevention.
        Journal of Community Psychology, 10, 142-150.

5-823   Mishara, B. L., Baker, A. H., & Mishara,
        T. T. (1976). The frequency of suicide attempts:
        A retrospective approach applied to college
        students. American Journal of Psychiatry, 133,
        841-844. (Abstracts: PA, 1976, 56, No. 10104,
        p. 1210; ACP, 1976, 16, No. 2815, p. 733)

5-824   Murray, D. C. (1973). Suicidal and depressive
        feelings among college students. Psychological
        Reports, 33, 175-181. (Abstract: PA, 1974, 51,
        No. 7305, p. 922)

5-825   Okasha, A., Lotaif, F., & Sadek, A. (1981).
        Prevalence of suicidal feelings in a sample of
        non-consulting medical students. Acta
        Psychiatrica Scandinavica, 63, 409-415.

5-826   Paykel, E. S., Myers, J. K., Lindenthal, J. J., &
        Tanner, J. (1974). Suicidal feelings in the
        general population: A prevalence study. British
        Journal of Psychiatry, 124, 460-469.

5-827   Ross, M. W., Clayer, J. R., & Campbell,
        R. L. (1983). Parental rearing patterns and
        suicidal thoughts. Acta Psychiatrica
        Scandinavica, 67, 429-433. (Abstract: PA, 1984,
        71, No. 4230, p. 449)

5-828   Schotte, D. E., & Clum, G. A. (1982). Suicide
        ideation in a college population: A test of a
        model. Journal of Consulting and Clinical
        Psychology, 50, 690-696.

5-829   Schwab, J. J., Warheit, G. J., & Holzer, C. E.
        (1972). Suicide ideation and behavior in a
        general population. Diseases of the Nervous
        System, 33, 745-748.

5-830   Schwab, J. J., Warheit, G. J., & Holzer, C. E.,
        III. (1977). Studies on suicidal ideation and
        behavior in a general population: I.
        Epidemiologic considerations. In B. L. Danto &
        A. H. Kutscher (Eds.), Suicide and bereavement
        (pp. 105-119). New York: MSS Information
        Corporation.

5-831   Vandivort, D. S., & Locke, B. Z. (1979). Suicide
        ideation: Its relation to depression, suicide
        and suicide attempt. Suicide and Life-
        Threatening Behavior, 9, 205-218.

5-832   Wright, L. S. (1982). Parental permission to date
        and its relationship to drug use and suicidal
        thoughts among adolescents. Adolescence, 17(66),
        409-418. (Abstract: PA, 1982, 68, No. 7993,
        p. 881)

See also: Beck et al. (1979, reference 6-041) for the Scale
for Suicide Ideation; Berman (1975, reference 5-086);
Flynn & McMahon (1983, reference 5-647); Lester (1983,
reference 1-042), pp. 89-90, "Suicidal ideation"; McBrien
(1983, reference 10-067); Minear & Brush (1980-81,
reference 7-035); Myers (1982, reference 6-421a); Saxon et
al. (1978, 1980, references 5-673 and 5-674); Wenz
(1978-79, reference 6-164).

5.14 Feelings and Cognitive Aspects of the Suicidal

5-833   Adams, R. L., Giffen, M. B., & Garfield, F. (1973).
Risk taking among suicide attempters. Journal of
Abnormal Psychology, 82, 262-267.

5-834   Alvarez, A. (1972). The savage god: A study of
suicide (pp. 120-137). New York: Random House,
"Feelings." (Reprinted in E. S. Shneidman
(Ed.) (1980), Death: Current perspectives (2nd
ed.) (pp. 435-445). (3rd ed., 1984,
pp. 286-296). Palo Alto, CA: Mayfield.)

5-835   Arffa, S. (1983). Cognition and suicide: A
methodological review. Suicide and Life-
Threatening Behavior, 13, 109-122.

5-836   Beck, A. T., Kovacs, M., & Weissman, A. (1975).
Hopelessness and suicidal behavior: An overview.
Journal of the American Medical Association, 234,
1146-1149.

5-837   Beck, A. T., Steer, R. A., & McElroy, M. G. (1982).
Relationships of hopelessness, depression and
previous suicide attempts to suicidal ideation in
alcoholics. Journal of Studies on Alcohol, 43,
1042-1046.

5-838   Beck, A. T., Weissman, A., & Kovacs, M. (1976).
Alcoholism, hopelessness and suicidal behavior.
Journal of Studies on Alcohol 37, 66-77.

5-839   Bedrosian, R. C., & Beck, A. T. (1979). Cognitive
aspects of suicidal behavior. Suicide and
Life-Threatening Behavior, 9, 87-96.

5-840   Boor, M. (1976). Relationship of internal-external
control and national suicide rates. Journal of
Social Psychology, 100, 143-144.

5-841   Boor, M. (1976). Relationship of internal-external
control and United States suicide rates,
1966-1973. Journal of Clinical Psychology, 32,
795-797.

5-842   Boor, M. (1979). Relationship of internal-external
control and United States suicide rates,
1973-1976. Journal of Clinical Psychology, 35,
513-516.

5-843   Boor, M. (1979). Anomie and United States suicide
rates, 1973-1976. Journal of Clinical
Psychology, 35, 703-706.

5-844a Dyer, J. A. T., & Kreitman, N. (1984).
Hopelessness, depression and suicidal intent in

parasuicide. British Journal of Psychiatry, 144, 127-133.

5-844b Emery, G. D., Steer, R. A., & Beck, A. T. (1981). Depression, hopelessness and suicidal intent among heroin addicts. International Journal of the Addictions, 16, 425-429.

5-845 Goldney, R. D. (1982). Locus of control in young women who have attempted suicide. Journal of Nervous and Mental Disease, 170, 198-201.

5-846 Goldsmith, L. A. (1979). Adaptive regression, humor, and suicide. Journal of Consulting and Clinical Psychology, 47, 628-630.

5-847 Goldstein, A. M., & Reznikoff, M. (1971). Suicide in chronic hemodialysis patients from an external locus of control framework. American Journal of Psychiatry, 127, 1204-1207.

5-848 James, N. (1977). Psychological states experienced by suicidal persons. In C. L. Hatton, S. M. Valente, & A. Rink (Eds.), Suicide: Assessment and intervention (pp. 21-33). New York: Appleton-Century-Crofts. [see also 4-054]

5-849 Kaplan, H. B., & Pokorny, A. D. (1976). Self-attitudes and suicidal behavior. Suicide and Life-Threatening Behavior, 6, 23-35.

5-850 Keith-Spiegel, P., Spiegel, D., & Gonska, J. (1971). Cartoon appreciation in suicidal and control groups. Journal of Psychiatric Research, 8, 161-165.

5-851 Kovacs, M., & Beck, A. T. (1977). The wish to die and the wish to live in attempted suicides. Journal of Clinical Psychology, 33, 361-365.

5-852 Kovacs, M., Beck, A. T., & Weissman, A. (1975). Hopelessness: An indicator of suicidal risk. Suicide, 5, 98-103.

5-853 Lambley, P., & Silbowitz, M. (1973). Rotter's internal-external scale and prediction of suicide contemplators among students. Psychological Reports, 33, 585-586. (Abstract: PA, 1974, 51, No. 9396, p. 1193)

5-854 Leonard, C. V. (1973). Self-ratings of alienation in suicidal patients. Journal of Clinical Psychology, 29, 423-428.

5-855 Lester, D. (1973, August). Suicide and internal-external orientation. Psychology,

10(3), 35-39.

5-856   Levenson, M. (1974). Cognitive correlates of
        suicidal risk. In C. Neuringer (Ed.),
        Psychological assessment of suicidal risk
        (pp. 150-163). Springfield, IL: Thomas.

5-857   Linehan, M. M., & Laffaw, J. A. (1982). Suicidal
        behaviors among clients at an outpatient
        psychology clinic versus the general population.
        Suicide and Life-Threatening Behavior, 12,
        234-239.

5-858   Linehan, M. M., & Nielsen, S. L. (1981).
        Assessment of suicide ideation and parasuicide:
        Hopelessness and social desirability. Journal of
        Consulting and Clinical Psychology, 49, 773-775.

5-859   Linehan, M. M., & Nielsen, S. L. (1983). Social
        desirability: Its relevance to the measurement
        of hopelessness and suicidal behavior. Journal
        of Consulting and Clinical Psychology, 51,
        141-143.

5-860   Lukianowicz, N. (1972). Suicidal behavior: An
        attempt to modify the environment. British
        Journal of Psychiatry, 121, 387-390.

5-861   Minkoff, K., Bergman, E., Beck, A. T., & Beck,
        R. (1973). Hopelessness, depression, and
        attempted suicide. American Journal of
        Psychiatry, 130, 455-459.

5-862   Nekanda-Trepka, C. J. S., Bishop, S., & Blackburn,
        I. M. (1983). Hopelessness and depression.
        British Journal of Clinical Psychology, 22,
        49-60. (Abstracts: PA, 1983, 70, No. 3560,
        p. 404; CPA, 1983, 23, No. 763, p. 158)

5-863   Neuringer, C. (1974). Attitudes toward self in
        suicidal individuals. Life-Threatening Behavior,
        4, 96-106.

5-864   Neuringer, C. (1976). Current developments in the
        study of suicidal thinking. In E. S. Shneidman
        (Ed.), Suicidology: Contemporary developments
        (pp. 234-256). New York: Grune & Stratton.

5-865   Neuringer, C., & Lettierri, D. J. (1971).
        Cognition, attitude, and affect in suicidal
        individuals. Life-Threatening Behavior, 1,
        106-124.

5-866   Neuringer, C., & Lettierri, D. J. (1982). Suicidal
        women: Their thinking and feeling patterns. New
        York: Gardner.

5-867   Nevid, J. S. (1983). Hopelessness, social
        desirability, and construct validity. Journal of
        Consulting and Clinical Psychology, 51, 139-140.

5-868   Olin, H. S. (1978). Dying without death: The
        third wish in suicide. American Journal of
        Psychotherapy, 32, 270-275.

5-869   Patsiokas, A., Clum, G., & Luscomb, R. (1979).
        Cognitive characteristics of suicide attemptors.
        Journal of Consulting and Clinical Psychology,
        47, 478-484.

5-870   Petrie, K., & Chamberlain, K. (1983). Hopelessness
        and social desireability as moderator variables
        in predicting suicidal behavior. Journal of
        Consulting and Clinical Psychology, 51, 485-487.
        (Abstract: PA, 1983, 70, No. 12939,
        pp. 1454-1455)

5-871   Pokorny, A. D., Kaplan, H. B., & Tsai,
        S. Y. (1975). Hopelessness and attempted
        suicide: A reconsideration. American Journal of
        Psychiatry, 132, 954-956.

5-872   Prociuk, T. J., Breen, L. J., & Lussier,
        R. J. (1976). Hopelessness, internal-external
        locus of control, and depression. Journal of
        Clinical Psychology, 32, 299-300.

5-873   Ringel, E. (1976). The presuicidal syndrome.
        Suicide and Life-Threatening Behavior, 6,
        131-149.

5-874   Rush, J., & Weissenburger, J. (1982). Depression
        and suicide. In R. Grieger & I. Z. Grieger
        (Eds.), Cognition and emotional disturbance
        (pp. 76-109). New York: Human Sciences Press.

5-875   Sendbuehler, J. M. (1973). Attempted suicide: A
        description of the pre and post suicidal states.
        Canadian Psychiatric Association Journal, 18,
        113-116.

5-876   Shneidman, E. S. (1969). Logical content analysis:
        An explication of styles of "concludifying." In
        G. Gerber, O. R. Holsti, K. Krippendorff,
        W. J. Paisley, & P. J. Stone (Eds.), The analysis
        of communication content: Developments in
        scientific theories and computer techniques
        (pp. 261-279). New York: Wiley. (Reprinted in
        Suicide and Life-Threatening Behavior, 1981,
        11(4), 300-324.)

5-877   Shneidman, E. S., & Farberow, N. L. (1957). The
        logic of suicide. In E. S. Shneidman &

N. L. Farberow (Eds.), <u>Clues to suicide</u>
(pp. 31-40). New York: McGraw-Hill. (Reprinted
in E. S. Shneidman, N. L. Farberow, &
R. E. Litman (Eds.) (1970), <u>The psychology of</u>
<u>suicide</u> (pp. 63-71). New York: Science House.)

5-878   Spiegel, D., Keith-Spiegel, P., Abrahams, J., &
Kranitz, L. (1969). Humor and suicide: Favorite
jokes of suicidal patients. <u>Journal of</u>
<u>Consulting and Clinical Psychology, 33,</u> 504-505.

5-879   Taylor, S. (1978). The confrontation with death
and the renewal of life. <u>Suicide and</u>
<u>Life-Threatening Behavior, 8,</u> 89-98.

5-880   Topol, P., & Reznikoff, M. (1982). Perceived peer
and family relationships, hopelessness, and locus
of control as factors in adolescent suicide
attempts. <u>Suicide and Life-Threatening Behavior,</u>
<u>12,</u> 141-150. (Abstract: <u>PA</u>, 1983, <u>69</u>,
No. 12968, p. 1432)

5-881   Weissman, A. N., Beck, A. T., & Kovacs, M. (1979).
Drug abuse, hopelessness and suicidal behavior.
<u>International Journal of the Addictions</u>, <u>14</u>,
451-464.

5-882   Wenz, F. V. (1975). Anomie and level of
suicidality in individuals. <u>Psychological</u>
<u>Reports</u>, <u>36</u>, 817-818.

5-883   Wenz, F. V. (1977). Subjective powerlessness, sex,
and suicide potential. <u>Psychological Reports</u>,
<u>40</u>, 927-928.

5-884   Wenz, F. V. (1978). Breadth of perspective and
suicide threats. <u>Psychological Reports</u>, <u>43</u>,
649-650.

5-885   Wetzel, R. D. (1975). Self-concept and suicide
intent. <u>Psychological Reports, 36</u>, 279-282.

5-886   Wetzel, R. D. (1976). Hopelessness, depression,
and suicide intent. <u>Archives of General</u>
<u>Psychiatry</u>, <u>33</u>, 1069-1073.

5-887   Wetzel, R. D., Margulies, T., Davis, R., & Karam,
E. (1980). Hopelessness, depression, and suicide
intent. <u>Journal of Clinical Psychiatry</u>, <u>41</u>,
159-160.

5-888   Williams, C. B., & Nickels, J. B. (1969).
Internal-external control dimension as related to
accident and suicide proneness. <u>Journal of</u>
<u>Consulting and Clinical Psychology</u>, <u>33</u>, 485-494.

5-889   Williams, C. L., Davidson, C. L., & Montgomery,
        I. (1980). Impulsive suicidal behavior. Journal
        of Clinical Psychology, 36, 90-94.

See also: For the measurement of hopelessness, Beck et
al. (1974, reference 6-044).

See also: Kazdin et al. (1983, reference 6-090); Lester
(1972, reference 1-041), Chapter 18, "The thought processes
of the suicidal individual" (pp. 203-207); Lester & Lester
(1971, reference 1-043), Chapter 11, "Thought processes of
the suicidal person" (pp. 82-87); Maris (1981, reference
5-104), Chapter 8, "The emotional context of suicide:
Depression and hopelessness" (pp. 205-235); Pretzel &
Riddle (1981, reference 5-175.05).

5.15 Biological Factors and Suicide

5-890   Asberg, M., Traskman, L., & Thoren, P. (1976).
        5-HIAA in the cerebrospinal fluid: A biochemical
        suicide predictor. Archives of General
        Psychiatry, 33, 1193-1197.

5-891   Banki, C. M., & Arato, M. (1983). Amine
        metabolites and neuroendocrine responses related
        to depression and suicide. Journal of Affective
        Disorders, 5, 223-232. [IM dec 1983]

5-892   Blath, R. A., McClure, J. N., Jr., & Wetzel,
        R. D. (1973). Familial factors and suicide.
        Diseases of the Nervous System, 34, 90-93.

5-893   Brown, G. L., Goodwin, F. K., & Bunney, W. E.,
        Jr. (1982). Human aggression and suicide: Their
        relationship to neuropsychiatric diagnoses and
        serotonin metabolism. Advances in Biochemical
        Psychopharmacology, 34, 287-307. [IM 1983 Feb]

5-894   Bunney, W. E., Jr., & Fawcett, J. A. (1968).
        Biochemical research in depression and suicide.
        In H. L. P. Resnik (Ed.), Suicide: Diagnosis and
        management (pp. 144-159). Boston: Little,
        Brown.

5-895   Coryell, W., & Schlesser, M. A. (1981). Suicide
        and the dexamethasone suppression test in
        unipolar depression. American Journal of
        Psychiatry, 138, 1120-1121. (Abstract: PA,
        1981, 66, No. 10411, p. 1086)

5-896   Dezelsky, T. L., & Toohey, J. V. (1978).
        Biorhythms and the prediction of suicide
        behavior. Journal of School Health, 48, 399-403.

5-897   Garvey, M. J., Tuason, V. B., Hoffmann, N., &
        Chastek, J. (1983). Suicide attempters,

nonattempters, and neurotransmitters.
Comprehensive Psychiatry, 24, 332-336.

5-898   Hankoff, L. D. (1979). Physiochemical correlates.
In L. D. Hankoff & B. Einsidler (Eds.), Suicide:
Theory and clinical aspects (pp. 105-110).
Littleton, MA: PSG Publishing.

5-899   Ostroff, R., Giller, E., Bonese, K., Ebersole, E.,
Harkness, L., & Mason, J. (1982). Neuroendocrine
risk factors of suicidal behavior. American
Journal of Psychiatry, 138, 1323-1325.

5-900   Pichot, P., & Menahem, R. (1972). Constitutional
factors in suicide. In J. Waldenstrom,
T. Larsson, & N. Ljungstedt (Eds.), Suicide and
attempted suicide (pp. 102-111). Stockholm:
Nordiska Bokhandelns Forlag.

5-901   Rockwell, D. A., Winget, C. M., Rosenblatt, L. S.,
Higgins, E. A., & Hetherington, N. W. (1978).
Biological aspects of suicide. Journal of
Nervous and Mental Disease, 166, 851-858.

5-902   Roy, A. (1983). Family history of suicide.
Archives of General Psychiatry, 40, 971-974.

5-903   Stanley, M., & Mann, J. J. (1983). Increased
serotonin-2 binding sites in frontal cortex of
suicide victims. Lancet, 1, 214-216.

5-904   Struve, F. A. (1979). Clinical
electroencephalography. In L. D. Hankoff &
B. Einsidler (Eds.), Suicide: Theory and
clinical aspects (pp. 111-129). Littleton, MA:
PSG Publishing.

5-905   Struve, F. A. (1983). Electoencephalographic
relationship to suicidal behavior: Qualitative
considerations and a report on a series of
completed suicides. Clinical
Electroencephalography, 14, 20-26.

5-906   Targum, S. D., Rosen, L., & Capodanno,
A. E. (1983). The dexamethasone suppression test
in suicidal patients with unipolar depression.
American Journal of Psychiatry, 140, 877-879.
(Abstract: PA, 1983, 70, No. 10436, p. 1169)

5-907   Tsuang, M. T. (1977). Genetic factors in suicide.
Diseases of the Nervous System, 38, 498-501.

5-908   Van Praag, H. M. (1982). Depression, suicide and
the metabolism of serotonin in the brain.
Journal of Affective Disorders, 4, 275-290.
(Abstract: PA, 1983, 70, No. 5830, p. 654)

5-909   Whitlock, F. A. (1982).   The neurology of affective
          disorder and suicide. Australia & New Zealand
          Journal of Psychiatry, 16, 1-12. (Abstract: PA,
          1983, 69, No. 3527, p. 380)

See also: Lester (1972, reference 1-041), Chapter 5, "The
inheritance of suicidal inclinations," pp. 25-27; Lester
(1983, reference 1-042), Chapters 1, "The inheritance of
suicidal inclinations," pp. 5-6, and Chapter 2,
"Physiological factors in suicidal inclinations," pp. 7-13;
Lester & Lester (1971, reference 1-043), Chapter 4,
"Heredity and environment in the causation of suicide,"
pp. 24-33; deCatanzaro (1980, 1981, references 4-073 and
4-074); Fink & Carpenter (1976, reference 6-072);   Krieger
(1970, 1975, references 6-096 and 6-097);   Petzel & Cline
(1978, reference 5-206).

5.16 Suggestion/Imitation/Epidemic/Media Aspects

5-910   Ashton, J. R., & Donnan, S. (1981). Suicide by
          burning as an epidemic phenomenon: An analysis
          of 82 deaths and inquests in England and Wales in
          1978-79. Psychological Medicine, 11, 735-739.

5-911   Barraclough, B., Shepherd, D., & Jennings,
          C. (1977). Do newspaper reports of coroners'
          inquests incite people to commit suicide?
          British Journal of Psychiatry, 131, 528-530.

5-912   Blumenthal, S., & Bergner, L. (1973). Suicide and
          newspapers: A replicated study. American
          Journal of Psychiatry, 130, 468-471.
          [Replication of Motto, 1970, reference 5-918]

5-913   Bollen, K. A., & Phillips, D. P. (1981). Suicidal
          motor vehicle fatalities in Detroit: A
          replication. American Journal of Sociology, 87,
          404-412.

5-914   Bollen, K. A., & Phillips, D. P. (1982). Imitative
          suicides: A national study of the effects of
          television news stories. American Sociological
          Review, 47, 802-809. (Abstract: PA, 1983, 70,
          No. 3590, p. 407)

5-915   Garner, H. G. (1975). An adolescent suicide, the
          mass media, and the educator. Adolescence,
          10(38), 241-246.

5-916   Holding, T. A. (1974). The B.B.C. 'Befriender'
          series and its effect. British Journal of
          Psychiatry, 124, 470-472. [See also Kreitman,
          1977, reference 2-038, pp. 133-136.]

5-917   Lester, D. (1981). Freedom of the press and
          personal violence: A cross-national study of

suicide and homicide. Journal of Social
Psychology, 114, 267-269.

5-918   Motto, J. A. (1970). Newspaper influence on
suicide: A controlled study. Archives of
General Psychiatry, 23, 143-148.

5-919   Pell, B., & Watters, D. (1982). Newspaper policies
on suicide. Canada's Mental Health, 30(4), 8-9.
(Abstract: PA, 1984, 71, No. 3605, p. 381)

5-920   Phillips, D. P. (1974). The influence of
suggestion on suicide: Substantive and
theoretical implications of the Werther effect.
American Sociological Review, 39, 340-354.

5-921   Phillips, D. P. (1977). Motor vehicle fatalities
increase just after publicized suicide stories.
Science, 196, 1464-1466.

5-922   Phillips, D. P. (1978). Airplane accident
fatalities increase just after newspaper stories
about murder and suicide. Science, 201, 748-750.

5-923   Phillips, D. P. (1979). Suicide, motor vehicle
fatalities, and the mass media: Evidence toward
a theory of suggestion. American Journal of
Sociology, 84, 1150-1174.

5-924   Phillips, D. P. (1980). Airplane accidents,
murder, and the mass media: Towards a theory of
imitation and suggestion. Social Forces, 58,
1001-1024.

5-925   Phillips, D. P. (1982). The impact of fictional
television stories on U.S. adult fatalities: New
evidence on the effect of the mass media on
violence. American Journal of Sociology, 87,
1340-1359. (Abstract: PA, 1983, 69, No. 2995,
pp. 319-320)

5-926   Robbins, D., & Conroy, R. C. (1983). A cluster of
adolescent suicide attempts: Is suicide
contagious? Journal of Adolescent Health Care,
3, 253-255.

5-927   Rounsaville, B. J., & Weissman, M. M. (1980). A
note on suicidal behavior among intimates.
Suicide and Life-Threatening Behavior, 10, 24-28.

5-928   Rubinstein, D. H. (1983). Epidemic suicide among
Micronesian adolescents. Social Science and
Medicine, 17, 657-665. (Abstract: PA, 1984, 71,
No. 7045, p. 745)

5-929   Shepherd, D., & Barraclough, B. M. (1978). Suicide

reporting [newspapers]: Information or
entertainment? <u>British Journal of Psychiatry</u>,
<u>132</u>, 283-287.

5-930   Stack, S. (1983, April). <u>The effect of imitation</u>
<u>on suicide: A reassessment</u>. Paper presented at
the annual meeting of the North Central
Sociological Association, Columbus, Ohio.
(Abstract: <u>Sociological Abstracts</u>, 1983, <u>31</u>,
Supplement 121, No. S15330, p. 22)

See also: Stack (1982, reference 4-035); Stack (1983,
reference 5-786); Lester (1972, reference 1-041), Chapter
16, "Suicide, suggestibility, and contagion," pp. 187-189;
Lester (1983, reference 1-042), Chapter 20, "Suicide and
suggestion," pp. 126-128.

Chapter 6
PREVENTION, INTERVENTION, TREATMENT, ASSESSMENT &
PREDICTION OF SUICIDAL BEHAVIOR

Prevention was suggested by Caplan to be possible at three levels--primary, secondary, and tertiary prevention. As applied to suicide, the terms "prevention," "intervention," and "postvention" are more commonly used, respectively. Prevention of suicide at the primary level is the most ideal, with suicidal behavior deterred before it ever is apparent. This is accomplished by eliminating or alleviating circumstances and societal practices which promote distress and suicidal crises, e.g., unemployment, prejudice, isolation, etc. Such prevention is the most pervasive but is also the slowest to effect because it often demands societal change, a notoriously gradual occurrence at best. As a result, most preventive efforts have been at the secondary or intervention level, after the behavior and distress are apparent. Methods to deal with suicidal crises have most commonly taken the form of crisis intervention or suicide prevention center telephone services in the U.S., 24-hour "lifelines" for those in distress (see Section 6.7). Once the behavior has occurred as expressed ideation, depressive symptomatology, or a non-fatal suicide attempt, medical and psychological/social interventions and management techniques may be employed (see Section 6.4), followed often by some form of therapy to alleviate the circumstances and problems leading to the distress and suicidal crisis (see Section 6.6). Another aspect of secondary prevention is the attempt to recognize or predict those in the population who are potentially or actively suicidal to allow early intervention and lessen the likelihood that the situation will progress to the point of a suicidal act. Major efforts have been made to find scales, tests, and other indicators that might identify or anticipate the high risk individuals (see Section 6.3).

Postvention, or "after the fact" prevention, will be discussed in greater detail in Chapter 9, but it refers here to efforts made to aid those who remain following a suicide, i.e., the family members, friends, etc., who are affected by the death (often called "survivor victims"). This level of preventive measures has only recently received increased attention.

6.1 Bibliographies on Prevention Issues

6-001   American Association of Suicidology. Suicide prevention centers [Annotated bibliography]. Denver: AAS.

6-002   Miller, M.   Intervention by phone [Non-annotated bibliography].   San Diego: Suicide Information Center, No. R-47 (listed in 1984 catalog).

6.2 Considerations of Suicide Prevention

6-003   Bagley, C. (1973).   Social policy and the prevention of suicidal behaviour. British Journal of Social Work, 3, 473-495.

6-004   Bennett, A. E. (1957).   Suggestions for suicide prevention.   In E. S. Shneidman & N. L. Farberow (Eds.), Clues to suicide (pp. 187-193).   New York: McGraw-Hill.

6-005   Bloom, V. (1970).   Prevention of suicide. Current Psychiatric Therapies, 10, 105-109.

6-006   Bloomberg, S. C. (1972).   The present state of suicide prevention--An African survey. International Journal of Social Psychiatry, 18, 104-108.

6-007   Choron, J. (1972).   Suicide (pp. 79-85).   New York: Scribner's, Chapter 8, "Suicide prevention."

6-008   Diggory, J. C. (1969).   Calculation of some costs of suicide prevention using certain predictors of suicidal behavior. Psychological Bulletin, 71, 373-386.

6-009   Draper, E., & Margolis, P. (1976).   A psychodynamic approach to suicide prevention. Community Mental Health Journal, 12, 376-382.

> A theory of suicide emphasizing unremitting psychological pain is presented.   See also Draper (1976, reference 4-075).

6-010   Dublin, L. I. (1963).   Suicide: A sociological and statistical study (pp. 194-206).   New York: Ronald Press, Chapter 21, "Toward sound mental health."

> Dublin outlines efforts which will promote mental health and lessen the likelihood of suicide (i.e., primary prevention).

6-011   Farber, M. L. (1968). Theory of suicide
        (pp. 82-95). New York: Funk & Wagnalls, Chapter
        8, "Social engineering and suicide prevention."

6-012   Farberow, N. L. (1980). Clinical developments in
        suicide prevention in the United States. Crisis,
        1, 16-26.

6-013   Gorman, M. L. (1971). Primary and secondary
        prevention: A frame of reference. In
        D. B. Anderson & L. J. McClean (Eds.),
        Identifying suicide potential (pp. 57-62). New
        York: Behavioral Publications.

6-014   Grollman, E. A. (1971). Suicide: Prevention,
        intervention, postvention (pp. 119-136). Boston:
        Beacon Press, Chapter 8, "A summons for community
        action."

6-015   Hendin, H. (1982). Suicide in America
        (pp. 177-187). New York: Norton, Chapter 9,
        "Suicide prevention."

6-016   Kiev, A. (1971). Suicide prevention. In
        D. B. Anderson & L. J. McClean (Eds.),
        Identifying suicide potential (pp. 3-14). New
        York: Behavioral Publications.

6-017   Kiev, A. (1978). The prevention of suicide.
        Current Psychiatric Therapies, 18, 91-95.

6-018   Lonnqvist, J., Achte, K., & Aalberg, V. (1977). On
        suicide prevention. In K. A. Achte &
        J. Lonnqvist (Eds.), Suicide research:
        Proceedings of the seminars of suicide research
        by Yrjo Jahnsson Foundation 1974-1977
        (pp. 59-66). Helsinki: Psychiatria Fennica
        (Psychiatria Fennica Supplementum 1976).

6-019   Lum, D. (1973). Economic and public health issues
        in suicide prevention. Hawaii Medical Journal,
        32, 391-394.

6-020   Maris, R. W. (1969). The sociology of suicide
        prevention: Policy implications of differences
        between suicidal patients and completed suicides.
        Social Problems, 17, 132-149.

6-021   McCulloch, J. W., & Philip, A. E. (1972). Suicidal
        behaviour (pp. 99-110). New York: Pergamon
        Press, Chapter 7, "Implications for prevention."

6-022   Miller, M. (1979). Suicide after sixty: The final
        alternative (pp. 91-94). New York: Springer,
        Chapter 15, "How we can decrease the number of
        geriatric suicides."

6-023 Morgan, H. G. (1979). Death wishes? The
       understanding and management of deliberate
       self-harm (pp. 75-84). New York: Wiley, Chapter
       7, "Suicide prevention."

6-024 Motto, J. A. (1976). Suicide prevention for
       high-risk persons who refuse treatment. Suicide
       and Life-Threatening Behavior, 6, 223-230.

6-025 Oast, S. P., III., & Zitrin, A. (1975). Public
       health approach to suicide prevention. American
       Journal of Public Health, 65, 144-147.

6-026 Pretzel, P. W. (1972). Understanding and
       counseling the suicidal person (pp. 87-135).
       Nashville, TN: Abingdon, Chapter 3, "Preventing
       suicide."

6-027 Rassell, J. A. (1968). Suicide. In
       F. C. R. Chalke & J. J. Day (Eds.), Primary
       prevention of psychiatric disorders: The
       Clarence M. Hincks memorial lectures, 1967
       (pp. 110-139). Toronto: University of Toronto
       Press.

6-028 Roberts, A. R. (1975). Self-destruction by one's
       own hand: Suicide and suicide prevention. In
       A. R. Roberts (Ed.), Self-destructive behavior
       (pp. 21-77). Springfield, IL: Thomas.

6-029 Ross, C. P. (1980). Mobilizing schools for suicide
       prevention. Suicide and Life-Threatening
       Behavior, 10, 239-243.

6-030 Shneidman, E. S. (1967, December). Some current
       developments in suicide prevention. Bulletin of
       Suicidology, pp. 31-34.

6-031 Shneidman, E. S., & Mandelkorn, P. (1967). How to
       prevent suicide. New York: Public Affairs
       Committee, Public Affairs Pamphlet No. 406.
       (Reprinted in E. S. Shneidman, N. L. Farberow, &
       R. E. Litman (Eds.) (1970), The psychology of
       suicide (pp. 125-143). New York: Science
       House.)

6-032 Sonneck, G., & Ringel, E. (1977). Suicide
       prevention and the community. Mental Health and
       Society, 4, 80-84.

6-033 Stengel, E. (1964). Suicide and attempted suicide
       (pp. 117-128). Baltimore, MD: Penquin Books,
       Chapter 15, "Prevention and prophylaxis."

6-034 Stengel, E. (1969). Recent progress in suicide
       research and prevention. Israel Annals of

Psychiatry, 7, 127-137.

6-035   Thomas, C. B. (1969). Suicide among us: Can we learn to prevent it? John Hopkins Medical Journal, 125, 276-285.

6-036   Welu, T. C., & Cam, O. S. (1972). Broadening the focus of suicide prevention activities utilizing the public health model. American Journal of Public Health, 62, 1625-1628.

6-037   World Health Organization. (1968). Prevention of suicide. World Health Organization (WHO) Public Health Papers, No. 35, pp. 1-84.

See also Shulman (1968, reference 8-157).

6.3 Assessment and Prediction of Suicidal Behavior

6-038   Arffa, S. (1982). Predicting adolescent suicidal behavior and the order of Rorschach measurement. Journal of Personality Assessment, 46, 563-568.

* 6-039   Bassuk, E. L. (1982). General principles of assessment. In E. L. Bassuk, S. C. Schoonover, & A. D. Gill (Eds.), Lifelines: Clinical perspectives on suicide (pp. 17-46). New York: Plenum Press.

            Materials for assessment (checklists, etc.) are presented for the clinician regarding interviewing and suicidal behavior. Especially helpful is an appendix which includes 6 rating scales: Scale for Suicide Ideation (Beck et al., 1979, reference 6-041); Hopelessness Scale (Beck et al., 1974, reference 6-044); Suicide Intent Scale (Beck et al., 1974, reference 6-042.01); Suicide Risk among Attempters (Tuckman & Youngman, 1968, reference 6-155); Scale for Assessing Suicide Potential [Los Angeles Suicide Prevention Center scale, from Beck et al., 1974, reference 6-042, pp. 76-78. Reprinted also in Miller, 1982, reference 10-038, pp. 57-60; Reprinted also in Vorkoper & Petty, 1980, reference 9-074, pp. 178-179; Reprinted also in Getz et al., 1983, reference 6-243, pp. 263-266].

6-040   Beck, A. T., Beck, R., & Kovacs, M. (1975). Classification of suicidal behaviors: I. Quantifying intent and medical lethality. American Journal of Psychiatry, 132, 285-287.

6-041   Beck, A. T., Kovacs, M., & Weissman, A. (1979). Assessment of suicidal intent: The scale for

suicidal ideation. Journal of Consulting and
Clinical Psychology, 47, 343-352.

* 6-042   Beck, A. T., Resnik, H. L. P., & Lettieri,
          D. J. (Eds.) (1974). The prediction of suicide
          Bowie, MD: Charles Press.

          Of the 14 articles in this excellent book, 11
          are on assessment and/or prediction and are
          listed below.

          6-042.01   Beck, A. T., Schuyler, D., & Herman,
                     I. Development of suicidal intent
                     scales. pp. 45-56.

          6-042.02   Diggory, J. C. Predicting suicide:
                     Will-o-the-wisp or reasonable
                     challenge? pp. 59-70.

          6-042.03   Lester, D. Demographic versus clinical
                     prediction of suicidal behaviors: A
                     look at some issues. pp. 71-84.

          6-042.04   Motto, J. A. Refinement of variables in
                     assessing suicide risk. pp. 85-93.

          6-042.05   Aitken, R. C. B. Assessment of mood by
                     analogue. pp. 94-105.

          6-042.06   Murphy, G. E. (1972). The clinical
                     identification of suicidal risk.
                     pp. 109-118. (Reprinted from Archives
                     of General Psychiatry, 27, 356-359.)

          6-042.07   Lettieri, D. J., & Nehemkis, A. M. A
                     socio-clinical scale for certifying
                     mode of death. pp. 119-140.

          6-042.08   Litman, R. E., Farberow, N. L., Wold,
                     C. I., & Brown, T. R. Prediction
                     models of suicidal behaviors.
                     pp. 141-159.

          6-042.09   Lettieri, D. J. Suicidal death
                     prediction scales. pp. 163-192.

          6-042.10   Weisman, A., & Worden, J. W. (1972).
                     Risk-rescue rating in suicide
                     assessment. pp. 193-213. (Reprinted
                     from Archives of General Psychiatry,
                     26, 553-556.)

          6-042.11   Zung, W. W. K. Index of potential
                     suicide (IPS): A rating scale for
                     suicide prevention. pp. 221-249.

6-043   Beck, A. T., Ward, C. H., Mendelson, M., Mock, J.,
        & Erbaugh, J. (1961). An inventory for measuring
        depression. Archives of General Psychiatry, 4,
        561-571.

        A discussion of the Beck Depression Inventory
        and its development. This is one of the most
        commonly employed scales for measuring
        depression. The scale is included in an
        appendix of this article (pp. 569-571). The
        scale also is reprinted in Getz et al. (1983,
        reference 6-243), pp. 259-262, and Beck et
        al., reference 6-229, pp. 398-399. The
        following articles also include information or
        revisions of the inventory.

        6-043.01   Beck, A. T. (1970). Depression: Causes
                   and treatment Philadelphia: University
                   of Pennsylvania Press. (Published
                   under the title Depression: Clinical,
                   experimental, and theoretical aspects,
                   1967.) [Scale appears on pp. 333-337.]

        6-043.02   Beck, A. T., & Beamesderfer, A. (1974).
                   Assessment of depression: The
                   Depression Inventory. In P. Pichot
                   (Ed.), Psychological measurements in
                   psychopharmacology, Volume 7 of Modern
                   problems of pharmacopsychiatry series
                   (pp. 151-169). New York: Basel. [The
                   short form of the inventory appears on
                   pp. 167-169.]

        6-043.03   Beck, A. T., Rial, W. Y., & Rickels,
                   K. (1974). Short form of Depression
                   Inventory: Cross-validation.
                   Psychological Reports, 34, 1184-1186.

6-044   Beck, A. T., Weissman, A., Lester, D., & Trexler,
        L. (1974). The measurement of pessimism: The
        hoplessness scale. Journal of Consulting and
        Clinical Psychology, 42, 861-865.

        Because of the strong relationship observed
        between hopelessness, suicide, and depression
        (see Chapter 5, references 5-836, 5-852,
        etc.), this scale citation is included here.

6-045   Beck, A. T., Weissman, A., Lester, D., & Trexler,
        L. (1976). Classification of suicidal behaviors:
        II. Dimensions of suicidal intent. Archives of
        General Psychiatry, 33, 835-837.

6-046   Beck, R. W., Morris, J. B., & Beck, A. T. (1974).
        Cross-validation of the suicidal intent scale.
        Psychological Reports, 34, 445-446.

6-047   Blatt, S. J., & Ritzler, B. A. (1974). Suicide and
         the representation of transparency and
         cross-sections on the Rorschach. Journal of
         Consulting and Clinical Psychology, 42, 280-287.

6-048   Borg, S. E., & Stahl, M. (1982). Prediction of
         suicide: A prospective study of suicides and
         controls among psychiatric patients. Acta
         Psychiatrica Scandinavica, 65, 221-232.

6-049   Braucht, G. N., & Wilson, L. T. (1970). Predictive
         utility of the revised suicide potential scale.
         Journal of Consulting and Clinical Psychology,
         35, 426.

* 6-050 Brown, T. R., & Sheran, T. J. (1972). Suicide
         prediction: A review. Life-Threatening
         Behavior, 2, 67-98.

6-051   Buglass, D., & Horton, J. (1974). A scale for
         predicting subsequent suicidal behavior. British
         Journal of Psychiatry, 124, 573-578.

6-052   Buglass, D., & McCulloch, J. W. (1970). Further
         suicidal behaviour: The development and
         validation of predictive scales. British Journal
         of Psychiatry, 116, 483-491.

6-053   Capodanno, A. E., & Targum, S. D. (1983, May).
         Assessment of suicide risk: Some limitations in
         the prediction of infrequent events. Journal of
         Psychosocial Nursing and Mental Health Services,
         21(5), 11-14.

6-054   Catalan, J. (1980). The assessment of patients
         following self-poisoning: A comparison of
         doctors and nurses. In R. D. T. Farmer &
         S. R. Hirsch (Eds.), The suicide syndrome
         (pp. 203-214). London: Croom Helm.

6-055   Catalan, J., Marsack, P., Hawton, K. E., Whitwell,
         D., Fagg, J., & Bancroft, J. H. J. (1980).
         Comparison of doctors and nurses in the
         assessment of deliberate self-poisoning patients.
         Psychological Medicine, 10, 483-491.

6-056   Cohen, E., Motto, J. A., & Seiden, R. H. (1966).
         An instrument for evaluating suicide potential:
         A preliminary study. American Journal of
         Psychiatry, 122, 886-891.

6-057a   Clopton, J. R. (1979). The MMPI and suicide. In
         C. S. Newmark (Ed.), MMPI: Clinical and research
         trends (pp. 149-166). New York: Praeger.

6-057b   Clopton, J. R., & Baucom, D. H. (1979). MMPI

ratings of suicide risk. _Journal of Personality Assessment_, _43_, 293-296.

6-058   Clopton, J. R., & Jones, W. C. (1975). Use of the MMPI in the prediction of suicide. _Journal of Clinical Psychology_, _31_, 52-54.

6-059a   Clopton, J. R., Pallis, D. J., & Birtchnell, J. (1979). Minnesota Multiphasic Personality Inventory profile patterns of suicide attempters. _Journal of Consulting and Clinical Psychology_, _47_, 135-139.

6-059b   Clopton, J. R., Post, R. D., & Larde, J. (1983). Identification of suicide attempters by means of MMPI profiles. _Journal of Clinical Psychology_, _39_, 868-871.

6-060   Colson, D. B., & Hurwitz, B. A. (1973). A new experimental approach to the relationship between color-shading and suicide attempts. _Journal of Personality Assessment_, _37_, 237-241.

6-061   Danto, B. L. (1971, Fall). Assessment of the suicidal person in the telephone interview. _Bulletin of Suicidology_, No. 8, pp. 48-56.

6-062   Devries, A. G. (1966). A potential suicide personality inventory. _Psychological Reports_, _18_, 731-738.

6-063   Diran, M. O. (1976, January). You can prevent suicide. _Nursing76_, _6_, 60-64. (Reprinted in M. Miller (Ed.) (1982), _Suicide intervention by nurses_ (pp. 52-56). New York: Springer.)

         Diran discusses suicide evaluation and recognition by nurses and includes a 13 item questionnaire to determine the possibility of suicide.

* 6-064 Engelsmann, F., & Ananth, J. (1981). Suicide rating scales. _Psychiatric Journal of the University of Ottawa_, _6_, 47-51. (Abstract: _PA_, 1982, _67_, No. 4721, p. 501)

         A review of rating scales and tests to predict suicidal behavior is presented.

6-065   Epstein, L. C., Thomas, C. B., Shaffer, J. W., & Perlin, S. (1973). Clinical prediction of physician suicide based on medical student data. _Journal of Nervous and Mental Disease_, _156_, 19-29.

6-066   Exner, J. E., & Wylie, J. (1977). Some Rorschach

data concerning suicide. Journal of Personality Assessment, 41, 339-348.

6-067   Farberow, N. L. (1974). Use of the Rorschach in predicting and understanding suicide. Journal of Personality Assessment, 38, 411-419.

6-068   Farberow, N. L., & MacKinnon, D. R. (1974). A suicide prediction schedule for neuropsychiatric hospital patients. Journal of Nervous and Mental Disease, 158, 408-419.

6-069   Farberow, N. L., & MacKinnon, D. R. (1975). Prediction of suicide: A replication study. Journal of Personality Assessment, 39, 497-501.

6-070   Farberow, N. L., & MacKinnon, D. R. (1977). Prediction of suicide: A replication study. In K. Achte & J. Lonnqvist (Eds.), Suicide research: Proceedings of the seminars of suicide research by Yrjo Jahnsson Foundation 1974-1977 (pp. 141-145). Helsinki: Psychiatria Fennica (Psychiatria Fennica Supplementum 1976).

6-071   Fawcett, J. (1974). Clinical assessment of suicidal risk. Postgraduate Medicine, 55, 85-89.

6-072   Fink, E. B., & Carpenter, W. T., Jr. (1976). Further examination of a biochemical test for suicide potential. Diseases of the Nervous System, 37, 341-343.

6-073   Garb, H. N. (1983). A conjoint measurement analysis of clinical predictions. Journal of Clinical Psychology, 39, 295-301.

        This article discusses how systems-oriented therapists predict the occurrence of suicide.

6-074   Garzotto, N., Siani, R., Tansella, C. Z., & Tansella, M. (1976). Cross-validation of a predictive scale for subsequent suicidal behaviour in an Italian sample. British Journal of Psychiatry, 128, 137-140.

6-075   Golden, K. M. (1978). Suicide assessment: A clinical model. Journal of Family Practice, 6, 1221-1227.

6-076   Goldney, R. D. (1979). Assessment of suicidal intent by a visual analogue scale. Australian and New Zealand Journal of Psychiatry, 13, 153-155.

6-077   Greist, J. H., Gustafson, D. H., Strauss, F. F., Rowse, G. L., Laughren, T. P., & Chiles,

J. A. (1973). A computer interview for suicide-risk prediction. American Journal of Psychiatry, 130, 1327-1332.

6-078   Greist, J. H., Gustafson, D. H., Strauss, F. F., Rowse, G. L., Laughren, T. P., & Chiles, J. A. (1974). Suicide risk prediction: A new approach. Life-Threatening Behavior, 4, 212-223.

This reference, the Greist et al., reference 6-077, preceding, and the two Gustafson et al., references 6-079 and 6-080, below, describe the use of computers in suicide prevention and especially in prediction.

6-079   Gustafson, D. H., Greist, J. H., Strauss, F. F., Erdman, H., & Laughren, T. (1977). A probabilistic system for identifying suicide attempters. Computers and Biomedical Research, 10, 83-89.

6-080   Gustafson, D. H., Tianen, B., & Greist, J. H. (1981). A computer-based system for identifying suicide attemptors. Computers and Biomedical Research, 14, 144-157.

6-081   Hamilton, M. (1960). A rating scale for depression. Journal of Neurology, Neurosurgery and Psychiatry, 23, 56-61.

Like Beck's (e.g., reference 6-043) and Zung's (1965, reference 6-171) scales, this commonly used scale for the assessment of depression is included because of the close relationship of depressive feelings and suicidal behavior.

6-082   Hartley, W., & Hartley, E. (1972, November). New test helps make suicide predictable: Index of Potential Suicide. Science Digest, 72, 25-31.

A discussion of Zung's Index of Potential Suicide (scale appears on pp. 30-31; see reference 6-042.11) and its predictive use for suicide.

* 6-083   Hatton, C. L., & Valente, S. M. (1984). Assessment of suicidal risk. In C. L. Hatton & S. M. Valente (Eds.), Suicide: Assessment and intervention (2nd ed.) (pp. 61-82). Norwalk, CT: Appleton-Century-Crofts.

* 6-084   Hatton, C. L., Valente, S. M., & Rink, A. (1977). Assessment of suicidal risk. In C. L. Hatton, S. M. Valente, & A. Rink (Eds.), Suicide: Assessment and intervention (pp. 39-61). New York: Appleton-Century-Crofts.

6-085   Hertz, M. R. (1965). Detection of suicidal risks
        with the Rorschach. In L. E. Abt & S. L.
        Weissman (Eds.), Acting out: Theoretical and
        clinical aspects (pp. 257-270). New York: Grune
        & Stratton.

6-086   Hipple, J., & Cimbolic, P. (1979). The counselor
        and suicidal crisis: Diagnosis and intervention
        (pp. 30-40). Springfield, IL: Thomas, Chapter
        3, "Diagnosis of the self-destructive
        personality."

6-087   Hoey, H. P. (1974). Lethality of suicidal behavior
        and the MMPI. Psychological Reports, 35, 942.

6-088   Jacobs, D. (1982-83). Evaluation and care of
        suicidal behavior in emergency settings.
        International Journal of Psychiatry in Medicine,
        12(4), 295-310. (Abstract: CPA, 1983, 23,
        No. 773, p. 160)

6-089   Kaplan, R. D., Kottler, D. B., & Frances,
        A. J. (1982). Reliability and rationality in the
        prediction of suicide. Hospital and Community
        Psychiatry, 33, 212-215.

6-090   Kazdin, A. E., French, N. H., Unis, A. S.,
        Esveldt-Dawson, K., & Sherick, R. B. (1983).
        Hopelessness, depression, and suicidal intent
        among psychiatrically disturbed inpatient
        children. Journal of Consulting and Clinical
        Psychology, 51, 504-510. (Abstract: PA, 1983,
        70, No. 12820, p. 1440)

        A hopelessness scale for children was
        developed and administered.

6-091   Kendra, J. M. (1979). Predicting suicide using the
        Rorschach Inkblot Test. Journal of Personality
        Assessment, 43, 452-456.

6-092   Kestenbaum, J. M., & Lynch, D. (1978). Rorschach
        suicide predictors: A crossvalidation study.
        Journal of Clinical Psychology, 34, 754-758.

6-093   Kiev, A. (1974). Prognostic factors in attempted
        suicide. American Journal of Psychiatry, 131,
        987-990.

6-094   Kovacs, M. (1982). Prediction of suicidal
        behaviors. In J. Wilmotte & J. Mendlewicz
        (Eds.), New trends in suicide prevention
        (pp. 61-76). New York: Karger (Bibliotheca
        Psychiatrica No. 162).

6-095   Kreitman, N. (1982). How useful is the prediction

of suicide following parasuicide? In J. Wilmotte
& J. Mendlewicz (Eds.), New trends in suicide
prevention (pp. 77-84). New York: Karger
(Bibliotheca Psychiatrica No. 162).

6-096   Krieger, G. (1970). Biochemical predictors of
        suicide. Diseases of the Nervous System, 31,
        478-482.

6-097   Krieger, G. (1975). Is there a biochemical
        predictor of suicide? Suicide, 5, 228-231.

6-098   Lambley, P., & Silbowitz, M. (1973). Rotter's
        Internal-External scale and prediction of suicide
        contemplators among students. Psychological
        Reports, 33, 585-586.

6-099   Larsen, K. S., Garcia, D., Langenberg, D. R., &
        Leroux, J. A. (1983). The Psychological
        Screening Inventory as a predictor of
        predisposition to suicide among patients at the
        Oregon State Hospital. Journal of Clinical
        Psychology, 39, 100-103. (Abstracts: PA, 1983,
        69, No. 11665, p. 1277; CPA, 1983, 23, No. 1752,
        p. 371)

6-100   Leonard, C. V. (1973). Bender-Gestalt as an
        indicator of suicidal potential. Psychological
        Reports, 32, 665-666.

6-101   Leonard, C. V. (1977). The MMPI as a suicide
        predictor. Journal of Consulting and Clinical
        Psychology, 45, 367-377. (Clopton, J. R. (1978).
        A note on the MMPI as a suicide predictor
        [Rejoinder]. 46, 335-336. Leonard,
        C. V. (1978). Reply to "A note on the MMPI as a
        suicide predictor. 46, 337-338.)

6-102   Lessey, R. A., & Reading, A. (1975). Evaluating
        suicide risk. Primary Care, 2, 57-63.

* 6-103   Lester, D. (1970). Attempts to predict suicidal
        risk using psychological tests. Psychological
        Bulletin, 74, 1-17.

        A review of the literature on the use of
        psychological tests to predict suicidal risk.

6-104   Lester, D. (1972). Why people kill themselves: A
        summary of research findings on suicidal behavior
        (pp. 301-307). Springfield, IL: Thomas, Chapter
        24, "Attempts to predict suicidal risk using
        psychological tests."

        A summary of Lester's (1970, reference 6-103),
        review.

6-105   Lester, D., Kendra, J. M., & Perdue, W. C. (1974).
        Distinguishing murderers from suicides with the
        Rorschach. Perceptual and Motor Skills, 39, 474.

6-106   Lester, D., Kendra, J. M., & Thisted, R. A. (1977).
        Prediction of homicide and suicide: A test in a
        healthy risk-taking group. Perceptual and Motor
        Skills, 44, 222.

6-107   Lester, D., & Perdue, W. C. (1972). Suicide,
        homicide, and color-shading response on the
        Rorschach. Perceptual and Motor Skills, 35, 562.

6-108   Lester, D., & Perdue, W. C. (1974). The detection
        of attempted suicides and murderers using the
        Rorschach. Journal of Psychiatric Research, 10,
        101-103.

6-109   Lettieri, D. J. (1973). Suicide in the aging:
        Empirical prediction of suicidal risk among the
        aging. Journal of Geriatric Psychiatry, 6, 7-42.

6-110   Linehan, M. M., Goodstein, J. L., Nielsen, S. L., &
        Chiles, J. A. (1983). Reasons for staying alive
        when you are thinking of killing yourself: The
        Reasons for Living Inventory. Journal of
        Consulting and Clinical Psychology, 51, 276-286.

6-111   Linehan, M. M., & Nielsen, S. L. (1981).
        Assessment of suicide ideation and parasuicide:
        Hopelessness and social desireability. Journal
        of Consulting and Clinical Psychology, 49,
        773-775.

6-112   Linehan, M. M., & Nielsen, S. L. (1983). Social
        desireability: Its relevance to the measurement
        of hopelessness and suicidal behavior. Journal
        of Consulting and Clinical Psychology, 51,
        141-143. (Abstract: PA, 1983, 69, No. 12939,
        p. 1429)

6-113   Litman, R. E., & Farberow, N. L. (1961). Emergency
        evaluation of self-destructive potentiality. In
        N. L. Farberow & E. S. Shneidman (Eds.), The cry
        for help (pp. 48-59). New York: McGraw-Hill.
        (Reprinted as "Emergency evaluation of suicide
        potential." in E. S. Shneidman, N. L. Farberow,
        & R. E. Litman (Eds.) (1970), The psychology of
        suicide (pp. 259-272). New York: Science
        House.)

6-114   MacKinnon, D. R., & Farberow, N. L. (1976). An
        assessment of the utility of suicide prediction.
        Suicide and Life-Threatening Behavior, 6, 86-91.

6-115   Mareth, T. R. (1977, October). Suicide and the

family physician: Clinical assessment of suicide
risk. Texas Medicine, 73(10), 57-63.

6-116   Margolin, C. (1977, May/June). Evaluating suicide
potential in the emergency department. Journal
of Emergency Nursing, 3, 21-25. (Reprinted as
"Evaluating suicide potential." In M. Miller
(Ed.) (1982), Suicide intervention by nurses
(pp. 46-52). New York: Springer.)

6-117   McIntire, M. S., & Angle, C. R. (1975). Evaluation
of suicide risk in adolescents. Journal of
Family Practice, 2, 339-341.

6-118   Miller, J. (1980). Helping the suicidal client:
Some aspects of assessment and treatment.
Psychotherapy: Theory, Research and Practice,
17, 94-100.

6-119   Mintz, J., O'Brien, C. P., Woody, G., & Beck,
A. T. (1979). Depression in treated narcotic
addicts, ex-addicts, nonaddicts, and suicide
attempters: Validation of a very Brief
Depression Scale. American Journal of Drug and
Alcohol Abuse, 6, 385-396.

6-120   Miskimins, R. W., & Wilson, L. T. (1969). Revised
suicide potential scale. Journal of Consulting
and Clinical Psychology, 33, 258.

6-121   Morgan, H. G. (1979). Death wishes? The
understanding and management of deliberate
self-harm (pp. 52-62, 139-149). New York:
Wiley, Chapter 5, "Assessment of the suicidal
individual," and Chapter 12, "Assessment,"
respectively.

6-122   Motto, J. A. (1977). Estimation of suicide risk by
the use of clinical models. Suicide and
Life-Threatening Behavior, 7, 236-245.

6-123   Motto, J. A., & Heelbron, D. C. (1976).
Development and validation of scales for
estimation of suicide risk. In E. S. Shneidman
(Ed.), Suicidology: Contemporary developments
(pp. 169-199). New York: Grune & Stratton.

6-124   Murphy, G. E. (1983). On suicide prediction and
prevention [Comment]. Archives of General
Psychiatry, 40, 343-344.

6-125   Neuringer, C. (1965). The Rorschach test as a
research device for the identification,
prediction, and understanding of suicidal
ideation and behavior. Journal of Projective
Techniques and Personality Assessment, 29, 71-82.

A review of the empirical literature on the
use of the Rorschach for suicide
identification.

6-126   Neuringer, C. (1972). Suicide attempt and social
isolation on the MAPS [Make-A-Picture Story]
Test. Life-Threatening Behavior, 2, 139-144.

6-127   Neuringer, C. (1974). Suicide and the Rorschach:
A rueful postscript. Journal of Personality
Assessment, 38, 535-539.

* 6-128   Neuringer, C. (Ed.) (1974). Psychological
assessment of suicidal risk. Springfield, IL:
Thomas.

11 chapters consider a variety of assessment
aspects and are listed below.

6-128.01   Neuringer, C. Problems of assessing
suicidal risk. pp. 3-17.

6-128.02   Freeman, D. J., Wilson, K., Thigpen, J.,
& McGee, R. K. Assessing intention to
die in self-injury behavior.
pp. 18-42.

6-128.03   Lettieri, D. J. Research issues in
developing prediction scales.
pp. 43-73.

6-128.04   Neuringer, C. Rorschach Inkblot Test
assessment of suicidal risk.
pp. 74-94.

6-128.05   McEvoy, T. L. Suicide risk via the
Thematic Apperception Test.
pp. 95-117.

6-128.06   Clopton, J. R. Suicidal risk assessment
via the Minnesota Mulitphasic
Personality Inventory (MMPI).
pp. 118-133.

6-128.07   Eisenthal, S. Assessment of suicide risk
using selected tests. pp. 134-149.

6-128.08   Levenson, M. Cognitive correlates of
suicidal risk. pp. 150-163.

6-128.09   Bagley, C., & Greer, S. (1971). Clinical
and social predictors of repeated
attempted suicide: A multivariate
analysis. (Reprinted from British
Journal of Psychiatry, 119, 515-521.)

6-128.10 Litman, R. E. Models for predicting
          suicide risk. pp. 177-185.

6-128.11 Farberow, N. L., & MacKinnon, D.
          Prediction of suicide in
          neuropsychiatric hospital patients.
          pp. 186-224.

6-129   Neuringer, C. (1975, July). Problems in predicting
        adolescent suicidal behavior. Psychiatric
        Opinion, 12(6), 27-31.

6-130   Newson-Smith, J. G. B. (1980). The use of social
        workers as alternatives to psychiatrists in
        assessing parasuicide. In R. D. T. Farmer &
        S. R. Hirsch (Eds.), The suicide syndrome
        (pp. 215-225). London: Croom Helm.

6-131   Obayuwana, A. O., Collins, J. L., Carter, A. L.,
        Rao, M. S., Mathura, C. C., & Wilson,
        S. B. (1982). Hope Index Scale: An instrument
        for the objective assessment of hope. Journal of
        the National Medical Association, 74, 761-765.

6-132a Pallis, D. J., Barraclough, B. M., Levey, A. B.,
        Jenkins, J. S., & Sainsbury, P. (1982).
        Estimating suicide risk among attempted suicides:
        I. The development of new clinical scales.
        British Journal of Psychiatry, 141, 37-44.
        (Abstract: PA, 1983, 69, No. 3693, p. 399)

6-132b Pallis, D. J., Gibbons, J. S., & Pierce,
        D. W. (1984). Estimating suicide risk among
        attempted suicides: II. Efficiency of predictive
        scales after the attempt. British Journal of
        Psychiatry, 144, 139-148.

6-133   Pallis, D. J., & Sainsbury, P. (1976). The value
        of assessing intent in attempted suicide.
        Psychological Medicine, 6, 487-492.

6-134   Patterson, W. M., Dohn, H. H., Bird, J., &
        Patterson, G. A. (1983). Evaluation of suicidal
        patients: The SAD PERSONS scale.
        Psychosomatics, 24, 343-352. (Abstract: PA,
        1984, 71, No. 217, p. 22)

        An easily learned scale based on 10 major risk
        factors is discussed, presented, and tested.

6-135   Pettifor, J., Perry, D., Plowman, B., & Pitcher,
        S. (1983). Risk factors predicting childhood and
        adolescent suicides. Journal of Child Care, 1,
        17-49. (Abstract: PA, 1983, 70, No. 8220,
        p. 921)

6-136   Pierce, D. W. (1977). Suicidal intent in
        self-injury. British Journal of Psychiatry, 130,
        377-385.

        A modified, objective form of Beck's suicide
        intent scale (reference 6-042.01) was
        developed and administered.

6-137   Pierce, D. W. (1981). The predictive validity of a
        suicide intent scale: A five year follow-up.
        British Journal of Psychiatry, 139, 391-396.

        Those who completed the Intent Score Scale, a
        modified version of Beck's suicide intent
        scale, were followed up. The scale is
        presented in an appendix of the paper.

6-138   Piotrowski, Z. A. (1968). Psychological test
        prediction of suicide. In H. L. P. Resnik (Ed.),
        Suicidal behaviors: Diagnosis and management
        (pp. 198-208). Boston: Little Brown.

6-139   Piotrowski, Z. A. (1970). Test differentiation
        between effected and attempted suicides. In
        K. Wolff (Ed.), Patterns of self-destruction:
        Depression and suicide (pp. 67-81). Springfield,
        IL: Thomas.

6-140   Poeldinger, W. J., Gehring, A., & Blaser,
        P. (1973). Suicide risk and MMPI scores,
        especially as related to anxiety and depression.
        Life-Threatening Behavior, 3, 147-154.

6-141   Pokorny, A. D. (1983). Prediction of suicide in
        psychiatric patients. Archives of General
        Psychiatry, 40, 249-257.

6-142   Resnick, J. H., & Kendra, J. M. (1973). Predictive
        value of the "Scale for Assessing Suicide Risk"
        (SASR) with hospitalized psychiatric patients.
        Journal of Clinical Psychology, 29, 187-190.

6-143   Rierdan, J., Lang, E., & Eddy, S. (1978). Suicide
        and transparency responses on the Rorschach: A
        replication. Journal of Consulting and Clinical
        Psychology, 46, 1162-1163.

        A replication of Blatt & Ritzler (1974,
        reference 6-047).

6-144   Robins, E. (1981). The final months: A study of
        the lives of 134 persons who committed suicide
        (pp. 407-421). New York: Oxford University
        Press, Chapter 8, "How predictable are predictors
        of suicide?"

6-145   Sendbuehler, J. M., Kincel, R. L., Nemeth, G., &
        Oertel, J. (1979). Dimensions of seriousness in
        attempted suicide: Significance of the MF scale
        in suicidal MMPI profiles. Psychological
        Reports, 44, 343-361.

6-146   Shaffer, J. W., Perlin, S., Schmidt, C. W., Jr., &
        Stephens, J. H. (1974). The prediction of
        suicide in schizophrenia. Journal of Nervous and
        Mental Disease, 159, 349-355.

6-147   Siani, R., Garzotto, N., Tansella, C. Z., &
        Tansella, M. (1979). Predictive scales for
        parasuicide repetition: Further results. Acta
        Psychiatrica Scandinavica, 59, 17-23.

6-148   Smith, K. (1981). Using a battery of tests to
        predict suicide in a long-term hospital: A
        quantitative analysis. Journal of Clinical
        Psychology, 37, 555-563. (Abstract: PA, 1983,
        70, No. 2468, p. 274)

        The Wechsler-Bellvue Intelligence Scales, the
        Rorschach, TAT, and the Word-Association Test
        were administered.

6-149   Stallone, F., Dunner, D. L., Ahern, J., & Fieve,
        R. R. (1980). Statistical predictors of suicide
        in depressives. Comprehensive Psychiatry, 21,
        381-387.

6-150   Tabachnick, N. D., & Farberow, N. L. (1961). The
        assessment of self-destructive potentiality. In
        N. L. Farberow & E. S. Shneidman (Eds.), The cry
        for help (pp. 60-77). New York: McGraw-Hill.

6-151   Thomas, C. B. (1974). Suicide among us:
        II. Habits of nervous tension as potential
        predictors. John Hopkins Medical Journal, 129,
        190-201.

6-152   Thomas, C. B., & Greenstreet, R. L. (1973).
        Psychobiological characteristics in youth as
        predictors of five disease states: Suicide,
        mental illness, hypertension, coronary heart
        disease, and tumor. John Hopkins Medical
        Journal, 132, 16-43.

6-153   Thomas, C. B., Ross, D. C., Brown, B. S., &
        Duszynski, K. R. (1973). A prospective study of
        the Rorschachs of suicides: The predictive
        potential of pathological content. John Hopkins
        Medical Journal, 132, 334-360.

6-154   Tuckman, J., & Youngman, W. F. (1968). Assessment
        of suicide risk in attempted suicides. In

H. L. P. Resnik (Ed.), Suicidal behaviors:
Diagnosis and management (pp. 190-197). Boston:
Little Brown.

6-155   Tuckman, J., & Youngman, W. F. (1968). A scale for
assessing suicide risk of attempted suicides.
Journal of Clinical Psychology, 24, 17-19.

6-156   Van de Loo, K. J., & Diekstra, R. W. (1970). The
construction of a questionnaire for the
prediction of subsequent suicide attempts.
Nederlands Tijdschrift voor de Psychologie en
Haar Grensgebieden, 25, 95-100.

6-157   Vanderplas, J. M., & Vanderplas, J. H. (1979).
Multiple- vs. single-index predictors of
dangerousness, suicide, and other rare behaviors.
Psychological Reports, 45, 343-349.

6-158   Van Praag, H. M. (1982). Biochemical and
psychopathological predictors of suicidality. In
J. Wilmotte & J. Mendlewicz (Eds.), New trends in
suicide prevention (pp. 42-60). New York:
Karger (Bibliotheca Psychiatrica No. 162).

6-159   Victoroff, V. M. (1983). The suicidal patient:
Recognition, intervention, management
(pp. 63-77). Oradell, NJ: Medical Economics
Books, Chapter 7, "Predictors of suicidal risk."

6-160   Waters, B. G., Sendbuehler, J. M., Kincel, R. L.,
Boodoosingh, C. A., & Marchenko, I. (1982). The
use of the MMPI for the differentiation of
suicidal and non-suicidal depressions. Canadian
Journal of Psychiatry, 27, 663-667. (Abstract:
PA, 1983, 70, No. 3585, pp. 406-407)

6-161   Watson, C. G., Klett, W. G., Walters, C., &
Laughlin, P. R. (1983). Identification of
suicidal episodes with the MMPI. Psychological
Reports, 53, 919-922.

6-162   Watson, C. G., Klett, W. G., Walters, C., & Vassar,
P. (1984). Suicide and the MMPI: A
cross-validation of predictors. Journal of
Clinical Psychology, 40, 115-119.

6-163   Weiss, A. A., & Dana, Y. (1977). Personality types
of suicidal persons as reflected in Rorschach's
test. Israel Annals of Psychiatry and Related
Disciplines, 15, 389-396.

6-164   Wenz, F. V. (1978-79). Suicide-related experiences
among blacks: An empirical test of a suicide
potential scale. Omega, 9, 183-191. (Abstract:
PA, 1980, 63, No. 3489, p. 400)

A 3 item suicide potential scale is developed
and administered.

6-165   Wetzel, R. D. (1976). Semantic differential
        ratings of concepts and suicide risk. Journal of
        Clinical Psychology, 32, 4-13.

6-166   Wetzel, R. D. (1977). Factor structures of Beck's
        suicide intent scales. Psychological Reports,
        40, 295-302.

6-167   Woolersheim, J. P. (1974). The assessment of
        suicide potential via interview methods.
        Psychotherapy: Theory, Research and Practice,
        11, 222-225.

6-168   Worden, J. W. (1976). Lethality factors and the
        suicide attempt. In E. S. Shneidman (Ed.),
        Suicidology: Contemporary developments
        (pp. 139-162). New York: Grune & Stratton.

6-169   Yufit, R. I., & Benzies, B. (1973). Assessing
        suicide potential by time perspective.
        Life-Threatening Behavior, 3, 270-282.

6-170   Yufit, R. I., Benzies, B., Fonte, M. E., & Fawcett,
        J. A. (1970). Suicide potential and time
        perspective. Archives of General Psychiatry, 23,
        158-163.

6-171   Zung, W. W. K. (1965). A self-rating depression
        scale. Archives of General Psychiatry, 12,
        63-70.

        The strong relationship between depression and
        depressive symptomatology and suicide prompt
        the inclusion of this much-utilized scale.

6-172   Zung, W. W. K. (1972). The Depression Status
        Inventory: An adjunct to the self-rating
        depression scale. Journal of Clinical
        Psychology, 28, 539-543.

See also Frederick (1968, reference 9-174). See also
Section 5.11a, personality and suicide.

6.4 Suicidal Intervention, Management & Medical Treatment

6-173   Barraclough, B. (1972). A medical approach to
        suicide prevention. Social Science and Medicine,
        6, 661-667.

* 6-174 Bassuk, E. L., Schoonover, S. C., & Gill,
        A. D. (Eds.) (1982). Lifelines: Clinical
        perspectives on suicide. New York: Plenum

Press.

The following 5 chapters are appropriate here.

6-174.01 Schoonover, S. C. Crisis therapies.
          pp. 49-57.

6-174.02 Schoonover, S. C. Pharmacotherapy of the
          suicidal patient. pp. 59-68.

6-174.03 Bassuk, E. L. Care of the suicidal
          patient in the emergency setting.
          pp. 103-114.

6-174.04 Silverman, D. Care, containment, and
          countertransference: Managing the
          suicidal patient in medical settings.
          pp. 115-136.

6-174.05 Schoonover, S. C. Intensive care for
          suicidal patients. pp. 137-153.

6-175   Benensohn, H., & Resnik, H. L. P. (1973).
        Guidelines for "suicide-proofing" a psychiatric
        unit. American Journal of Psychotherapy, 27,
        204-212.

6-176   Bocker, F. (1981). Treatment and follow-up care
        after suicide attempts. Crisis, 2, 37-40.

6-177   Boman, B., Streimer, G., & Perkins, M. (1981).
        Crisis intervention and pharmacotherapy. Crisis,
        2, 41-49.

6-178   Farberow, N. L. (1972). Prevention and therapy in
        crisis. In J. Waldenstrom, T. Larsson, &
        N. Ljungstedt (Eds.), Suicide and attempted
        suicide (pp. 303-316). Stockholm: Nordiska
        Bokhandlens Forlag.

6-179   Farberow, N. L. (1981). Suicide prevention in the
        hospital. Hospital and Community Psychiatry, 32,
        99-104.

6-180   Frederick, C. J. (1977). Crisis intervention and
        emergency mental health. In W. R. Johnson (Ed.),
        Health in action (pp. 376-411; esp. pp. 387-398,
        "The crisis of suicide"). New York: Holt,
        Rinehart & Winston.

6-181   Frederick, C. J. (1981). Suicide prevention and
        crisis intervention in mental health emergencies.
        In C. E. Walker (Ed.), Clinical practice of
        psychology: A guide for mental health
        professionals (pp. 189-213). New York: Pergamon
        Press.

6-182   Frederick, C. J., & Resnik, H. L. P. (1970).
        Interventions with suicidal patients. Journal of
        Contemporary Psychotherapy, 2(2), 103-109.

6-183   Goldney, R. D., & Burvill, P. W. (1980). Trends in
        suicidal behaviour and its management.
        Australian & New Zealand Journal of Psychiatry,
        14, 1-15.

6-184   Grollman, E. A. (1971). Suicide: Prevention,
        intervention, postvention (pp. 85-106). Boston:
        Beacon Press, Chapter 6, "Helping the potential
        suicide: Intervention."

* 6-185 Hatton, C. L., Valente, S. M., & Rink, A. (1977).
         Intervention. In C. L. Hatton, S. M. Valente, &
         A. Rink (Eds.), Suicide: Assessment and
         intervention (pp. 62-112). New York:
         Appleton-Century-Crofts.

         The process of intervention is discussed,
         illustrative interventions, and a description
         of the services offered by various services
         are presented. The second edition version of
         this well done chapter is Valente & Hatton,
         reference 6-218 below.

6-186   Hawton, K. (1980). Domiciliary and out-patient
        treatment following deliberate self-poisoning.
        In R. D. T. Farmer & S. R. Hirsch (Eds.), The
        suicide syndrome (pp. 246-258). London: Croom
        Helm.

6-187   Hillard, J. R. (1983). Emergency management of the
        suicidal patient. In J. I. Walker (Ed.),
        Psychiatric emergencies: Intervention and
        resolution (pp. 101-123). Philadelphia:
        Lippincott.

6-188   Hipple, J., & Cimbolic, P. (1979). The counselor
        and suicidal crisis: Diagnosis and intervention.
        Springfield, IL: Thomas.

        Several chapters are appropriate here:
        Chapter 4, "Counseling with the suicidal
        client" (pp. 41-64); Chapter 5, "Contracts to
        stay alive and get well" (pp. 65-73); Chapter
        6, "The life line" (pp. 74-81); and Chapter
        10, "Medical and chemotherapeutic
        interventions" (pp. 101-114).

* 6-189 Hirsch, S. R., Walsh, C., & Draper, R. (1982).
         Parasuicide: A review of treatment
         interventions. Journal of Affective Disorders,
         4, 299-311. (Abstract: PA, 1983, 70, No. 6072,
         p. 682)

6-190   Jacobs, D. (1982-83). Evaluation and care of
        suicidal behavior in emergency settings.
        International Journal of Psychiatry in Medicine,
        12, 295-310. (Abstract: PA, 1983, 70,
        No. 10909, p. 1220)

6-191   Kiev, A. (1974). The role of chemotherapy in
        managing potentially suicidal patients. Diseases
        of the Nervous System, 35, 108-111.

6-192   Kiev, A. (1976). Crisis intervention and suicide
        prevention. In E. S. Shneidman (Ed.),
        Suicidology: Contemporary developments
        (pp. 454-478). New York: Grune & Stratton.

6-193   Kiev, A. (1981). The management of suicidal
        patients. Current Psychiatric Therapies, 20,
        183-187.

6-194   Kirkstein, L., Weissman, M. M., & Prusoff,
        B. (1975). Utilization review and suicide
        attempts: Exploring discrepancies between
        experts' criteria and clinical practice. Journal
        of Nervous and Mental Disease, 160, 49-56.

6-195   Kreitman, N. (1979). Reflections on the management
        of parasuicide. British Journal of Psychiatry,
        135, 275-277.

6-196   Krieger, G. (1976). The management and
        mismanagement of a suicidal patient. Hospital
        and Community Psychiatry, 27, 411-413.

6-197   Litman, R. E. (1970). Management of suicidal
        patients in medical practice. In
        E. S. Shneidman, N. L. Farberow, & R. E. Litman
        (Eds.), The psychology of suicide (pp. 449-459).
        New York: Science House. (Reprinted from
        California Medicine, 1966, 104, 168-174.)

6-198   Litman, R. E., & Farberow, N. L. (1970). Suicide
        prevention in hospitals. In E. S. Shneidman,
        N. L. Farberow, & R. E. Litman (Eds.), The
        psychology of suicide (pp. 461-473). New York:
        Science House. (Reprinted from Zeitschrift fur
        Preventiv Medizin, 1965, 10, 488-498.)

6-199   Lum, D. (1974). Responding to suicidal crisis:
        For church and community (pp. 83-96). Grand
        Rapids, MI: Eerdmans, Chapter 5, "Understanding
        suicidal crisis intervention."

6-200   Miller, M. (1982). Suicide intervention by nurses.
        New York: Springer.

        While many of the articles reprinted here are

appropriate in this section, the following 3
are especially so (see also reference 10-038).

6-200.01   Horoshak, I. (1977, September). How to
handle high-risk patients. pp. 63-68.
(Reprinted from "How to spot and handle
high-risk patients," RN, 40, 59-63.)

6-200.02   Diran, M. O. (1976). How to intervene in
a suicidal episode. pp. 68-71.
(Reprinted from "You can prevent
suicide," Nursing76, 6, 60-64.)

6-200.03   Kalkman, M. (1967). Responding to a
suicidal patient. pp. 71-80.
(Reprinted from "The problem of
suicide," in M. Kalkman, Psychiatric
nursing (3rd ed.) (pp. 193-195). New
York: McGraw-Hill.)

6-201   Montgomery, S. A., & Montgomery, D. (1982).
Pharmacological prevention of suicidal behavior.
Journal of Affective Disorders, 4, 291-298.
(Abstract: PA, 1983, 70, No. 6270, p. 704)

6-202   Montgomery, S. A., & Montgomery, D. B. (1982).
Drug treatment of suicidal behaviours. Advances
in Biochemical Psychopharmacology, 32, 347-355.

6-203   Monto, A., Ross, C., Heymann, C., & Rosenthal,
H. (1975). A survey of hospital services for
suicidal persons. Suicide, 5, 169-176.

6-204   Morgan, H. G. (1979). Death wishes? The
understanding and management of deliberate
self-harm. New York: Wiley.

Chapters dealing with "Management of suicide
risk" (pp. 63-74) and "Management and
prevention of non-fatal deliberate self-harm"
(pp. 150-158) are included in this book.

6-205   Morgan, H. G. (1981). Management of suicidal
behaviour. British Journal of Psychiatry, 138,
259-260.

6-206   Paykel, E. S. (1982). Psychopharmacology of
suicide. Journal of Affective Disorders, 4,
271-273.

6-207   Paykel, E. S., Hallowell, C., Dressler, D. M.,
Shapiro, D. L., & Weissman, M. M. (1974).
Treatment of suicide attempters: A descriptive
study. Archives of General Psychiatry, 31,
487-491.

6-208 Poldinger, W. J. (1972). Drug therapy in
       depressive states with special reference to
       suicide prevention. In J. Waldenstrom,
       T. Larsson, & N. Ljungstedt (Eds.), Suicide and
       attempted suicide (pp. 263-278). Stockholm:
       Nordiska Bokhandlens Forlag.

6-209 Resnik, H. L. P. (Ed.) (1968). Suicidal behaviors:
       Diagnosis and management. Boston: Little Brown.

       Among the included chapters are the following
       which are appropriate here.

       6-209.01 Harris, J. R., & Myers, J. M. Hospital
                 management of the suicidal patient.
                 pp. 297-305.

       6-209.02 Kalinowsky, L. B. Somatotherapy of
                 suicidal patients. pp. 306-312.

       6-209.03 Kline, N. S. Pharmacotherapy of the
                 depressed and suicidal patient.
                 pp. 313-327.

6-210 Ruben, H. L. (1979, January 19). Managing suicidal
       behavior. Journal of the American Medical
       Association, 241, 282-284.

6-211 Singh, A. N. (1974). Use of chemotherapy as
       anti-suicidal prophylaxis. International Journal
       of Clinical Pharmacology, 9, 32-36.

6-212 Sletten, I. W., & Barton, J. L. (1979). Suicidal
       patients in the emergency room: A guide for
       evaluation and disposition. Hospital and
       Community Psychiatry, 30, 407-411.

6-213 Snyder, J. A. (1971, Fall). The use of gatekeepers
       in crisis management. Bulletin of Suicidology,
       No. 8, pp. 39-44.

6-214 Sonneck, G. (1982). [Crisis intervention and
       suicide prevention.] Psychiatria Clinica,
       15(1/2), 5-96. (In German)

6-215 Spero, M. H. (1980-81). Bracketing and
       stabilization: Interventative steps in
       counseling the suicidal client. Omega, 11,
       325-339.

6-216 Stone, M. H. (1980). The suicidal patient: Points
       concerning diagnosis and intensive treatment.
       Psychiatric Quarterly, 52, 52-70.

6-217 Tabachnick, N. (1970, June). The crisis treatment
       of suicide. California Medicine, 112(6), 1-8.

* 6-218   Valente, S. M., & Hatton, C. L. (1984).
          Intervention. In C. L. Hatton & S. M. Valente
          (Eds.), Suicide: Assessment and intervention
          (2nd ed.) (pp. 83-148). Norwalk, CT:
          Appleton-Century-Crofts.

  6-219   Victoroff, V. M. (1983). The suicidal patient:
          Recognition, intervention, management. Oradell,
          NJ: Medical Economics Books.

          Part 3 of this book, "Management of the
          suicidal patient" is particularly relevant
          here (pp. 79-145).

  6-220   Waltzer, H. (1979). The medical practitioner. In
          L. D. Hankoff & B. Einsidler (Eds.), Suicide:
          Theory and clinical aspects (pp. 353-361).
          Littleton, MA: PSG Publishing.

  6-221   Wekstein, L. (1979). Handbook of suicidology:
          Principles, problems and practice (pp. 94-127;
          187-213). New York: Brunner/Mazel, Chapters 6,
          "Intervention in suicidology," and 9,
          "Management," respectively.

6.5 How & Where to Find Help/Community Resources

  6-222   Coleman, W. L. (1979). Understanding suicide
          (pp. 109-118). Elgin, IL: David C. Cook,
          Chapter 13, "How can I get help for him?"

  6-223   Giffin, M., & Felsenthal, C. (1983). A cry for
          help (pp. 264-285). Garden City, NY: Doubleday,
          Chapter 12, "Finding help in your community."

  6-224   Lester, G., & Lester, D. (1971). Suicide: The
          gamble with death (pp. 159-166). Englewood
          Cliffs, NJ: Prentice-Hall, Chapter 20,
          "Resources for preventing suicide."

See also the citation for the American Association of
Suicidology, reference 1-001, which maintains a current
listing of Suicide Prevention Centers across the country.
See also the telephone yellow pages under "Suicide
Prevention," "Crisis Intervention," and "Mental Health."
See also Shneidman et al. (1961, reference 7-062).

6.6 Therapy and the Suicidal

  6-225   Alanen, Y. O., Rinne, R., & Paukkonen, P. (1981).
          On family dynamics and family therapy in suicidal
          attempts. Crisis, 2, 20-26.

  6-226   Alfaro, R. R. (1970, Spring). A group therapy
          approach to suicide prevention. Bulletin of
          Suicidology, No. 6, pp. 56-59.

6-227   Asimos, C. T., & Rosen, D. H. (1978). Group
        treatment of suicidal and depressed persons:
        Indications for an open-ended group therapy
        program. Bulletin of the Menninger Clinic, 42,
        515-519.

* 6-228   Bassuk, E. L., Schoonover, S. C., & Gill,
        A. D. (1982). Lifelines: Clinical perspectives
        on suicide. New York: Plenum Press.

            Many articles on therapeutic issues are
            included, with the 4 below most appropriate
            here.

        6-228.01 Gill, A. D. Outpatient therapies for
                  suicidal patients. pp. 71-82.

        6-228.02 Kahn, A. The moment of truth:
                  Psychotherapy with the suicidal person.
                  pp. 83-92.

        6-228.03 Kahn, A. The stress of therapy [on the
                  therapist]. pp. 93-100.

        6-228.04 Fuchs, R. Suicidal patients and the
                  therapist-in-training. pp. 181-192.

6-229   Beck, A. T., Rush, A. J., Shaw, B. F., & Emery,
        G. (1979). Cognitive therapy of depression
        (pp. 209-224; 225-243). New York: Guilford
        Press, Chapter 10, "Specific techniques for the
        suicidal patient," Chapter 11, "Interview with a
        depressed suicidal patient."

6-230   Billings, J. H., Rosen, D. H., Asimos, C., & Motto,
        J. A. (1974). Observations on long-term group
        therapy with suicidal and depressed persons.
        Life-Threatening Behavior, 4, 160-170.

6-231   Birtchnell, J. (1975). The special place of
        psychotherapy in the treatment of attempted
        suicide, and the special type of psychotherapy
        required. Observations derived from the
        experience of treating by psychotherapy. A
        research series of young married suicide
        attempters. Psychotherapy & Psychosomatics, 25,
        3-6.

6-232   Birtchnell, J. (1983). Psychotherapeutic
        considerations in the management of the suicidal
        patient. American Journal of Psychotherapy, 37,
        24-36. (Abstract: PA, 1983, 70, No. 1503,
        p. 174)

6-233   Clayton, P. J., & Barrett, J. E. (Eds.) (1983).
        Treatment of depression: Old controversies and

new approaches. New York: Raven Press.

> This recent source is included because of the
> close relationship of suicide and depression
> and the similarity that often results in their
> treatment. Included in this edited book are
> articles on biological predictors of treatment
> response, somatic and drug therapies, and
> psychotherapies.

6-234   Clum, G. A., Patsiokas, A. T., & Luscomb,
        R. L. (1979). Empirically based comprehensive
        treatment programs for parasuicide. Journal of
        Consulting and Clinical Psychology, 47, 937-945.

6-235   Comstock, B. S., & McDermott, M. (1975). Group
        therapy for patients who attempt suicide.
        International Journal of Group Psychotherapy, 25,
        44-49.

6-236   de Martis, D. (1973). Problems of psychotherapy of
        attempted suicide in teen-agers. Psihotherapija,
        2, 111-129.

6-237   Elliott, T. N., Smith, R. D., & Wildman, R. W.,
        II. (1972). Suicide and systematic
        desensitization: A case study. Journal of
        Clinical Psychology, 28, 420-423.

6-238   Farberow, N. L. (1957). The suicidal crisis in
        psychotherapy. In E. S. Shneidman &
        N. L. Farberow (Eds.), Clues to suicide
        (pp. 119-130). New York: McGraw-Hill.
        (Reprinted in E. S. Shneidman, N. L. Farberow, &
        R. E. Litman (Eds.) (1970), The psychology of
        suicide (pp. 415-428). New York: Science
        House.)

6-239a Farberow, N. L. (1972). Vital process in suicide
        prevention: Group psychotherapy as a community
        of concern. Life-Threatening Behavior, 2,
        239-251.

6-239b Farberow, N. L. (1976). Group psychotherapy for
        self-destructive persons. In H. J. Parad,
        H. L. P. Resnik, & L. G. Parad (Eds.), Emergency
        and disaster management: A mental health
        sourcebook (pp. 169-185). Bowie, MD: Charles
        Press.

* 6-240 Fawcett, J., Comstock, E. G., Hendin, H.,
        Jagodinski, J. P., Litman, R. E., May, M., Mintz,
        R. S., & Motto, J. A. (1973). Priorities for
        improved treatment approaches. In H. L. P.
        Resnik & B. C. Hathorne (Eds.), Suicide
        prevention in the 70s (pp. 91-97). Washington,

D.C.:   USGPO, DHEW Publication No. (HSM) 72-9054.

6-241 Frederick, C. J., & Farberow, N. L. (1970).   Group
       psychotherapy with suicidal persons: A
       comparison with standard group methods.
       International Journal of Social Psychiatry, 16,
       103-111.

6-242 Frey, D. H., Motto, J. A., & Ritholz, M. D. (1983).
       Group therapy for persons at risk for suicide:
       An evaluation using the intensive design.
       Psychotherapy: Theory, Research and Practice,
       20, 281-293.

6-243 Getz, W. L., Allen, D. B., Myers, R. K., & Lindner,
       K. C. (1983).   Brief counseling with suicidal
       persons. Lexington, MA: Lexington Books.

6-244 Glaser, K. (1978).   The treatment of depressed and
       suicidal adolescents. American Journal of
       Psychotherapy, 32, 252-269. (Abstracts: ACP,
       1979, 19, No. 288, p. 64; PA, 1979, 62,
       No. 3999, p. 409)

6-245 Hackel, J., & Asimos, C. T. (1980)/(1981).
       Resistances encountered in starting a group
       therapy program for suicide attempters in varied
       administrative settings. Suicide and
       Life-Threatening Behavior, 10, 100-105, & 11,
       93-98.

           The same article appears in both volumes of
           this journal.

6-246 Halperin, D. A. (1979).   Psychodynamic strategies
       with outpatients. In L. D. Hankoff &
       B. Einsidler (Eds.), Suicide: Theory and
       clinical aspects (pp. 363-372). Littleton, MA:
       PSG Publishing.

6-247 Hendin, H. (1981).   Psychotherapy and suicide.
       American Journal of Psychotherapy, 35, 469-480.
       (Abstract: PA, 1982, 67, No. 10299, p. 1109)
       (Reprinted in H. Hendin (1982). Suicide in
       America (pp. 160-174). New York: Norton.)

6-248 Hipple, J. (1982).   Group treatment of suicidal
       clients. Journal for Specialists in Group Work,
       7, 245-250. (Abstract: PA, 1983, 69, No. 13193,
       p. 1458)

6-249 Hirsch, S. R., Walsh, C., & Draper, R. (1983).   The
       concept and efficacy of the treatment of
       parasuicide. British Journal of Clinical
       Pharmacology, 15(Supplement 2), 189S-194S.

6-250   Kiev, A. (1975). Psychotherapeutic strategies in
        the management of depressed and suicidal
        patients. American Journal of Psychotherapy, 29,
        345-354.

6-251   Kovacs, M., Beck, A. T., & Weissman, A. (1975).
        The use of suicidal motives in the psychotherapy
        of attempted suicides. American Journal of
        Psychotherapy, 29, 363-368.

6-252   Krieger, G. (1978). Common errors in the treatment
        of suicidal patients. Journal of Clinical
        Psychiatry, 39, 649-651. (Abstract: PA, 1980,
        63, No. 12142, p. 1352)

6-253   Leonard, C. V. (1975, March-April). Treating the
        suicidal patient: A communication approach.
        Journal of Psychiatric Nursing, 13(2), 19-22.

6-254   Lesse, S. (1975). The range of therapies in the
        treatment of severely depressed suicidal
        patients. American Journal of Psychotherapy, 29,
        308-326.

6-255   Liberman, R. P., & Eckman, T. (1981). Behavior
        therapy vs. insight-oriented therapy for repeated
        suicide attempters. Archives of General
        Psychiatry, 38, 1126-1130.

6-256   Litman, R. E. (1957). Some aspects of the
        treatment of the potentially suicidal patient.
        In E. S. Shneidman & N. L. Farberow (Eds.), Clues
        to suicide (pp. 111-118). New York:
        McGraw-Hill. (Reprinted as "Treatment of the
        potentially suicidal patient," in
        E. S. Shneidman, N. L. Farberow, & R. E. Litman
        (Eds.) (1970), The psychology of suicide
        (pp. 405-413). New York: Science House.)

6-257   Maltsberger, J. T., & Buie, D. H. (1974).
        Countertransference hate [on the part of the
        therapist] in the treatment of suicidal patients.
        Archives of General Psychiatry, 30, 625-633.

6-258   Mayer, D. Y. (1971). A psychotherapeutic approach
        to the suicidal patient. British Journal of
        Psychiatry, 119, 629-633.

6-259   Miller, D. (1981). Adolescent suicide: Etiology
        and treatment. Adolescent Psychiatry, 9,
        327-342.

6-260   Mintz, R. S. (1971). Basic considerations in the
        psychotherapy of the depressed suicidal patient.
        American Journal of Psychotherapy, 25, 56-73.

6-261   Morris, J., Selkin, J., & Yost, J. F. (1970). A
        home treatment program by an indigenous
        professional, the visiting nurse, with a group of
        adolescents who have attempted suicide. American
        Journal of Orthopsychiatry, 40, 340-342.
        (Abstract: ACP, 1971, 11, No. 287, p. 85)

6-262   Moss, L. M., & Hamilton, D. M. (1957).
        Psychotherapy of the suicidal patient (with
        discussion by O. S. English). In E. S. Shneidman
        & N. L. Farberow (Eds.), Clues to suicide
        (pp. 99-110). New York: McGraw-Hill.
        (Reprinted from American Journal of Psychiatry,
        1956, 112, 814-820.)

6-263   Motto, J. A. (1975, July). Treatment and
        management of suicidal adolescents. Psychiatric
        Opinion, 12(6), 14-20.

6-264   Nidiffer, F. D. (1978). Combining cognitive and
        behavioral approaches to suicidal depression: A
        42-month follow-up. Psychological Reports, 47,
        539-542.

6-265   Novak, W. J. (1976). Suicidal preoccupation and
        psychoanalytic technique. Comprehensive
        Psychiatry, 17, 81-97.

6-266   Olin, H. S. (1976). Psychotherapy of the
        chronically suicidal patient. American Journal
        of Psychotherapy, 30, 570-575.

6-267   Pfeffer, C. R. (1978). Psychiatric hospital
        treatment of suicidal children. Suicide and
        Life-Threatening Behavior, 8, 150-160.

6-268   Pfeffer, C. R. (1982). Interventions for suicidal
        children and their parents. Suicide and
        Life-Threatening Behavior, 12, 240-248.
        (Abstract: PA, 1983, 70, No. 13219, p. 1486)

6-269   Radwan, R., & Davidson, S. (1977). Short-term
        treatment in a general hospital following a
        suicide attempt. Hospital and Community
        Psychiatry, 28, 537-538.

6-270   Resnik, H. L. P. (Ed.) (1968). Suicidal behaviors:
        Diagnosis and management. Boston: Little Brown.

        This excellent book contains many articles on
        treatment, including especially the 3 listed
        below.

        6-270.01 Mintz, R. S. Psychotherapy of the
                  suicidal patient. pp. 271-296.

6-270.02   Farberow, N. L.   Group psychotherapy with
           suicidal persons. pp. 328-340.

6-270.03   Speck, R. V. Family therapy of the
           suicidal patient. pp. 341-347.

6-271   Resnik, H. L. P., Davison, W. T., Schuyler, D., &
        Christopher, P. (1973). Videotape confrontation
        after attempted suicide. American Journal of
        Psychiatry, 130, 460-463.

6-272   Richman, J. (1978). Symbiosis, empathy, suicidal
        behavior, and the family. Suicide and
        Life-Threatening Behavior, 8, 139-149.

6-273   Richman, J. (1979). The family therapy of
        attempted suicide. Family Process, 18, 131-142.

6-274   Richman, J. (1981). Suicide and the family:
        Affective disturbances and their implications for
        understanding, diagnosis, and treatment. In
        M. R. Lansky (Ed.), Family therapy and major
        psychopathology (pp. 145-160). New York: Grune
        & Stratton.

6-275   Rosen, H. (1981). Therapies of depression.
        Current Psychiatric Therapies, 20, 301-311.

           An overview of psychotherapies, group
           therapies, pharmacotherapy, and ECT as used
           for depression.

6-276   Rush, A. J., & Beck, A. T. (1978). Cognitive
        therapy of depression and suicide. American
        Journal of Psychotherapy, 32, 201-219.

6-277   Schmidt, C. (1976, November-December). Treating
        the suicidal patient: A psychologist's view.
        Part II. Respiratory Therapy, 6(6), 70-73.

6-278a Schwartz, D. A., Flinn, D. E., & Slawson,
        P. F. (1974). Treatment of the suicidal
        character. American Journal of Psychotherapy,
        28, 194-207.

6-278b Selkin, J., & Braucht, A. N. (1976). Home
        treatment of suicidal persons. In H. J. Parad,
        H. L. P. Resnik, & L. G. Parad (Eds.), Emergency
        and disaster management: A mental health
        sourcebook (pp. 45-53). Bowie, MD: Charles
        Press.

6-279   Shneidman, E. S. (1971). The role of psychotherapy
        in the treatment of suicidal persons: On the
        deromanticization of death. American Journal of
        Psychotherapy, 25, 4-17.

6-280   Shneidman, E. S. (1980). Psychotherapy with
        suicidal patients. In T. B. Karasu & L. Bellak
        (Eds.), Specialized techniques in individual
        psychotherapy (pp. 305-313). New York:
        Brunner/Mazel. (Reprinted in Suicide and
        Life-Threatening Behavior, 1981, 11(4), 341-348.)

6-281   Toolan, J. M. (1978). Therapy of depressed and
        suicidal children. American Journal of
        Psychotherapy, 32, 243-251.

6-282   Wolff, K. (1971, July). The treatment of the
        depressed and suicidal geriatric patient.
        Geriatrics, 26, 65-69.

6.7 Suicide Prevention Centers (SPCs)/Telephone Intervention

6-283   Aalberg, V. (1977). SOS-Service, the suicide
        prevention center in Helsinki. In K. Achte &
        J. Lonnqvist (Eds.), Suicide research:
        Proceedings of the seminars of suicide research
        by Yrjo Jahnsson Foundation, 1974-1977
        (pp. 67-68). Helsinki: Psychiatria Fennica
        (Psychiatria Fennica Supplementum 1976).

6-284   Bartholomew, A. A., & Olijnyk, E. (1972, October
        21). An analysis of suicide calls received by a
        personal emergency telephone advisory service
        after ten years of operation. Medical Journal of
        Australia, 2, 929-932.

6-285   Benningfield, M. F. (1966, January). Review of
        suicide prevention centers in the United States.
        Pastoral Psychology, 16, 41-45.

6-286   Brunt, H. H., Jr. (1969, February). Organization
        of a suicide prevention center. Journal of the
        Medical Society of New Jersey, 66, 62-65.

6-287   Brunt, H. H., Jr., Rotov, M., & Glenn, T. (1968).
        A suicide prevention center in a public mental
        hospital. Mental Hygiene, 52, 254-262.

6-288   Cherico, D. J., & Beirne, J. (1977). A brief
        analysis: Calls to a suicide prevention service
        line. In B. L. Danto & A. H. Kutscher (Eds.),
        Suicide and bereavement (pp. 249-252). New York:
        MSS Information Corporation.

6-289   Danto, B. L. (1970). How to start a suicide
        prevention center without really trying.
        Michigan Medicine, 69, 119-121.

6-290   Danto, B. L. (1977). Crisis and death
        intervention: Recruitment, training, and
        supervision of the volunteer. In B. L. Danto &

A. H. Kutscher (Eds.), Suicide and bereavement
(pp. 240-248). New York: MSS Information
Corporation.

6-291   Delworth, U., Rudow, E. H., & Taub,
        J. (Eds.) (1972). Crisis center/Hotline: A
        guidebook to beginning and operating.
        Springfield, IL: Thomas.

        This book describes the establishment,
        administration, and training for crisis
        intervention centers. Included also is the
        Los Angeles Suicide Prevention Center's 1968
        training manual (see also reference 7-082, and
        Farberow et al., 1970, reference 6-297). The
        specific chapters are listed below.

        6-291.01 Smart, D. W. Volunteers: Who are they?
                  pp. 3-17.

        6-291.02 Delworth, U. Selection: Who can be
                  helpful? pp. 18-35.

        6-291.03 Delworth, U. Training: Making sure the
                  helper is helpful. pp. 36-45.

        6-291.04 Rudow, E. H., & Gebhardt, B. Financing
                  tips for crisis centers and hotlines.
                  pp. 46-54.

        6-291.05 Tate, P., & Greenfield, C. Legal
                  considerations in crisis center
                  operations. pp. 55-61.

        6-291.06 Taub, J. The nitty-gritty of center
                  operations. pp. 62-73.

        6-291.07 Taub, J. Getting it together: Group
                  cohesion. pp. 74-81.

        6-291.08 Hinkle, J. E. Evaluation: Let us do
                  what we said we would. pp. 82-88.

        6-291.09 Moore, M. Drugs: The role of the crisis
                  center. pp. 89-103.

        6-291.10 Farberow, N. L., Heilig, S. M., & Litman,
                  R. E. Techniques in crisis
                  intervention: A training manual.
                  pp. 104-122. [A reprint of the 1968
                  LASPC training manual.]

6-292   Dennis, R. E., & Kirk, A. (1976). Survey of the
        use of crisis intervention centers by the black
        population. Suicide and Life-Threatening
        Behavior, 6, 101-105.

6-293   Dixon, M. C., & Burns, J. (1975). The training of
         telephone crisis intervention volunteers.
         American Journal of Community Psychology, 3,
         145-150.

6-294   Dublin, L. I. (1963). Suicide: A sociological and
         statistical study (pp. 179-193). New York:
         Ronald Press, Chapter 20, "Efforts to prevent
         suicide."

6-295   Eastwood, M. R., Brill, L., & Brown, J. H. (1976).
         Suicide and prevention centres. Canadian
         Psychiatric Association Journal, 21, 571-575.

6-296   Elkins, R. L., Jr., & Cohen, C. R. (1982). A
         comparison of the effects of prejob training and
         job experiences on nonprofessional telephone
         crisis counselors. Suicide and Life-Threatening
         Behavior, 12, 84-89.

* 6-297 Farberow, N. L., Heilig, S. M., & Litman,
         R. E. (1970). Evaluation and management of
         suicidal persons. In E. S. Shneidman,
         N. L. Farberow, & R. E. Litman (Eds.), The
         psychology of suicide (pp. 273-291). New York:
         Science House. (Reprinted from Techniques in
         crisis intervention: A training manual. (1968).
         Los Angeles: Suicide Prevention Center, Inc.)

         A reprint of the 1968 Los Angeles Suicide
         Prevention Center training manual.

6-298   Farberow, N. L., & Shneidman, E. S. (1961). A
         survey of agencies for the prevention of suicide.
         In N. L. Farberow & E. S. Shneidman (Eds.), The
         cry for help (pp. 136-149). New York:
         McGraw-Hill.

         A historical and contemporary (to 1960)
         presentation of the suicide prevention
         agencies worldwide.

6-299   Finlay-Jones, R. A., & Kidd, C. B. (1972, April 1).
         The clients of the telephone samaritan service in
         Western Australia. Medical Journal of Australia,
         1, 690-694.

6-300   Fisher, S. A. (1973). Suicide and crisis
         intervention: Survey and guide to services. New
         York: Springer.

         Fisher surveys various aspects of the
         operation of suicide prevention centers in the
         U.S.

6-301   Frederick, C. J. (1972). Organizing and funding

suicide prevention and crisis services. Hospital and Community Psychiatry, 23, 346-348.

6-302   Furth, M. S. (1973). Relationship between poison information centers and suicide prevention centers. Life-Threatening Behavior, 3, 131-136.

6-303   Gordon, R. A. (1974). Social class bias of suicide prevention volunteers. American Journal of Community Psychiatry, 2, 393-398.

6-304   Greaves, G., & Ghent, L. (1972). Comparison of accomplished suicides with persons contacting a crisis intervention clinic. Psychological Reports, 31, 290.

6-305   Greer, F. L., & Weinstein, R. S. (1979). Suicide prevention center outreach: Callers and noncallers compared. Psychological Reports, 44, 387-393.

6-306   Hankoff, L. D., & Waltzer, H. (1968). A suicide prevention service in a psychiatric receiving hospital setting. In H. L. P. Resnik (Ed.), Suicidal behaviors: Diagnosis and management (pp. 391-398). Boston: Little Brown.

* 6-307   Hatton, C. L., Valente, S. M., & Rink, A. (1977). What to do in an emergency. In C. L. Hatton, S. M. Valente, & A. Rink (Eds.), Suicide: Assessment and intervention (pp. 182-186). New York: Appleton-Century-Crofts.

        Specific instructions are presented for an emergency (suicide-in-progress) caller or client. This material is included on pages 141-147 of the 2nd edition of this book (see reference 1-068 and 6-218 above).

6-308   Haughton, A. (1968, July). Suicide prevention programs in the U.S.--An overview. Bulletin of Suicidology, pp. 25-29.

6-309   Haughton, A. (1968). Suicide prevention programs: The current scene. American Journal of Psychiatry, 124, 1692-1696.

6-310   Heilig, S. M., Farberow, N. L., Litman, R. E., & Shneidman, E. S. (1968). The role of non-professional volunteers in a suicide prevention center. Community Mental Health Journal, 4, 287-295. (Reprinted as "Nonprofessional volunteers in a suicide prevention center," in E. S. Shneidman, N. L. Farberow, & R. E. Litman (Eds.) (1970), The psychology of suicide (pp. 109-123). New York:

Science House.)

6-311   Hinson, J. (1982).   Strategies for suicide
        intervention by telephone. Suicide and
        Life-Threatening Behavior, 12, 176-184.
        (Abstracts: PA, 1983, 69, No. 13355, p. 1475;
        CPA, 1982, 22, No. 2721, p. 581)

6-312   Hipple, J., & Cimbolic, P. (1979). The counselor
        and suicidal crisis: Diagnosis and intervention
        (pp. 86-93). Springfield, IL: Thomas, Chapter
        8, "The use of the telephone in treatment."

6-313   Hirsch, S. (1981). A critique of volunteer-staffed
        suicide prevention centres. Canadian Journal of
        Psychiatry, 26, 406-410.

6-314   Jarmusz, R. T. (1969). Some considerations in
        establishing a suicide prevention center. Mental
        Hygiene, 53, 351-356.

6-315   Kiev, A. (1970). New directions for suicide
        prevention centers. American Journal of
        Psychiatry, 127, 87-88.

6-316   Kiev, A. (1972). New directions for suicide
        prevention centers. Life-Threatening Behavior,
        2, 189-193.

6-317   Lester, D. (1971). The suicide prevention
        contribution to mental health. Psychological
        Reports, 28, 903-905.

6-318   Lester, D. (1974). The unique qualities of
        telephone therapy. Psychotherapy: Theory,
        Research and Practice, 11, 219-221.

* 6-319   Lester, D., & Brockopp, G. W. (Eds.) (1973).
        Crisis intervention and counseling by telephone.
        Springfield, IL: Thomas.

        An excellent coverage of a large variety of
        topics related to crisis intervention and the
        use of telephones by such services.

        6-319.01 Brockopp, G. W. An emergency telephone
                  service: The development of a
                  presence. pp. 9-23.

        6-319.02 McGee, R. K., Richard, W. C., & Bercun,
                  C. (1972). A survey of telephone
                  answering systems in suicide prevention
                  and crisis intervention agencies.
                  pp. 24-40. (A shortened version of
                  this chapter appeared in Life-
                  Threatening Behavior, 2, 42-47.)

6-319.03   Roth, H. S., Palmer, C., & Schut, A. J.
            Community youth line: A hotline
            program for troubled adolescents.
            pp. 41-57.

6-319.04   MacKinnon, R. A., & Michels, R. (1970).
            The role of the telephone in the
            psychiatric interview. pp. 58-76.
            (Reprinted from Psychiatry, 33, 82-93.)

6-319.05   Williams, T., & Douds, J. The unique
            contribution of telephone therapy.
            pp. 80-88.

6-319.06   Brockopp, G. W. Crisis intervention:
            Theory, process and practice.
            pp. 89-104.

6-319.07   Lamb, C. W. (1969-1970). Telephone
            therapy: Some common errors and
            fallacies. pp. 105-110. (Reprinted
            from Voices: The art and Science of
            Psychotherapy, 5(4), 42-46. Abstract:
            PA, 1971, 45, No. 6923, pp. 753-754)

6-319.08   Brockopp, G. W. The telephone call:
            Conversation or therapy. pp. 111-116.

6-319.09   Brockopp, G. W., & Oughterson, E. D.
            Legal and procedural aspects of
            telephone emergency services.
            pp. 117-131.

6-319.10   Hoff, L. A. Beyond the telephone
            contact. pp. 132-148.

6-319.11   Richard, W. C., & McGee, R. K. CARE
            team: An answer to need for suicide
            prevention center outreach program.
            pp. 149-154.

6-319.12   Brockopp, G. W., & Lester, D. The
            obscene caller. pp. 157-174.

6-319.13   Lester, D., Brockopp, G. W., & Blum, D.
            The chronic caller. pp. 175-192.
            (Includes a reprint of Lester, D., &
            Brockopp, G. W. (1970). Chronic
            callers to a suicide prevention center.
            Community Mental Health Journal, 6,
            246-250. Appears on pp. 175-182 of
            this book.)

6-319.14   Brockopp, G. W. The covert cry for help.
            pp. 193-198.

6-319.15   Brockopp, G. W., & Lester, D.   The silent
           caller.   pp. 199-205.

6-319.16   Brockopp, G. W.   The nuisance caller.
           pp. 206-210.

6-319.17   Brockopp, G. W.   The "one counselor"
           caller.   pp. 211-218.

6-319.18   McGee, R. K., & Jennings, B.   Ascending
           to "lower" levels: The case for
           nonprofessional crisis workers.
           pp. 223-237.

6-319.19   McColskey, A. S.   The use of the
           professional in telephone counseling.
           pp. 238-251.

6-319.20   Brockopp, G. W.   Selecting the telephone
           counselor.   pp. 252-261.

6-319.21   Brockopp, G. W.   Training the telephone
           counselor.   pp. 262-272.

6-319.22   Lester, D.   The evaluation of telephone
           counseling services.   pp. 276-286.

6-319.23   Fowler, D. E., & McGee, R. K.   Assessing
           the performance of telephone crisis
           workers: The development of Technical
           Effectiveness scale.   pp. 287-297.
           [Scale appears on p. 291.]

6-319.24   Knickerbocker, D. A., & McGee, R. K.
           Clinical effectivness of
           nonprofessional and professional
           telephone workers in a crisis
           intervention center.   pp. 298-309.

6-319.25   Williamson, J. W., Goldberg, E., &
           Packard, M.   Use of simulated patients
           in evaluating patient management skills
           of telephone counselors--A proposal.
           pp. 310-322.

6-320   Litman, R. E. (1972).   Experiences in a suicide
        prevention center.   In J. Waldenstrom,
        T. Larsson, & N. Ljungstedt (Eds.), Suicide and
        attempted suicide (pp. 217-230).   Stockholm:
        Nordiska Bokhandlens Forlag.

6-321   McClean, L. J. (1971).   What can we learn from the
        low-risk caller to a suicide prevention center?
        In D. B. Anderson & L. J. McClean (Eds.),
        Identifying suicide potential (pp. 81-84).   New
        York: Behavioral Publications.

6-322   McGee, R. K. (1974). <u>Crisis intervention in the</u>
        <u>community</u>. Baltimore: University Park Press.

        This book includes a history of crisis
        intervention services in the United States
        (pp. 3-20) as well as descriptions of 10
        programs and practical information regarding
        the establishing and conducting of a crisis
        intervention service.

6-323   McGee, R. K. (1975).   To be, or not to be--
        certified. <u>Suicide</u>, <u>5</u>, 194-206.

6-324   McGee, R. K. (1976).   The volunteer suicidologist:
        Current status and future prospects.   In
        E. S. Shneidman (Ed.), <u>Suicidology: Contemporary</u>
        <u>developments</u> (pp. 482-498).   New York: Grune &
        Stratton.

* 6-325 McGee, R. K., Berg, D., Brockopp, G. W., Harris,
        J. R., Haughton, A. B., Rachlis, D., Tomes, H., &
        Hoff, L. A. (1972).   The delivery of suicide and
        crisis intervention services.   In H. L. P. Resnik
        & B. C. Hathorne (Eds.), <u>Suicide prevention in</u>
        <u>the 70s</u> (pp. 81-89).   Washington, D.C.:   USGPO,
        DHEW Publication No. (HSM) 72-9054.

6-326   McGee, R. K., Knickerbocker, D. A., Fowler, D. E.,
        Jennings, B., Ansel, E. L., Zelenka, M. H., &
        Marcus, S. (1972).   Evaluation of crisis
        intervention programs and personnel: A summary
        and critique. <u>Life-Threatening Behavior</u>, <u>2</u>,
        42-47.

6-327   McGee, R. K., & McGee, J. P. (1968).   A total
        community response to the cry for help: WE CARE
        Inc., of Orlando, Florida.   In H. L. P. Resnik
        (Ed.), <u>Suicidal behaviors: Diagnosis and</u>
        <u>management</u> (pp. 441-452).   Boston: Little Brown.

6-328   Miller, H. L., Coombs, D. W., Murkhertee, D., &
        Barton, S. N. (1979).   Suicide prevention centers
        in America. <u>Alabama Journal of Medical Sciences</u>,
        <u>16</u>, 26-31.

6-329   Motto, J. A. (1969, March).   Developments of
        standards for suicide prevention centers.
        <u>Bulletin of Suicidology</u>, pp. 33-37.

6-330   Motto, J. A. (1973).   On standards for suicide
        prevention and crisis centers. <u>Life-Threatening</u>
        <u>Behavior</u>, <u>3</u>, 251-260.

6-331   Motto, J. A. (1979).   Starting a therapy group in a
        suicide prevention and crisis center. <u>Suicide</u>
        <u>and Life-Threatening Behavior</u>, <u>9</u>, 47-56.

6-332   Motto, J. A. (1979). New approaches to crisis
         intervention. Suicide and Life-Threatening
         Behavior, 9, 173-184.

* 6-333 Motto, J. A., Brooks, R. M., Ross, C. P., & Allen,
         N. H. (1974). Standards for suicide prevention
         and crisis centers New York: Behavioral
         Publications.

6-334   Murphy, G. E., Wetzel, R. D., Swallow, C. S., &
         McClure, J. N., Jr. (1969). Who calls the
         suicide prevention center: A study of 55 persons
         calling on their own behalf. American Journal of
         Psychiatry, 126, 314-324.

6-335   Neimeyer, R. A., & Diamond, R. J. (1983). Suicide
         management skills and the medical student.
         Journal of Medical Education, 58, 562-567.
         (Abstract: PA, 1984, 71, No. 7825, pp. 821-822)

6-336   Neimeyer, R. A., & MacInnes, W. D. (1981).
         Assessing paraprofessional competence with the
         Suicide Intervention Response Inventory. Journal
         of Counseling Psychology, 28, 176-179.

6-337   Neimeyer, R. A., & Oppenheimer, B. (1983).
         Concurrent and predictive validity of the Suicide
         Intervention Response Inventory. Psychological
         Reports, 52, 594. (Abstract: PA, 1984, 71,
         No. 210, p. 21)

         In these 3 publications (i.e., references
         6-335--6-337), Neimeyer and associates report
         the results of an instrument to assess the
         skill and ability of individuals to respond to
         suicidal clients in an effective fashion.

6-338   Nelson, G., McKenna, J., Koperno, M., Chatterson,
         J., & Brown, J. H. (1975). The role of anonymity
         in suicidal contacts with a crisis intervention
         centre. Canadian Psychiatric Association
         Journal, 20, 455-459.

6-339   Powell, E. R. (1976). Worker and caller variety in
         three crisis centers. Suicide and
         Life-Threatening Behavior, 6, 202-208.

6-340   Powell, E. R., Heaton, M. E., & Ashton,
         P. T. (1974). Systematic observation of crisis
         center telephone interactions. Life-Threatening
         Behavior, 4, 224-239.

6-341   Resnik, H. L. P. (1968). A community antisuicide
         organization: The FRIENDS of Dade County,
         Florida. In H. L. P. Resnik (Ed.), Suicidal
         behaviors: Diagnosis and management

(pp. 418-440). Boston: Little Brown.

6-342   Roberts, A. R. (1970, May-June). An organizational study of suicide prevention agencies in the United States. Police, 14(5), 64-72. (Reprinted as "Organization of suicide prevention agencies," in L. D. Hankoff & B. Einsidler (Eds.) (1979), Suicide: Theory and clinical aspects (pp. 391-399). Littleton, MA: PSG Publishing.)

6-343a Roberts, A. R., & Grau, J. J. (1970). Procedures used in crisis intervention by suicide prevention agencies. Public Health Reports, 85, 691-697.

* 6-343b Rosenbaum, A., & Calhoun, J. F. (1977). The use of the telephone hotline in crisis intervention: A review. Journal of Community Psychology, 5, 325-339. [see also 6-351b]

6-344   Ross, C. P., & Motto, J. A. (1971, Fall). Implementation of standards for suicide prevention centers. Bulletin of Suicidology, No. 8, pp. 18-21.

6-345   Sawyer, J. B., & Jameton, E. M. (1979). Chronic callers to a suicide prevention center. Suicide and Life-Threatening Behavior, 9, 97-104.

6-346   Shneidman, E. S. (1970, Spring). Special Issue: Commemorating the tenth anniversary of the Los Angeles Suicide Prevention Center [1968]. Bulletin of Suicidology, No. 6.

        In commemoration of the LASPC's important role in the suicide prevention movement, this issue contained a number of articles related to SPCs.

6-346.01 Farberow, N. L. Ten years of suicide prevention--Past and future. pp. 6-11.

6-346.02 Litman, R. E. Suicide prevention center patients: A follow-up study. pp. 12-17.

6-346.03 Wold, C. I. Characteristics of 26,000 suicide prevention center patients. pp. 24-28.

6-346.04 Pretzel, P. W. The volunteer clinical worker at the suicide prevention center. pp. 29-34.

6-346.05 Randell, J. H. The nightwatch program in a suicide prevention center. pp. 50-55.

6-347   Shneidman, E. S., & Farberow, N. L. (1965).   The
        Los Angeles Suicide Prevention Center: A
        demonstration of public health feasibilities.
        American Journal of Public Health, 55, 21-26.
        (Reprinted as "Feasibilities of the Los Angeles
        Suicide Prevention Center," in E. S. Shneidman,
        N. L. Farberow, & R. E. Litman (Eds.) (1970),
        The psychology of suicide (pp. 97-107). New
        York: Science House.)

6-348   Shneidman, E. S., & Farberow, N. L. (1968).   The
        suicide prevention center of Los Angeles.   In
        H. L. P. Resnik (Ed.), Suicidal behaviors:
        Diagnosis and management (pp. 367-380).   Boston:
        Little Brown.

6-349   Shneidman, E. S., Farberow, N. L., & Litman,
        R. E. (1961).   The suicide prevention center [of
        Los Angeles].   In N. L. Farberow & E. S.
        Shneidman (Eds.), The cry for help (pp. 6-18).
        New York: McGraw-Hill.   (Reprinted with the
        first 2 authors reversed, in Pastoral Psychology,
        January 1966, 16, 30-40.)

6-350   Shore, J. H., Bopp, J. F., Dawes, J. W., & Waller,
        T. R. (1972).   A suicide prevention center on an
        Indian reservation.   American Journal of
        Psychiatry, 128, 1086-1091.   (Abstract: ACP,
        1972, 12, No. 1925, p. 598)

6-351a Slaikeu, K., Lester, D., & Tulkin, S. R. (1973).
        Show versus no show: A comparison of referral
        calls to a suicide prevention and crisis service.
        Journal of Consulting and Clinical Psychology,
        40, 481-486.

* 6-351b Stein, D. M., & Lambert, M. J. (1984).   Telephone
        counseling and crisis intervention: A review.
        American Journal of Community Psychology, 12,
        101-126.   [see also 6-343b]

6-352   Stelmachers, Z. T. (1976).   Current status of
        program evaluation efforts.   Suicide and
        Life-Threatening Behavior, 6, 67-78.

6-353   Stelmachers, Z. T., Baxter, J. W., & Ellenson,
        G. M. (1978).   Auditing the quality of care of a
        crisis center.   Suicide and Life-Threatening
        Behavior, 8, 18-31.

6-354   Sudak, H. S., Hall, S. R., & Sawyer, J. B. (1970,
        Fall).   The suicide prevention center as a
        coordinating facility.   Bulletin of Suicidology,
        No. 7, pp. 17-22.

6-355   Tabachnick, N., & Klugman, D. (1970).   Anonymous

suicidal telephone calls: A research critique. *Psychiatry*, 33, 526-532.

6-356   Tarrant, B. (1970).   Report on the crisis intervention and suicide prevention centre for Greater Vancouver. *Canadian Journal of Public Health*, 61, 66-67.

6-357   Tarrant, B. (1970).   A suicide prevention center in Vancouver. *Canada's Mental Health*, 18, 3-4, 11-14.

6-358   Thigpen, J. D., & Jones, E. (1979).   A comprehensive client management system for crisis intervention services. *Suicide and Life-Threatening Behavior*, 9, 227-234.

6-359   Trowell, I. (1979).   Telephone services. In L. D. Hankoff & B. Einsidler (Eds.), *Suicide: Theory and clinical aspects* (pp. 401-409). Littleton, MA: PSG Publishing.

6-360   Tuckman, J. (1970).   Suicide and the suicide prevention center.   In K. Wolff (Ed.), *Patterns of self-destruction: Depression and suicide* (pp. 3-17). Springfield, IL: Thomas.

6-361   Wilkins, J. (1969).   Suicide prevention centers: Comparison of clients in several cities. *Comprehensive Psychiatry*, 10, 443-451.

6-362   Wilkins, J. (1972, October 21).   Suicide calls and identification of suicidal callers. *Medical Journal of Australia*, 2, 923-929.

6-363   Zusman, J., & Davidson, D. L. (Eds.) (1971). *Organizing the community to prevent suicide*. Springfield, IL: Thomas.

Several chapters on suicide prevention center issues are presented in this book and are listed below.

6-363.01 McGee, R. K.   Selection and training of nonprofessionals and volunteers. pp. 37-42.

6-363.02 McGee, R. K.   Development of "We Care, Inc." pp. 59-73.

6-363.03 Brockopp, G. W.   The manpower problem in suicide prevention centers or programming the suicide prevention center for extinction. pp. 75-83.

6-363.04 Zusman, J.   Suicide prevention, crisis

                              intervention, and community mental
                              health services. pp. 85-93.

See also the AAS training manual for suicide prevention,
reference 7-082. See also Danto (1971, reference 6-061).

6.8 Other Prevention Agencies

6-364 Barraclough, B., & Shea, M. (1970, October 24).
       Suicide and Samaritan clients. Lancet, 2,
       868-870. [Barlow, S. M. (1970, November 21).
       Suicide and Samaritan clients [Letter]. Lancet,
       2, 1091.]

6-365 Cutter, F. (1979). The relationship of new
       Samaritan clients and volunteers to high risk
       people in England and Wales (1965-1977). Suicide
       and Life-Threatening Behavior, 9, 245-250.

6-366 Day, G. (1974). The Samaritan movement in Great
       Britain. Perspectives in Biology and Medicine,
       17, 507-512.

6-367 Fox, R. (1977). Suicide prevention in Great
       Britain. Mental Health and Society, 4, 74-79.

6-368 Kreitman, N., & Chowdhury, N. (1973). Distress
       behaviour: A study of selected Samaritan clients
       and parasuicides ('attempted suicide' patients).
       Part I.: General aspects. British Journal of
       Psychiatry, 123, 1-8. Part II.: Attitudes and
       choice of action. British Journal of Psychiatry,
       123, 9-14.

6-369 Norris, M. (1979). Paradoxical Samaritans:
       Techniques in a suicide prevention agency.
       Social Science and Medicine (Medical Psychology
       and Medical Sociology), 13A, 487-490.

6-370 Resnik, H. L. P. (Ed.) (1968). Suicidal behaviors:
       Diagnosis and management. Boston: Little Brown.

          This book includes descriptions of several
          suicide prevention agencies which are not
          exclusively suicide prevention centers (i.e.,
          primarily performing telephone therapy/crisis
          intervention).

       6-370.01 Ringel, E. Suicide prevention in Vienna.
                 pp. 381-390.

       6-370.02 Garrard, R. L., Mrs. [first name not
                 given]. Community suicide-prevention
                 activities: Greensboro, North
                 Carolina. pp. 399-404.

6-370.03 Fox, R. The Samaritans. pp. 405-417.

6-371 Varah, C. (1966). The Samaritans. New York: Macmillan.

6.9 Effectiveness and Outcome of SPCs

6-372 Achte, K. (1976). Present status and evaluation of suicide prevention and crisis intervention services in Europe. Mental Health and Society, 3, 169-174.

6-373 Achte, K. (1981). Evaluation of suicide prevention and crisis programs in Finland. Crisis, 2, 50-57.

* 6-374 Auerback, S. M., & Kilmann, P. R. (1977). Crisis intervention: A review of outcome research. Psychological Bulletin, 84, 1189-1217 (esp. pp. 1191-1194).

6-375 Bagley, C. (1968). The evaluation of a suicide prevention scheme [Samaritans] by an ecological method. Social Science and Medicine, 2, 1-14.

6-376 Bagley, C. (1971). An evaluation of suicide prevention agencies. Life-Threatening Behavior, 1, 245-259.

6-377 Barraclough, B. M., Jennings, C., & Moss, J. R. (1977, July 30). Suicide prevention by the Samaritans: A controlled study of effectiveness. Lancet, 2, 237-239. [Bagley, C. R. (1977, August 13). Suicide prevention by the Samaritans [Letter]. Lancet, 2, 348-349. Birtchnell, J. (1977, August 27). Suicide prevention by the Samaritans [Letter]. Lancet, 2, 460.]

6-378 Barraclough, B. M., & Shea, M. (1972). A comparison between "Samaritan suicides' and living Samaritan clients. British Journal of Psychiatry, 120, 79-84.

6-379 Bridge, T. P., Potkin, S. G., Zung, W. W. K., & Soldo, B. J. (1977). Suicide prevention centers: Ecological study of effectiveness. Journal of Nervous and Mental Disease, 164, 18-24.

6-380 Greer, S., & Anderson, M. (1979). Samaritan contact among 325 parasuicide patients. British Journal of Psychiatry, 135, 263-268.

6-381 Jennings, C., & Barraclough, B. M. (1978). Have the Samaritans lowered the suicide rate? A controlled study. Psychological Medicine, 8,

413-422.

6-382   Jennings, C., & Barraclough, B. M. (1980). The
        effectiveness of the Samaritans in the prevention
        of suicide. In R. D. T. Farmer & S. R. Hirsch
        (Eds.), The suicide syndrome (pp. 194-200).
        London: Croom Helm.

6-383   Lester, D. (1971). Geographic location of callers
        to a suicide prevention center: Note on the
        evaluation of suicide prevention programs.
        Psychological Reports, 28, 421-422.

6-384   Lester, D. (1971). The evaluation of suicide
        prevention centers. International Behavioral
        Scientist, 3, 40-47.

6-385   Lester, D. (1972). The myth of suicide prevention.
        Comprehensive Psychiatry, 13, 555-560.

6-386   Lester, D. (1974). Effect of suicide prevention
        centers on suicide rates in the United States.
        Health Services Report, 89, 37-39.

6-387   Litman, R. E. (1971). Suicide prevention:
        Evaluating effectiveness. Life-Threatening
        Behavior, 1, 155-162.

6-388   Malleson, A. (1973). Suicide prevention: A myth
        or a mandate? [Letter]. British Journal of
        Psychiatry, 122, 238-239. [A reply is made by
        C. Bagley, 1973, 123, 130.]

6-389a McKenna, J., Nelson, G., Chatterson, J., Koperno,
        M., & Brown, J. H. (1975). Chronically and
        acutely suicidal persons one month after contact
        with a crisis intervention centre. Canadian
        Psychiatric Association Journal, 20, 451-454.

6-389b Miller, H. L., Coombs, D. W., Leeper, J. D., &
        Barton, S. N. (1984). An analysis of the effects
        of suicide prevention facilities on suicide rates
        in the United States. American Journal of Public
        Health, 74, 340-343.

6-390   Motto, J. A. (1971). Evaluation of a suicide
        prevention center by sampling the population at
        risk. Life-Threatening Behavior, 1, 18-22.

6-391   Sawyer, J. B., Sudak, H. S., & Hall, S. R. (1972).
        A follow-up study of 53 suicides known to a
        suicide prevention center. Life-Threatening
        Behavior, 2, 227-238.

6-392   Singh, A. N., & Brown, J. H. (1973). Suicide
        prevention: Review and evaluation. Canadian

Psychiatric Association Journal, 18, 117-121.

6-393   Weiner, I. W. (1969). The effectiveness of a
        suicide prevention program. Mental Hygiene, 53,
        357-363.

6-394   Wilkins, J. (1970). A follow-up study of those who
        called a suicide prevention center. American
        Journal of Psychiatry, 127, 155-161.

6-395   Wold, C. I.. (1973). A two-year follow-up of
        suicide prevention center patients.
        Life-Threatening Behavior, 3, 171-183.

6-396   Wold, C. I., & Litman, R. E. (1973). Suicide after
        contact with a suicide prevention center.
        Archives of General Psychiatry, 28, 735-739.

See also Hirsch et al. (1982, reference 6-410), especially
pp. 300-301, Litman (1970, reference 6-346.02), Stelmachers
(1976, reference 6-352), especially pp. 68-72, and
Barraclough (1972, reference 6-173), pp. 662-665.

6.10 Follow-up of the Suicidal and Outcome Studies

6-397a Achte, K. A., Lonnqvist, J., Niskanen, P., Ginman,
        L., & Karlsson, M. (1972). Attempted suicides by
        poisoning, and eight-year follow-up. Psychiatria
        Fennica, 3, 321-340.

6-397b Adam, K. S., Valentine, J., Scarr, G., & Streiner,
        D. (1983). Follow-up of attempted suicide in
        Christchurch. Australia and New Zealand Journal
        of Psychiatry, 17, 18-25. (Abstract: PA, 1984,
        71, No. 4188, p. 444)

6-398   Angle, C. R., O'Brien, T. P., & McIntire,
        M. S. (1983). Adolescent self-poisoning: A
        nine-year followup. Journal of Developmental &
        Behavioral Pediatrics, 4, 83-87. (Abstract: PA,
        1983, 70, No. 10446, p. 1170)

6-399   Bogard, H. M. (1970). Follow-up study of suicidal
        patients seen in emergency room consultation.
        American Journal of Psychiatry, 126, 1017-1020.

6-400   Buglass, D., & Horton, J. (1974). The repetition
        of parasuicide: A comparison of three cohorts.
        British Journal of Psychiatry, 125, 168-174.

6-401a Chowdhury, N., Hicks, R. C., & Kreitman, N. (1973).
        Evaluation of an aftercare service for
        parasuicide patients. Social Psychiatry, 8,
        67-81.

6-401b Cohen-Sandler, R., Berman, A. L., & King,

R. A. (1982). A follow-up study of hospitalized suicidal children. _Journal of the American Academy of Child Psychiatry, 21_, 398-403.

6-402   Dahlgren, K. G. (1977). Attempted suicide--35 years afterward. _Suicide and Life-Threatening Behavior, 7_, 75-79.

6-403   Ettlinger, R. (1975). Evaluation of suicide prevention after attempted suicide. _Acta Psychiatrica Scandinavica_, Supplement 260, 5-135.

6-404a Ettlinger, R. (1980). A follow-up investigation of patients after attempted suicide. In R. D. T. Farmer & S. R. Hirsch (Eds.), _The suicide syndrome_ (pp. 167-172). London: Croom Helm.

6-404b Evenson, R. C. (1983). Community adjustment of patients who threaten and attempt suicide. _Psychological Reports, 52_, 127-132. (Abstracts: _PA_, 1983, _70_, No. 12906, p. 1450; _CPA_, 1983, _23_, No. 1249, p. 264)

6-405   Fleer, J., & Pasework, R. A. (1982). Prior public health agency contacts of individuals committing suicide. _Psychological Reports, 50_, 1319-1324. (Abstract: _PA_, 1983, _69_, No. 4143, p. 447)

6-406a Gardner, R. (1980). Medical-psychiatric consultation and liaison: An evaluation of its effectiveness. In R. D. T. Farmer & S. R. Hirsch (Eds.), _The suicide syndrome_ (pp. 226-234). London: Croom Helm.

6-406b Gharagozlou, H., & Hadjmohammadi, M. (1977). Report on a three-year follow-up of 100 cases of suicidal attempts in Shiraz, Iran. _International Journal of Social Psychiatry, 23_, 209-210.

6-407   Goldney, R. D. (1975). Out-patient follow-ups of those who have attempted suicide: Fact or fantasy? _Australian & New Zealand Journal of Psychiatry, 9_, 111-113.

6-408   Greer, S., & Bagley, C. R. (1971, February 6). Effect of psychiatric intervention in attempted suicide: A controlled study. _British Medical Journal, 1_, 310-312.

6-409   Hawton, K., O'Grady, J., Osborn, M., & Cole, D. (1982). Adolescents who take overdoses: Their characteristics, problems, and contacts with helping agencies. _British Journal of Psychiatry, 140_, 118-123.

* 6-410   Hirsch, S. R., Walsh, C., & Draper, R. (1982).

Parasuicide: A review of treatment
interventions. Journal of Affective Disorders,
4, 299-311 (esp. pp. 301-305). (Abstract: PA,
1983, 70, No. 6072, p. 682)

6-411   Jokinen, K., & Lehtinen, V. (1977). Poisoning
patients followed up 5 to 6 years later. In
K. Achte & J. Lonnqvist (Eds.), Suicide research:
Proceedings of the seminars of suicide research
by Yrjo Jahnsson Foundation, 1974-1977
(pp. 147-148). Helsinki: Psychiatria Fennica
(Psychiatria Fennica Supplementum 1976).

6-412   Jones, D. R. (1977). A follow-up of self-poisoned
patients. Journal of the Royal College of
General Practitioners, 27, 717-719.

6-413   Kennedy, P. (1972). Efficacy of a regional
poisoning treatment centre in preventing futher
suicidal behaviour. British Medical Journal, 4,
255-257.

6-414   Knesper, D. J. (1982). A study of referral
failures for potentially suicidal patients: A
method of medical care evaluation. Hospital and
Community Psychiatry, 33, 49-52.

6-415   Koller, K., & Slaghuis, W. (1978). Suicide
attempts 1973-1977--Urban Hobart. A further five
year follow-up reporting a decline. Australian &
New Zealand Journal of Psychiatry, 12, 169-173.

6-416   Kraft, D. P., & Babigian, H. M. (1976). Suicide by
persons with and without psychiatric contacts.
Archives of General Psychiatry, 33, 209-215.

6-417   Lester, D., & Beck, A. T. (1976). Completed
suicides and their previous attempts. Journal of
Clinical Psychology, 32, 553-555.

6-418   Lonnqvist, J., Niskanen, T., Achte, K. A., &
Ginman, L. (1975). Self-poisoning with follow-up
considerations. Suicide, 5, 39-46.

6-419   Mayo, J. A. (1974). Psychopharmacological
roulette: A follow-up study of patients
hospitalized for drug overdose. American Journal
of Public Health, 64, 616-617.

6-420   Morgan, H. G., Barton, J., Pottle, S., Pocock, H.,
& Burns-Cox, C. J. (1976). Deliberate self-harm:
A follow-up study of 279 patients. British
Journal of Psychiatry, 128, 361-368.

6-421a Myers, E. D. (1982). Subsequent deliberate
self-harm in patients referred to a psychiatrist:

A prospective study. <u>British Journal of</u>
<u>Psychiatry</u>, <u>140</u>, 132-137.

6-421b Nardini-Maillard, D., & Ladame, F. G. (1980).   The
       results of a follow-up study of suicidal
       adolescents. <u>Journal of Adolescence</u>, <u>3</u>, 253-260.

6-422 Nelson, S. H., & Grunebaum, J. (1971).   A follow-up
       study of wrist slashers. <u>American Journal of</u>
       <u>Psychiatry</u>, <u>127</u>, 1345-1349

6-423 Niskanen, P., Koskinen, T., Lepola, U., &
       Venalainen, E. (1975).   A study of attempted
       suicides in urban versus rural areas, with a
       follow-up. <u>Acta Psychiatrica Scandinavica</u>, <u>52</u>,
       283-291.

6-424 Niskanen, P., Rinta-Manty, R., & Olikainen,
       L. (1977).   A comparison of hospitalized suicidal
       and non-suicidal psychiatric patients, with a
       long-term follow-up. In K. Achte & J. Lonnqvist
       (Eds.), <u>Suicide research: Proceedings of the</u>
       <u>seminars of suicide research by Yrjo Jahnsson</u>
       <u>Foundation, 1974-1977</u> (pp. 159-166). Helsinki:
       Psychiatria Fennica (<u>Psychiatria Fennica</u>
       Supplementum 1976).

6-425 Paerregaard, G. (1975).   Suicide among attempted
       suicides: A 10-year follow-up. <u>Suicide</u>, <u>5</u>,
       140-144.

6-426 Retterstol, N. (1970).   <u>Long-term prognosis after</u>
       <u>attempted suicide: A personal follow-up</u>
       <u>examination</u>. Springfield, IL: Thomas.

* 6-427 Retterstol, N. (1974).   The future fate of suicide
       attempters. <u>Life-Threatening Behavior</u>, <u>4</u>,
       203-211.

6-428 Retterstol, N., & Strype, B. (1973).   Suicide
       attempters in Norway: A personal follow-up
       examination. <u>Life-Threatening Behavior</u>, <u>3</u>,
       283-297.

6-429 Rosen, D. H. (1970).   The serious suicide attempt:
       Epidemiological and follow-up study of 886
       patients. <u>American Journal of Psychiatry</u>, <u>127</u>,
       764-770.

6-430a Rosen, D. H. (1976, May 10).   The serious suicide
       attempt: Five-year follow-up of 886 patients.
       <u>Journal of the American Medical Association</u>, <u>235</u>,
       2105-2109.

6-430b Seiden, R. H. (1978).   Where are they now? A
       follow-up study of suicide attempters from the

Golden Gate Bridge. Suicide and Life-Threatening Behavior, 8, 203-216.

6-431   Spaulding, R. C., & Edwards, D. E. (1975). Suicide attempts: An examination of occurrence, psychiatric intervention, and outcome. Military Medicine, 140, 263-267.

6-432a   Stengel, E. (1972). A survey of follow-up examinations of attempted suicides. In J. Waldenstrom, T. Larsson, & N. Ljungstedt (Eds.), Suicide and attempted suicide (pp. 250-256). Stockholm: Nordiska Bojkhandelns Forlag.

6-432b   Termansen, P. E., & Bywater, C. (1975). S.A.F.E.R.: A follow-up service for attempted suicide in Vancouver. Canadian Psychiatric Association Journal, 20, 29-34.

6-433   Turner, R. J. (1980). The use of health services prior to non-fatal deliberate self-harm. In R. D. T. Farmer & S. R. Hirsch (Eds.), The suicide syndrome (pp. 173-186). London: Croom Helm.

6-434   Weiss, J. M., & Scott, K. F., Jr. (1974). Suicide attempters ten years later. Comprehensive Psychiatry, 15, 165-171.

6-435   Welu, T. C. (1977). A follow-up program for suicide attempters: Evaluation of effectiveness. Suicide and Life-Threatening Behavior, 7, 17-30.

See also Fowler et al. (1979) and Tsuang & Kronfol (1979), references 7-102 and 7-114, respectively.

See also McCulloch & Philip (1972, pp. 89-90, reference 1-044).

Much like the topic of sexuality in the near past, suicide and death and dying in general are "taboo" topics (see Shneidman, 1963, reference 7-005). People are reluctant to discuss such matters with others and are often uncomfortable if the issue is raised. Prejudice, stigma, and disgrace often surround the topic and exposure to suicidal behavior. This taboo is part of a more general phenomenon regarding attitudes toward suicide. Attitudes toward suicide, suicide attempters, and survivors of suicide are frequently observed to be negative.

The reasons for negative ideas with respect to suicide are undoubtedly multiple in nature. However, the belief in various myths (i.e., false assumptions regarding suicide, see Pokorny, 1968, reference 7-059) and the limited knowledge about suicide that have been observed (see Section 7.3) undoubtedly promote and maintain such negative attitudes. Such misinformation and lack of knowledge suggest a great need for education of the public and especially those in contact with the potentially suicidal (often called "gatekeepers," e.g., personnel in the medical and helping professions). Widespread dissemination of accurate information about suicide should create more positive, caring attitudes as well as increased recognition of the suicidal and the availability of resources to contact when suicidal intentions or likelihood are encountered.

One of the primary components of such education would be the clues or warning signs of suicidal ideation or intention. Evidence suggests that virtually all suicidal individuals provide multiple clues to many people around them on several occassions (see e.g., Bernstein, 1978-79, reference 7-097). Shneidman (e.g., 1965, reference 7-093) proposes that these signs of suicidal ideation can be seen in the verbal statements, the behavior, and the situation of the individual. While some of these clues are obvious and quite direct, others can be subtle and easily missed or ignored. Most people do not recognize the danger signs, however, and often would not know where to turn or what to

do even if they did. One optimistic suggestion has been
that "If suicidal patients could be recognized early and
handled properly, maybe 50% of them could be saved"
(Bennett, 1967, reference 7-119, p. 175). The message then,
is that if families, friends, professionals, and the general
public were more knowledgeable about suicide, its warning
signs, and available treatment services, perhaps many or
most suicides could be prevented before they ever had a
chance to occur.

7.1 The Taboo of Suicide

7-001   Battin, M. P. (1982). Ethical issues in suicide
        (pp. 20-23, "The suicide taboo"). Englewood
        Cliffs, NJ: Prentice-Hall.

7-002   Frederick, C. J. (1971). The present suicide taboo
        in the United States. Mental Hygiene, 55,
        178-183.

7-003   Menninger, K. (1938). Man against himself
        (pp. 13-16, "The taboo"). New York: Harcourt,
        Brace & World.

7-004   Noyes, R., Jr. (1968). The taboo of suicide.
        Psychiatry, 31, 173-183.

7-005   Shneidman, E. S. (1963). Suicide. In
        N. L. Farberow (Ed.), Taboo topics (pp. 33-43).
        New York: Atherton Press. (Reprinted as
        "Suicide as a taboo topic" in E. S. Shneidman,
        N. L. Farberow, & R. E. Litman (Eds.) (1970),
        The psychology of suicide (pp. 541-549). New
        York: Science House.)

7-006   Van de Rijt, P. J. A. (1974). The suicide taboo in
        Western life and science. In N. Speyer,
        R. F. W. Diekstra, & K. J. M. Van de Loo (Eds.),
        Proceedings: 7th international conference for
        suicide prevention (Amsterdam, The Netherlands,
        August 27-30, 1973) (pp. 324-329). Amsterdam:
        Swets & Zeitlinger.

7.2 Attitudes Toward Suicide and the Suicidal

7-007   Ansel, E. L., & McGee, R. K. (1971, Fall).
        Attitudes toward suicide attempters. Bulletin of
        Suicidology, No. 8, pp. 22-28.

        Attitudes toward attempters are assessed among
        psychiatric residents, psychiatric nursing
        personnel, emergency room personnel, social
        workers, police, and the lay public and are
        found to be negative among all groups.

7-008   Barber, J. H., Hodgkin, G. K., Patel, A. R., &
        Wilson, G. M. (1975, May 24). Effect of teaching
        on students' attitudes to self-poisoning.
        British Medical Journal, 2(5968), 431-434.

        The attitudes of medical students, residents,
        and medical social workers are assessed and
        compared.

7-009   Bascue, L. O., & Epstein, L. (1980). Suicide
        attitudes and experiences of hospitalized
        alcoholics. Psychological Reports, 47,
        1233-1234.

7-010   Bell, D. E. (1978). Sex and chronicity as
        variables affecting attitudes of undergraduates
        towards peers with suicidal behaviors (Doctoral
        dissertation, University of Georgia, 1977).
        Dissertation Abstracts International, 38, 3380B.
        (University Microfilms No. 77-29,742)

7-011   Boldt, M. (1982-83). Normative evaluations of
        suicide and death: A cross-generational study.
        Omega, 13, 145-157. (Abstract: PA, 1983, 69,
        No. 8076, p. 885)

        A more accepting attitude toward suicide among
        youthful vs. parental generation subjects was
        observed and suggested as a possible
        explanation for increased youth suicide.

7-012   Domino, G. (1980). Altering attitudes toward
        suicide in an abnormal psychology course.
        Teaching of Psychology, 7, 239-240.

7-013   Domino, G. (1981). Attitudes toward suicide among
        Mexican American and Anglo youth. Hispanic
        Journal of Behavioral Sciences, 3, 385-395.
        (Abstract: PA, 1982, 68, No. 5612, p. 615)

7-014   Domino, G., Gibson, L., Poling, S., & Westlake,
        L. (1980). Students' attitudes toward suicide.
        Social Psychiatry, 15, 127-130. (Abstract: PA,
        1981, 66, No. 4356, p. 456)

7-015   Domino, G., Moore, D., Westlake, L., & Gibson,
        L. (1982). Attitudes toward suicide: A factor
        analytic approach. Journal of Clinical
        Psychology, 38, 257-262. (Abstract: PA, 1982,
        68, No. 2461, p. 266)

        A 100-item Suicide Opinion Questionnaire is
        presented.

7-016   Dressler, D. M., Prusoff, B., Mark, H., & Shapiro,
        D. (1975). Clinician attitudes toward the

suicide attempter. Journal of Nervous and Mental Disease, 160, 146-155.

7-017   Droogas, A., Siiter, R., & O'Connell, A. N. (1982-83). Effects of personal and situational factors on attitudes toward suicide. Omega, 13, 127-144. (Abstract: PA, 1983, 69, No. 8083, p. 886)

7-018   Farberow, N. L. (Ed.) (1975). Suicide in different cultures. Baltimore: University Park Press.

This book contains 17 chapters on suicide in various cultures. See the citation in chapter 5, reference 5-430, for specific chapter titles and authors. Most of the book's chapters include discussions of attitudes and historical aspects related to suicide in the culture under consideration. Attitudes are specifically discussed by Reynolds et al., reference 5-430.01; Yampey, reference 5-430.02, esp. pp. 67-71; Retterstol, reference 5-430.03, esp. pp. 78-79; Achte & Lonnqvist, reference 5-430.04, esp. pp. 109-112; Atkinson, reference 5-430.06; Speijer, reference 5-430.07; Noomen, reference 5-430.08, esp. pp. 170-172; Rin, reference 5-430.14, esp. pp. 245-248; Iga & Tatai, reference 5-430.15, esp. pp. 270-275.

7-019   Frederick, C. J. (1971). The present suicide taboo in the United States. Mental Hygiene, 55, 178-183.

Following a discussion of the taboo of suicide, the attitudes of 80 people toward suicide are studied.

7-020   Ginsburg, G. P. (1971). Public conceptions and attitudes about suicide. Journal of Health and Social Behavior, 12, 200-207.

7-021   Goldney, R. D., & Bottrill, A. (1980). Attitudes to patients who attempt suicide. Medical Journal of Australia, 2, 717-720.

7-022   Gurrister, L., & Kane, R. A. (1978). How therapists perceive and treat suicidal patients. Community Mental Health Journal, 14, 3-13.

The opinions of therapists are assessed. Those who had experienced a suicide in their practice had different opinions than those who had not.

7-023   Hansen, L. C., & McAleer, C. A. (1983-84).
        Terminal cancer and suicide: The health care
        professional's dilemma. Omega, 14, 241-248.

7-024   Hawton, K., Marsack, P., & Fagg, J. (1981). The
        attitudes of psychiatrists to deliberate
        self-poisoning: Comparison with physicians and
        nurses. British Journal of Medical Psychology,
        54, 341-348. (Abstract: PA, 1982, 68, No. 1371,
        p. 153)

7-025   Hipple, J., & Cimbolic, P. (1979). The counselor
        and suicidal crisis: Diagnosis and intervention
        (pp. 82-85). Springfield, IL: Thomas, Chapter
        7, "The therapist's personal reaction to
        suicide."

✓ 7-026   Hoelter, J. W. (1979). Religiosity, fear of death
        and suicide acceptability. Suicide and
        Life-Threatening Behavior, 9, 163-172.
        (Abstract: PA, 1980, 64, No. 10428, p. 1122)

        A 6-item Suicide Acceptability Scale is also
        presented.

7-027   Johnson, D., Fitch, S., Alston, J. P., & McIntosh,
        W. A. (1980). Acceptance of conditional suicide
        and euthanasia among adult Americans. Suicide
        and Life-Threatening Behavior, 10, 157-166.
        (Abstracts: PA, 1981, 66, No. 3705, p. 392;
        CPA, 1981, 21, No. 697, p. 162)

7-028   Kalish, R. A., Reynolds, D. K., & Farberow,
        N. L. (1974). Community attitudes toward
        suicide. Community Mental Health Journal, 10,
        301-308.

7-029   Kastenbaum, R. (1976). Suicide as the preferred
        way of death. In E. S. Shneidman (Ed.),
        Suicidology: Contemporary developments
        (pp. 425-441). New York: Grune & Stratton.

        Kastenbaum considers our changing orientation
        toward suicide and his feeling that it will
        become the preferred way of death in our
        society.

7-030   Kearl, M. C., & Harris, R. (1981-82).
        Individualism and the emerging "modern" ideology
        of death. Omega, 12, 269-280. (Abstract: PA,
        1982, 67, No. 12108, p. 1299)

        Attitudes toward suicide, abortion, and the
        right to die were assessed in 2 national
        samples of 3064 individuals.

7-031   Leshem, A., & Leshem, Y. (1977). Attitudes of
        college students toward men and women who commit
        suicidal acts (Doctoral dissertation, University
        of Northern Colorado, 1976). Dissertation
        Abstracts International, 37, 7042A. (University
        Microfilms No. 77-11,070)

7-032   Lester, D. (1971). Attitudes toward death and
        suicide in a non-disturbed population.
        Psychological Reports, 29, 386.

7-033   Litman, R. E. (1968). Psychotherapists'
        orientations toward suicide. In H. L. P. Resnik
        (Ed.), Suicidal behaviors: Diagnosis and
        management (pp. 357-363). Boston: Little,
        Brown.

7-034   Menninger, K. (1969). Expression and punishment.
        In E. S. Shneidman (Ed.), On the nature of
        suicide (pp. 68-73). San Francisco:
        Jossey-Bass.

        Menninger suggests that the times often
        determine how suicide will be viewed and that
        as a result, contemporary feelings have not
        been seen historically.

7-035   Minear, J. D., & Brush, L. R. (1980-81). The
        correlations of attitudes toward suicide with
        death anxiety, religiosity, and personal
        closeness to suicide. Omega, 11, 317-324.
        (Abstract: PA, 1981, 66, No. 13631, p. 1416)

        A 29-item attitudinal scale developed by the
        authors was administered. The scale included
        10 items measuring Suicide Beliefs, 11 items
        on Suicide Values, and 8 items on Belief in an
        Afterlife.

7-036   Nichol, D. S. (1976). Factors affecting the
        negativity of attitudes toward suicide (Doctoral
        dissertation, York University, Canada, 1973).
        Dissertation Abstracts International, 36,
        5235-5236B.

7-037   O'Brien, S. E., & Stoll, K. A. (1977). Attitudes
        of medical and nursing staff toward
        self-poisoning patients in a London hospital.
        International Journal of Nursing Studies, 14,
        29-35.

7-038   Ostheimer, J. M., & Moore, C. L., Jr. (1982). "The
        correlates of attitudes toward euthanasia"
        revisited. Social Biology, 28, 145-148.
        (Abstract: PA, 1983, 69, No. 10296, p. 1130)

Suicide attitudes were also measured and its correlation with religious affiliation determined. (A follow-up and reanalysis of the same data of Singh, 1979, reference 7-048 below).

7-039   Patel, A. R. (1975, May 24). Attitudes toward self-poisoning. British Medical Journal, 2(5968), 426-429.

The attitudes of physicians and senior nurses are assessed and generally unfavorable attitudes were observed.

7-040   Ramon, S. (1980). Attitudes of doctors and nurses to self-poisoning patients. Social Science and Medicine [Medical Psychology and Medical Sociology], 14, 317-324.

7-041   Ramon, S., & Breyter, C. E. (1978). Attitudes towards self-poisoning among British and Israeli doctors and nurses in a psychiatric hospital. Israel Annals of Psychiatry and Related Disciplines, 16, 206-218. (Abstract: PA, 1980, 64, No. 1943, pp. 213-214)

7-042   Ramon, S., Bancroft, J. H., & Skrimshire, A. M. (1975). Attitudes toward self-poisoning among physicians and nurses in a general hospital. British Journal of Psychiatry, 127, 257-264.

7-043   Rockwell, D. A., & O'Brien, W. (1973). Physicians' knowledge and attitudes about suicide. Journal of the American Medical Association, 225, 1347-1349. (Abstract: PA, 1974, 51, No. 7223, p. 912)

7-044   Rosenthal, N. R. (1983). Death education and suicide potentiality. Death Education, 7, 39-51.

Courses on death education are found to attract students with greater acceptance of suicide (which is unaffected by taking the course), but such education does not increase suicide potentiality. A 12-item Suicide Attitude Questionnaire is also developed and employed.

7-045   Sale, I., Williams, C. L., Hons, B. A., Clark, J., & Mills, J. (1975). Suicide behavior: Community attitudes and beliefs. Suicide, 5, 158-168.

7-046   Selby, J. W., & Calhoun, L. G. (1975). Social perception of suicide: Effects of three factors on causal attributions. Journal of Consulting and Clinical Psychology, 43, 431.

7-047   Shneidman, E. S. (1970, August).   You & death: A
        Psychology Today questionnaire.   Psychology
        Today, pp. 67-72.   Results are reported in
        Psychology Today, June 1971, pp. 43-45, 74-80,
        and are reprinted in E. S. Shneidman (Ed.)
        (1973), Deaths of man (pp. 201-224, "A national
        survey of attitudes toward death").   New York:
        Quandrangle.

        A 75-item questionnaire that includes several
        items on suicide appears and was returned by a
        large number of PT readers.

7-048   Singh, B. K. (1979).   Correlation of attitudes
        toward euthanasia.   Social Biology, 26, 247-253.

7-049   Stengel, E. (1964).   Suicide and attempted suicide
        (pp. 55-63).   Baltimore: Penquin Books, Chapter
        6, "The attitudes of society to suicide."

7-050   Weigand, J. (1972).   Physicians view death and
        suicide.   Life-Threatening Behavior 2, 163-167.

7-051   Weiss, J. M. A., & Perry, M. E. (1975).
        Transcultural attitudes toward homicide and
        suicide.   Suicide, 5, 223-227.

7-052   Wekstein, L. (1979).   Handbook of suicidology:
        Principles, problems, and practice (pp. 35-37,
        "Attitudes toward suicide").   New York:
        Brunner/Mazel.

See also Chapter 9 for attitudes and reactions of others to
family members who survive a suicide.   See Calhoun et
al. (1979, reference 9-013), Calhoun et al. (1980, reference
9-014), Calhoun et al. (1981, reference 9-018), and Rudestam
& Imbroll (1983, reference 9-059).

See also Davis (1983, reference 3-005) for the history of
social attitudes toward suicide.

7.3 Myths and Knowledge About Suicide

7-053   Alvarez, A. (1972).   The savage god: A study of
        suicide (pp. 79-89).   New York: Random House,
        Part 3, Chapter 1, "Fallacies."

7-054   Giffin, M., & Felsenthal, C. (1983).   A cry for
        help (pp. 17-38).   Garden City, NY: Doubleday,
        Chapter 2, "The deadly myths."

7-055   Gordon, S. E. L. (1979).   An analysis of the
        knowledge and attitudes of secondary school
        teachers concerning suicide among adolescents and

intervention in adolescent suicide (Doctoral dissertation, North Texas State University, 1979). Dissertation Abstracts International, 40, 1393-1394A. (University Microfilms No. 7919723)

7-056   Heimburger, E. M., McCallum, R. N., & Pratt, M. (1980). Facts about suicide: How knowledgeable is the primary care physician? Minnesota Medicine, 77, 295-298.

A 20-item Suicide Knowledge Questionnaire is included.

7-057   Klagsbrun, F. (1977). Too young to die: Youth and suicide (pp. 17-24). New York: Pocket Books, Chapter 1, "Myths and realities: What is true and what is false?" (Originally published, 1976, Boston: Houghton Mifflin.)

7-058   McIntosh, J. L., Hubbard, R. W., & Santos, J. F. (1983, April). Suicide facts and myths: A compilation and study of prevalence. Paper presented at the annual meeting of the American Association of Suicidology, Dallas, Texas.

A 32-item and a 16-item factual questionnaire are included. Copies are available from the first author. A later draft is under journal review.

* 7-059   Pokorny, A. D. (1968). Myths about suicide. In H. L. P. Resnik (Ed.), Suicidal behaviors: Diagnosis and management (pp. 57-72). Boston: Little, Brown.

A large number of myths about suicide and the documentation for the facts are presented.

7-060   Reid, P., & Smith, H. (1980). Knowledge about suicide among members of helping agencies in Ireland. Irish Medical Journal, 73, 117-119.

7-061   Rockwell, D. A., & O'Brien, W. (1973). Physicians' knowledge and attitudes about suicide. Journal of the American Medical Association, 225, 1347-1349. (Abstract: PA, 1974, 51, No. 7223, p. 912)

7-062   Shneidman, E. S., Farberow, N. L., & Leonard, C. V. (1961). Some facts about suicide: Causes and prevention (pp. 3-5). Washington, D.C.: USGPO, Public Health Service Publication No. 852, Health Information Services No. 101. Supt. of Documents No. HE 20.10: 101.

This pamphlet presents 8 myths about suicide

and the matching "facts." This booklet also
includes information on clues to suicide and
where to turn for help.

7.4 Education About Suicide

7-063   Allen, N. H. (1976). The health educator as a
suicidologist. Suicide and Life-Threatening
Behavior, 6, 195-201.

Suggestions and steps to be taken in a public
health program on suicide education and
prevention are outlined.

7-064   Cohen, E. (1974). Suicide and self-assault: An
introductory course for medical students.
Journal of Medical Education, 49, 383-385.

7-065   Comstock, B. S. (1979). Suicide in the 1970s: A
second look. Suicide and Life-Threatening
Behavior, 9, 3-13.

This article reviews the outcome of goals and
recommendations put forth in the document
Suicide prevention in the 70's (Resnik &
Hathorne, 1973, especially reference 7-075
below). Included in those recommendations
were many regarding education and training.
Comstock feels most of these suggestions have
been achieved, but more remains to be done.

7-066   Danto, B. L. (1976). Practical aspects of the
training of psychiatrists in suicide prevention.
Omega, 7, 69-74.

7-067   Farberow, N. L. (1969). Training in suicide
prevention for professional and community agents.
American Journal of Psychiatry, 125, 1702-1705.

Training available at the Los Angeles Suicide
Prevention Center is described.

7-068   Frederick, C. J., & Lague, L. (1972). Dealing with
the crisis of suicide. Public Affairs Pamphlet
No. 406A. New York: Public Affairs Committee.

A pamphlet intended for public education. A
brief overview of suicide, high-risk groups,
motivations, recognition of clues, where and
how to seek help are presented.

7-069   Heilig, S. M. (1970, Spring). Training in suicide
prevention. Bulletin of Suicidology, No. 6,
pp. 41-44.

Training and courses available through the Los
Angeles Suicide Prevention Center are
discussed.

7-070   Leviton, D. (1969). The need for education on
death and suicide. Journal of School Health, 39,
270-274. (Reprinted in B. Q. Hafen & E. J. Faux
(Eds.) (1972), Self-destructive behavior: A
national crisis (pp. 242-248). Minneapolis, MN:
Burgess.)

7-071   Leviton, D. (1971). Death, bereavement and suicide
education. In D. A. Read (Ed.), New directions
in health education: Some contemporary issues
for the emerging age (pp. 179-203,
esp. pp. 190-196, "Suicide and suicide
prevention"). New York: Macmillan.

7-072   Leviton, D. (1971). A course on death education
and suicide prevention: Implications for health
education. Journal of the American College
Health Association, 19, 217-220.

7-073   Leviton, D., & Leviton, S. (1969). Education for
death: Health education at the University of
Maryland. Journal of Health, Physical Education,
Recreation, 40, 46-51.

7-074   Light, D., Jr. (1976). Professional problems in
treating suicidal persons. Omega, 7, 59-68.

Light describes the generally inadequate
training of clinicians regarding the suicidal.

* 7-075   Maris, R. W., Dorpat, T. L., Hathorne, B. C.,
Heilig, S. M., Powell, W. J., Stone, H., & Ward,
H. P. (1973). Education and training in
suicidology for the seventies. In
H. L. P. Resnik & B. C. Hathorne (Eds.), Suicide
prevention in the 70's (pp. 23-44). Washington,
D.C.: USGPO, DHEW Publication No. (HSM) 72-9054.
[SuDoc No. HE 20.2402: Su 3]

Recommendations regarding curriculum and
training for professionals, non-professionals,
and paraprofessionals are outlined.

7-076   Peck, M. L. (1970, Spring). Research and training
in prevention of suicide in adolescents and
youths. Bulletin of Suicidology, No. 6,
pp. 35-40 (esp. pp. 39-40).

Training programs for various agencies and
groups encountering suicidal youths are
briefly discussed.

7-077   Perlin, S., & Schmidt, C. W. (1971). A fellowship
         program for the study of suicide and suicide
         prevention. In J. Zusman & D. L. Davidson
         (Eds.), Organizing the community to prevent
         suicide (pp. 43-51). Springfield, IL: Thomas.

         A description is presented of a late
         1960's-1970's government-funded fellowship
         program in suicidology and especially its
         curriculum.

7-078   Phillips, W. C. (1983). Suicide education for
         residence staff: Identification, intervention,
         and referral. Journal of College Student
         Personnel, 24, 376-378.

         To heighten awareness and sensitivity to
         suicide on resident campuses, a specific model
         is presented for training residence hall
         staff.

* 7-079 Resnik, H. L. P., & Hathorne, B. C. (1974).
         Teaching outlines in suicide studies and crisis
         intervention. Bowie, MD: Charles Press.

         In addition to its bibliographic potentials as
         outlined in Chapter 1, though now dated this
         source provides outlines of lectures/
         presentations on topics representing a broad
         and comprehensive coverage of the field of
         suicidology.

7-080   Sanborn, D. E., III, Sanborn, C. J., & Niswander,
         G. D. (1971). Role of education in reporting
         attempted suicide. Diseases of the Nervous
         System, 32, 467-471.

7-081   Shein, H. (1976). Suicide care: Obstacles in the
         education of psychiatric residents. Omega, 7,
         75-81.

* 7-082 Suicide prevention training manual. (1978).
         Dallas: American Association of Suicidology [in
         cooperation with Health Information Services,
         West Point, PA: Merck, Sharp, & Dohm, a division
         of Merck & Co., Inc.].

7-083   Wallace, M. A., & Morley, W. E. (1970). Teaching
         crisis intervention. American Journal of
         Nursing, 70, 1484-1487.

         This article includes some specific
         suggestions regarding the training of
         personnel to deal with suicidal consultees.

7.5 Clues to Suicide

7-084   Davis, P. A. (1983). Suicidal adolescents
        (pp. 41-43). Springfield, IL: Thomas, Chapter
        5, "Prodomal clues."

7-085   Giffin, M., & Felsenthal, C. (1983). A cry for
        help (pp. 39-74). Garden City, NY: Doubleday,
        Chapter 3, "Distress signals." [Popular Press]

        Sixteen "clues" or potential warning signs to
        suicide are discussed in this book about child
        and adolescent suicide.

7-086   Grollman, E. A. (1971). Suicide: Prevention,
        intervention, postvention (pp. 71-84). Boston:
        Beacon Press, Chapter 5, "Clues to suicide:
        Prevention."

7-087   Grollman, E. A. (1974). What you should know about
        suicide. In E. A. Grollman (Ed.), Concerning
        death: A practical guide for the living
        (pp. 313-332, esp. pp. 319-322, "How do you know
        if a person is suicide prone?"). Boston: Beacon
        Press.

7-088   Hersh, S. P. (1975). Suicide: Youth's high
        vulnerability to it/Signs to look for/How can you
        help. MH, 59(3), 23-25.

7-089   Kiev, A. (1979). The courage to live (pp. 9-22).
        New York: Crowell, Chapter 2, "Signs of
        depression."

7-090   Mason, S. (1979). Warning signs of impending
        suicide. Carolina Law, 29, 28-33.

7-091   Miller, M. (1979). Protecting your family and
        friends from suicide. Long Term Care & Health
        Service Administration Quarterly, 3, 98-101.

        Miller discusses numerous clues to suicide
        potential and action to be taken to prevent
        suicide.

7-092   Osgood, N. J. (1982). Suicide in the elderly: Are
        we heeding the warnings. Postgraduate Medicine,
        72, 123-130.

        Osgood provides a number of potential clues to
        suicide among the elderly.

* 7-093 Shneidman, E. S. (1965, May). Preventing suicide.
        American Journal of Nursing, 65(5), 111-116.
        (Reprinted in J. P. Gibbs (Ed.) (1968), Suicide
        (pp. 255-266). New York: Harper & Row.

Reprinted in Bulletin of Suicidology, December
1968, No. 4, pp. 19-25. Reprinted in
E. S. Shneidman, N. L. Farberow, & R. E. Litman
(Eds.) (1970), The psychology of suicide
(pp. 429-440). New York: Science House.
Reprinted in B. Q. Hafen & E. J. Faux (Eds.)
(1971), Self-destructive behavior: A national
crisis (pp. 256-265). Minneapolis, MN: Burgess.
Reprinted in R. F. Weir (Ed.) (1977), Ethical
issues in death and dying (pp. 363-373). New
York: Columbia University Press. Reprinted as
"The warning signs of suicide." In M. Miller
(Ed.) (1982), Suicide intervention by nurses
(pp. 31-45). New York: Springer.)

A highly-recommended and outstanding
presentation of possible suicide warning
signs. Although originally written for
nurses, this article is easily generalized.
Shneidman proposes four categories of clues
and provides examples of each: verbal,
behavioral, situational, syndromatic.

7-094   Singer, R. G., & Blumenthal, I. J. (1969).
Suicidal clues in psychotic patients. Mental
Hygiene, 53, 346-350.

14 patterns of behavior which could be suicide
clues among psychotic individuals are
described.

7-095   Victoroff, V. M. (1983). The suicidal patient:
Recognition, intervention, management
(pp. 49-62). Oradell, NJ: Medical Economics
Books, Chapter 6, "Clues to suicide."

Victoroff discusses aspects of patients'
histories which may be of use to the physician
in recognizing the suicidal.

7-096   Wekstein, L. (1979). Handbook of suicidology:
Principles, problems, and practice (pp. 53-56,
"Prodromal signs and clues"). New York:
Brunner/Mazel.

7.6 Communication of Suicide Clues and Warning Signs

* 7-097   Bernstein, M. (1978-79). The communication of
suicidal intent by completed suicides. Omega, 9,
175-182.

A review of the literature is presented.

7-098   Cowgell, V. G. (1977). Interpersonal effects of a
suicidal communication. Journal of Consulting
and Clinical Psychology, 45, 592-599.

7-099   Delong, W. B., & Robins, E. (1961). The
         communication of suicidal intent prior to
         psychiatric hospitalization: A study of 87
         patients. American Journal of Psychiatry, 117,
         695-705.

7-100   Dorpat, T. L., & Boswell, J. W. (1963). An
         evaluation of suicidal intent in suicide
         attempts. Comprehensive Psychiatry, 4, 117-125.

         It was observed that completed suicides
         communicate their intent more than do
         attempters and that those who make serious
         attempts communicate more than those who make
         gestures.

7-101   Fawcett, J., Leff, M., & Bunney, W. E., Jr. (1969).
         Suicide: Clues from interpersonal communication.
         Archives of General Psychiatry, 21, 129-137.

7-102   Fowler, R. C., Tsuang, M. T., & Kronfol, Z. (1979).
         Communication of suicidal intent and suicide in
         unipolar depression: A forty year follow-up.
         Journal of Affective Disorders, 1, 219-225.

7-103   Hudgens, R. W. (1974). Psychiatric disorders in
         adolescents (pp. 90-107). Baltimore: Williams &
         Wilkins, Chapter 5, "Suicide communications and
         attempts."

         The results of a study of 60 adolescent
         psychiatric inpatients for the incidence of
         various types of communications of suicidal
         intent (i.e., clues) are presented. Of the 60
         adolescents, 40 (67%) had communicated clues
         at some time in their lives. In addition,
         adolescent communications are compared to
         non-communicators on several dimensions.

7-104   Kovacs, M., Beck, A., & Weissman, A. (1976). The
         communication of suicidal intent: A
         reexamination. Archives of General Psychiatry,
         33, 198-201.

* 7-105 Lester, D. (1972). Why people kill themselves: A
         summary of research findings on suicidal behavior
         (pp. 238-241). Springfield, IL: Thomas, Chapter
         21, "Communication and the suicidal act."

7-106   Lester, D. (1983). Why people kill themselves: A
         1980's summary of research findings on suicidal
         behavior (2nd ed.) (pp. 101-105,
         esp. pp. 102-104, "Communication of intent").
         Springfield, IL: Thomas, Chapter 17,
         "Communication and the suicidal act."

7-107   Lester, G., & Lester, D. (1971). Suicide: The
         gamble with death (pp. 74-81, esp. pp. 74-76).
         Englewood Cliffs, NJ: Prentice-Hall, Chapter 10,
         "Suicidal communications and the suicide note."

* 7-108 Murphy, G. E., & Robins, E. (1968). Communication
         of suicidal ideas. In H. L. P. Resnik (Ed.),
         Suicidal behaviors: Diagnosis and management
         (pp. 163-170). Boston: Little, Brown.

7-109   Robins, E., Gassner, S., Kayes, J., Wilkinson,
         R. H., Jr., & Murphy, G. E. (1959). The
         communication of suicidal intent: A study of 134
         consecutive cases of successful (completed)
         suicides. American Journal of Psychiatry, 115,
         724-733. (Reprinted in W. A. Rushing (Ed.)
         (1969), Deviant behavior and social process
         (pp. 251-259). Chicago: Rand McNally.
         Reprinted in A. Giddens (Ed.) (1971), The
         sociology of suicide: A selection of readings
         (pp. 359-374). London: Cass.)

7-110   Rudestam, K. E. (1971). Stockholm and Los Angeles:
         A cross-cultural study of the communication of
         suicidal intent. Journal of Consulting and
         Clinical Psychology, 36, 82-90.

7-111   Rudestam, K. E. (1972). The "noncommunicating
         suicide": Does he exist? Omega, 3, 97-102.

7-112   Stevenson, E., Hudgens, R., Held, C., Meredith, C.,
         Hendrix, M., & Carr, D. (1972). Suicidal
         communication by adolescents: A study of two
         matched groups of 60 teenagers. Diseases of the
         Nervous System, 33, 112-122. (Abstract: PA,
         1972, 48, No. 11855, p. 1290)

7-113   Tayal, S. S. (1969). The communication of suicidal
         ideation in art therapy. Psychiatry & Art, 2,
         205-209.

7-114   Tsuang, M. T., & Kronfol, Z. (1979). Communication
         of suicidal intent and suicide in unipolar
         depression: A forty-year follow-up. Journal of
         Affective Disorders, 1, 219-225.

7-115   Wekstein, L. (1979). Handbook of suicidology:
         Principles, problems, and practice (pp. 62-64,
         "Communication of intent"). New York:
         Brunner/Mazel.

7-116   Yessler, P. G., Gibbs, J. J., & Becker,
         H. A. (1960). On the communication of suicidal
         ideas: I. Some sociological and behavioral
         considerations. Archives of General Psychiatry,
         3, 612-631.

7-117   Yessler, P. G., Gibbs, J. J., & Becker,
        H. A. (1961). On the communication of suicidal
        ideas: II. Some medical considerations.
        Archives of General Psychiatry, 5, 12-29.

See also Ansbacher (1969, 1970, references 4-049 and 4-050)
for a coverage of Adler's theory of suicide as
communication.

See also Farberow & Simon (1975, reference 5-430.10),
pp. 190-191 and Rudestam (1975, reference 5-430.05),
pp. 125-131 for cultural differences in the communication of
suicidal intent.

7.7 Recognition of Suicide Risk and Potential

7-118   Bascue, L. O., Inman, D. J., & Kahn, W. J. (1982).
        Recognition of suicidal lethality factors by
        psychiatric nursing assistants. Psychological
        Reports, 51, 197-198. (Abstract: CPA, 1982, 22,
        No. 2712, p. 579)

        Suicidal attitudinal items and a lethality
        scale (to assess the ability to predict
        potential suicide) were administered.

7-119   Bennett, A. E. (1967, May). Recognizing the
        potential suicide. Geriatrics, 22, 175-181.

7-120   Burdick, B. M., Holmes, C. B., & Waln,
        R. F. (1983). Recognition of suicide signs by
        physicians in different areas of specialization.
        Journal of Medical Education, 58, 716-721.

7-121   Burstein, A. G., Adams, R. L., & Giffen,
        M. B. (1973). Assessment of suicidal risk by
        psychology and psychiatry trainees. Archives of
        General Psychiatry, 29, 792-793.

7-122   Holmes, C. B., & Gilbert, J. F. (1983). Comparison
        of master's and doctoral level psychologists in
        recognizing signs of potential suicide.
        Psychological Reports, 53, 516-518.

7-123   Holmes, C. B., & Howard, M. E. (1980). Recognition
        of suicide lethality factors by physicians,
        mental health professionals, ministers, and
        college students. Journal of Consulting and
        Clinical Psychology, 48, 383-387. (Abstract:
        PA, 1980, 64, No. 4015, p. 436)

7-124   Holmes, C. B., & Wurtz, P. J. (1981). Counselor's
        recognition of factors in lethality of suicide.
        Psychological Reports, 49, 183-186. (Abstract:
        CPA, 1982, 22, No. 2722, p. 581)

7-125   Kaplan, R. D., Kottler, D. B., & Frances,
        A. J. (1982). Reliability and rationality in the
        prediction of suicide. Hospital and Community
        Psychiatry, 33, 212-215. (Abstract: SWRA, 1983,
        19, No. 1132, p. 77)

7-126   Patterson, W. M., Dohn, H. H., Bird, J., &
        Patterson, G. A. (1983). Evaluation of suicidal
        patients: The SAD PERSONS scale.
        Psychosomatics, 24, 343-352.

        An acronym for 10 suicide risk factors is
        presented that are employed and taught as a
        scale. This acronym is suggested as teachable
        in a single lecture and increases one's
        ability to recognize suicidal individuals.

7-127   Shochet, B. R. (1969). Recognizing the suicidal
        patient. Maryland Medical Journal, 18, 65-67.

7-128   Steele, T. E. (1975). Evaluation of first-year
        medical student's ability to recognize suicidal
        potential. Journal of Medical Education, 50,
        203-205.

7-129   West, D. A., & DiVasto, P. V. (1982). Suicide
        potential evaluation by nonpsychiatrists.
        Postgraduate Medicine, 72, 203-205, 208-212.

7-130   Zee, H. J. (1972). Blindspots in recognizing
        serious suicidal intentions. Bulletin of the
        Menninger Clinic, 36, 551-555.

Chapter 8
ETHICS OF SUICIDE:
MORAL, PHILOSOPHICAL, RELIGIOUS, AND LEGAL ASPECTS

Controversy over the ethics of suicide have long raged
among philosophers and in the religious community (see
Sections 8.3 and 8.4). For example, Camus in The Myth of
Sysiphus stated that: "There is but one philosophical
problem: whether or not to commit suicide." Recently,
those controversies have been brought to the fore by many
forces: changes in resuscitation and life-preserving
technologies, longer life expectancies, publicized
"rational" suicides, and "how-to" manuals (providing
explicit and specific information regarding methods of
suicide) which have been published in several countries.
The media and literature also provide us with examples of
easy and accepted suicide (see, e.g., Kurt Vonnegut's short
story "Welcome to the Monkey House," a futuristic portrayal
of an overpopulated world in which people are encouraged to
go to suicide centers to be assisted in dying; A 1970s
movie with Charlton Heston and Edward G. Robinson entitled
"Soylent Green" presented a similar theme; A 1980 PBS
presentation of "Rational Suicide" which presented Jo
Roman's suicide is another example, see references 8-003,
8-062, 8-044 and 8-045).

These moral, philosophical and religious arguments are
joined also by legal discussions regarding issues such as
the right to intervene by suicide prevention services, the
right of the individual to commit suicide, assisted suicide
and euthanasia, and failure to prevent suicides (e.g.,
malpractice suits). Suicide shares the ranks of topics such
as the determination of the point of death and life,
abortion, and euthanasia in polarity, disagreement,
controversy, and uncertainty. This can be seen most clearly
by the fact that there exists in our cultures both suicide
prevention agencies as well as suicide assisting
organizations (e.g., EXIT in Great Britain, and HEMLOCK in
the U.S.). Society has been generally unable or unwilling
to resolve or consider these problems. As can be seen by
the number of references (some of them quite recent, e.g.,
Battin, 1982, Battin & Mayo, 1980, Battin & Maris, 1983,

references 8-005, 8-007, 8-006), on this aspect of suicide, much has been said and written on both sides of the arguments but the morality of suicide remains an unresolved issue.

8.1 Ethics of Suicide: Bibliographies

8-001   American Association of Suicidology. Legal aspects of suicide [Annotated bibliography]. Denver, CO: AAS.

8-002   Miller, M. Non-annotated bibliographies. San Diego, CA: Center for Information on Suicide. 1984 Catalog includes:

8-002.01   Ethics of intervention. Bibliography No. R-19.
8-002.02   Religion and suicide. Bibliography No. R-26.
8-002.03   Malpractice and suicide. Bibliography No. R-46.
8-002.04   Suicide/Right to die. Bibliography No. R-48.

See also Farberow et al. (1961, reference 1-004), sections on "Medical-Legal" and "Religious-Philosophical."

8.2 Ethics/Morality/Rationality of Suicide

8-003   Backer, B. A., Hannon, N., & Russell, N. A. (1982). Death and dying: Individuals and institutions (pp. 304-308, "Rational suicide"). New York: Wiley.

Public reaction to the PBS special on Jo Roman's suicide is presented and discussed (see references 8-044, 8-045, & 8-062).

8-004   Barnard, C. (1980). Good life, good death: A doctor's case for euthanasia and suicide (esp. pp. 105-114). Englewood Cliffs, NJ: Prentice-Hall.

* 8-005   Battin, M. P. (1982). Ethical issues in suicide. Englewood Cliffs, NJ: Prentice-Hall. (Chapter 4 reprinted as "The concept of rational suicide," In E. S. Shneidman (Ed.), Death: Current perspectives (3rd ed.) (pp. 297-320). Palo Alto, CA: Mayfield.)

Discussions of rational suicide (Chapter 4, pp. 131-153) and suicide as a right (Chapter 6, pp. 176-191) are presented as are paternalism (Chapter 5, pp. 154-175), social arguments (Chapter 2, pp. 76-111), and the value of life (Chapter 3, pp. 112-128).

8-006 Battin, M. P., & Maris, R. W. (Eds.) (1983).
Suicide and ethics (A special issue of Suicide
and Life-Threatening Behavior, 13(4).). New
York: Human Sciences Press.

8-006.01 Maris, R. W. Suicide: Rights and
rationality. pp. 223-230.

8-006.02 Battin, M. P. Suicide and ethical theory.
pp. 231-239.

8-006.03 Narveson, J. Self-ownership and the ethics
of suicide. pp. 240-253.

8-006.04 Hill, T. E., Jr. Self-regarding suicide:
A modified Kantian view. pp. 254-275.

8-006.05 Regan, D. H. Suicide and the failure of
modern moral theory. pp. 276-292.

8-006.06 Sartorius, R. Coercive suicide prevention:
A libertian perspective. pp. 293-303.

8-006.07 Motto, J. A. Clinical implications of
moral theory regarding suicide.
pp. 304-312.

8-006.08 Mayo, D. J. Contemporary philosophical
literature on suicide: A review.
pp. 313-345.

* 8-007 Battin, M. P., & Mayo, D. J. (1980). Suicide: The
philosophical issues. New York: St. Martin's
Press.

A collection of excellent articles on the
morality and rationality of suicide as well as
suicide and psychiatry and suicide as a right.
The articles are listed below.

8-007.01 Lebacqz, K., & Engelhardt, H. T.,
Jr. (1977). Suicide and covenant.
pp. 84-89. (Adapted from "Suicide." In
D. J. Horan & D. Mall (Eds.), Death,
dying and euthanasia (pp. 669-705).
Washington, D.C.: University
Publications of America.)

8-007.02 Barrington, M. R. (1969). Apologia for
suicide. pp. 90-103. (Abridged from
A. B. Downing (Ed.), Euthanasia and the
right to death (pp. 152-172). London:
Peter Owen, and Los Angeles: Nash.)
(Reprinted in S. Gorovitz,

A. L. Jameton, R. Macklin,
J. M. O'Connor, E. V. Perrin,
B. P. St. Clair, & S. Sherwin (Eds.)
(1976), Moral problems in medicine
(pp. 396-401). Englewood Cliffs, NJ:
Prentice-Hall. Reprinted in
J. Rubinstein & B. D. Slife (Eds.) (in
press). Taking sides: Clashing views
on controversial psychological issues
(3rd ed.). Guilford, CT: Dushkin.)

8-007.03 Clements, C. D. The ethics of not-being:
Individual options for suicide.
pp. 104-114.

8-007.04 Brandt, R. B. (1975). The rationality of
suicide. pp. 117-132. (From "The
morality and rationality of suicide."
In S. Perlin (Ed.), see reference 8-012
below.)

8-007.05 Mayo, D. J. Irrational suicide.
pp. 133-137.

8-007.06 Devine, P. E. (1978). On choosing death.
pp. 138-143. (Adapted from Devine,
P. E. The ethics of homicide
(pp. 193-202). Ithaca, NY: Cornell
University Press.)

8-007.07 Martin, R. M. Suicide and false desires.
pp. 144-150.

8-007.08 Wood, D. Suicide as instrument and
expression. pp. 151-160.

8-007.09 Oates, J. C. (1979). The art of suicide.
pp. 161-168. (Adapted from The
re-evaluation of existing values and the
search for absolute values (pp. 183-190)
(Proceedings of the Seventh
International Conference on the Unity of
the Sciences, Boston, 1978). New York:
International Cultural Foundation.)

8-007.10 Battin, M. P. Manipulated suicide.
pp. 169-182. (Reprinted in Bioethics
Quarterly, 1980, 2, 123-134.)

8-007.11 Szasz, T. S. (1971). The ethics of
suicide. pp. 185-198. (Reprinted from
The Antioch Review, 31, 7-17. Reprinted
also in R. F. Weir (Ed.) (1977), Ethical
issues in death and dying (pp. 374-386).
New York: Columbia University Press.
Excerpt reprinted in T. L. Beauchamp &

S. Perlin (Eds.) (1978), Ethical issues
in death and dying (pp. 134-138).
Englewood Cliffs, NJ: Prentice-Hall.)

8-007.12 Slater, E. (1970). Choosing the time to
die. pp. 199-204. (From R. Fox (Ed.),
Proceedings of the fifth international
conference for suicide prevention
(London, 1969). Vienna: International
Association for Suicide Prevention,
1970.)

8-007.13 Ringel, E. Suicide prevention and the
value of human life. pp. 205-211.

8-007.14 Motto, J. A. (1972). The right to
suicide: A psychiatrist's view.
pp. 212-220. (Reprinted in S. Gorovitz,
A. L. Jameton, R. Macklin,
J. M. O'Connor, E. V. Perrin,
B. P. St. Clair, & S. Sherwin
(Eds.) (1976), Moral problems in
medicine (pp. 392-396). Englewood
Cliffs, NJ: Prentice-Hall. Reprinted
in J. P. Carse & A. B. Dallery
(Eds.) (1977), Death and society: A
book of readings and sources
(pp. 225-231). New York: Harcourt
Brace Jovanovich.)

8-007.15 Feinberg, J. (1980). Suicide and the
inalienable right to life. pp. 223-228.
(Abridged and revised from
S. M. McMurrin (Ed.), The Tanner
lectures on human values, Volume 1
(pp. 221-257). Salt Lake City:
University of Utah Press. Appears also
as "Voluntary euthanasia and the
inalienable right to life," in
Philosophy and Public Affairs, 1978, 7,
93-123, and reprinted in M. Cohen,
T. Nagel, & T. Scanlon (Eds.) (1981),
Medicine and moral philosophy
(pp. 245-275). Princeton, NJ:
Princeton University Press.)

8-007.16 Sullivan, A. L. A constitutional right to
suicide. pp. 229-253.

8-007.17 Battin, M. P. Suicide: A fundamental
right? pp. 267-285.

8-007.18 Bogen, J. Suicide and virtue.
pp. 286-292.

8-008 Bender, D. L. (Ed.) (1981). Problems of death:

Opposing viewpoints (2nd ed.) (pp. 105-142).
St. Paul, MN: Greenhaven Press, Chapter 3, "Is
suicide ever justified?" (1st ed., 1974, Chapter
4, "Suicide," pp. 114-125.)

This 1981 book includes 6 articles on suicide,
5 of which relate to the justification of
suicide. Three are listed here and two are
listed in section 8.4.

8-008.01   Tonne, H. A. (1979). Suicide as a sign of
civilization. pp. 106-111. (Reprinted
from "Suicide: Is it autoeuthanasia?"
Humanist, 39(4), 44-45.)

8-008.02   Barrington, M. R. (1969). Suicide is our
right. pp. 117-122. (Reprinted from
"Apologia for suicide." See reference
8-007.02 above. Appeared in Bender
(1974), pp. 114-119.)

8-008.03   Portwood, D. (1978). Common-sense suicide
for the elderly. pp. 128-132.
(Reprinted from reference 8-056 below.)

8-009   Bernard, M. L., & Bernard, J. L. (1980).
Institutional responses to the suicidal student:
Ethical and legal considerations. Journal of
College Student Personnel, 21(2), 109-113.

8-010   Beskow, J. (1972). Inevitable suicides? In
J. Waldenstrom, T. Larsson, & N. Ljungstedt
(Eds.), Suicide and attempted suicide
(pp. 293-302). Stockholm: Nordiska Bokhandlens
Forlag.

8-011   Blake, P. (1983, March 21). Going gentle into that
good night: Do suicide manuals create a bias
toward death? Time, p. 85.

A discussion of the controversial suicide
"how-to" manuals that have been published in
Europe. Manuals from Britain and France are
mentioned as are publications of the
U. S. HEMLOCK Society which support "the
option of active voluntary euthanasia for the
terminally ill." The "how-to" manuals and
HEMLOCK publications are:

8-011.01   Guillon, C., & Le Bonniec, Y. (1982).
Suicide mode d'emploi: Histoire,
technique, actualite [Suicide:
Operating instructions]. Paris:
Editions Alain Moreau.

8-011.02   Koestler, A. (1981). EXIT: A guide to

self- deliverance. London: EXIT
(British Voluntary Euthanasia Society).
This book is available only to EXIT
members over 25 and was distributed to
over 8000 members.

8-011.03   Humphrey, D. (1983). Let me die before I
wake: Hemlock's book of self-
deliverance for the dying. Los
Angeles: Hemlock.

8-011.04   Humphrey, D. (Ed.). (1982). Assisted
suicide: The compassionate crime [A
compilation of famous euthanasia
cases]. Los Angeles: Hemlock.

8-011.05   Humphrey, D., & Wickett, A. (1978).
Jean's way. New York: Quartet Books.
(2nd ed., 1981)

8-012   Brandt, R. B. (1975). The morality and rationality
of suicide. In S. Perlin (Ed.), A handbook for
the study of suicide (pp. 61-76). New York:
Oxford University Press. (Reprinted in
T. L. Beauchamp & S. Perlin (Eds.) (1978),
Ethical issues in death and dying (pp. 122-133).
Englewood Cliffs, NJ: Prentice-Hall. Reprinted
in J. Rachels (Ed.) (1979), Moral problems: A
collection of philosophical essays (3rd ed.)
(pp. 460-489) [2nd ed., 1975, pp. 363-387.] New
York: Harper & Row. Reprinted in T. A. Mappes &
J. S. Zembaty (Eds.) (1981). Biomedical ethics
(pp. 312-319). New York: McGraw-Hill. See also
references 8-007.04 above and 8-013 below.)

8-013   Brandt, R. B. (1976). The morality and rationality
of suicide. In E. S. Shneidman (Ed.),
Suicidology: Contemporary developments
(pp. 378-399). New York: Grune & Stratton.
(Parts of this paper appeared in Perlin, 1975,
reference 8-012 above.)

8-014a Brandt, R. B. (1979). A suicide attempt and
emergency room ethics: Commentary. Hastings
Center Report, 9(4), 12-13.

8-014b Bromberg, S., & Cassel, C. K. (1983). Suicide in
the elderly: The limits of paternalism. Journal
of the American Geriatrics Society, 31, 698-703.

8-015   Brown, J. H. (1981, March 21). Is suicide ever
rational [Letter]? Lancet, 1(8221), 660-661.

8-016a Burke, A. W. (1982). Last exit--Analysis of a
guide to suicide. Midwife Health Visitor and
Community Nurse, 18, 438, 440, 442.

A discussion of whether "how-to" guides to suicide are humane.

8-016b Childress, J. F., Roettinger, R. L., Siegler, M., & Thorup, O. A., Jr. (1982, Fall). Voluntary exit: Is there a case for rational suicide?--A panel discussion. The Pharos, 45(4), 25-31.

8-017 Choron, J. (1972). Suicide (pp. 96-101). New York: Charles Scribner's Sons, Chapter 11, "The problem of 'rational suicide'."

8-018 Clements, C. D., Sider, R. C., & Perlmutter, R. A. (1982). The ethics of suicide: Act and intervention. In D. Teichler-Zallen & C. D. Clements (Eds.), Science and morality: New directions in bioethics (pp. 239-251). Lexington, MA: Lexington Books.

8-019 Clements, C. D., Sider, R. C., & Perlmutter, R. (1983). Suicide: Bad act or good intervention. Suicide and Life-Threatening Behavior, 13, 28-41.

These authors critique the "rational suicide" notion as inappropriate and instead focus on the ethical justification of intervention.

8-020 Cutter, F. (1983). Art and the wish to die (pp. 223-248). Chicago: Nelson-Hall, Chapter 10, "Suicide: The right to commit versus the right to prevent."

8-021 Death my only love. (1977). Journal of Medical Ethics, 3, 93-97.

The presentation of a case history of a suicide and discussions of it by a philosopher, a barrister, and a general practitioner.

8-022 deCatanzaro, D. (1981). Suicide and self-damaging behavior: A sociobiological perspective (pp. 139-146). New York: Academic Press, Chapter 11, "Ethics and suicide."

8-023 Decker, N. (1977). The wish to die: Pathological depression or rational decision? In W. E. Fann, I. Karacan, A. D. Pokorny & R. L. Williams (Eds.), Phenomenonlogy and treatment of depression (pp. 187-195). New York: Spectrum Publications.

8-024 Diggory, J. C. (1968). Suicide and value. In H. L. P. Resnik (Ed.), Suicidal behaviors:

Diagnosis and management (pp. 3-18). Boston:
Little Brown.

8-025   Donnelly, J. (1978). Suicide and rationality. In
J. Donnelly (Ed.), *Language, metaphysics, and*
death (pp. 88-105). New York: Fordham
University Press.

8-026   Grisez, G. (1977). Suicide and euthanasia. In
D. J. Horan & D. Mall (Eds.), *Death, dying and*
euthanasia (pp. 742-817). Washington, D.C.:
University Publications of America.

8-027   Hauerwas, S. (1981). Rational suicide and reasons
for living. In M. D. Basson (Ed.), *Rights and*
responsibilities in modern medicine: The second
volume in a series on ethics, humanism, and
medicine (pp. 185-199). New York: Liss.
[Published also as part of volume 50 of *Progress*
in Clinical and Biological Research, see
reference 8-060.]

8-028   Heifetz, M. D. (1975). *The right to die: A*
neurosurgeon speaks of death with candor
(pp. 73-98). New York: Putnam, Chapter 7,
"Suicide: A right?"

8-029   Heilig, S. M. (1977). Suicide prevention: A
personal statement. In C. L. Hatton,
S. M. Valente, & A. Rink (Eds.), *Suicide:*
Assessment and intervention (pp. 205-211). New
York: Appleton-Century-Crofts. (2nd ed., Hatton
& Valente, 1984, pp. 256-261.)

          The right to suicide and the ethicality of
          suicide prevention are discussed.

8-030   Hendin, H. (1982). *Suicide in America*
(pp. 209-228). New York: Norton, Chapter 11,
"The right to suicide." (Reprinted in
J. Rubinstein & B. D. Slife (Eds.) (in press).
Taking sides: Clashing views on controversial
psychological issues (3rd ed.). Guilford, CT:
Dushkin.)

8-031   Heyd, D., & Bloch, S. (1981). The ethics of
suicide. In S. Bloch & P. Chodoff (Eds.),
Psychiatric ethics (pp. 185-202). New York:
Oxford University Press.

8-032   Hillman, J. (1964). *Suicide and the soul.* New
York: Harper & Row. (Reprinted, New York:
Harper, 1973; Zurich, Switzerland: Spring
Publications, 1976; Irving, TX: Spring
Publications, 1978.)

The ethics of suicide are discussed and
chapter 2 includes viewpoints on suicide
prevention of the law, theology, and medicine.

8-033   Hipple, J., & Cimbolic, P. (1979). The counselor
and suicidal crisis: Diagnosis and intervention
(pp. 94-100). Springfield, IL: Thomas, Chapter
9, "Legal and ethical considerations for the
suicidal crisis."

8-034   Holland, R. F. (1975). Suicide. In J. Rachels
(Ed.), Moral problems: A collection of
philosophical essays (2nd ed.) (pp. 388-400).
[1st ed., 1971, pp. 345-359.] New York: Harper &
Row.

8-035   Hook, S. (1975). The ethics of suicide. In
M. Kohl (Ed.), Beneficient euthanasia
(pp. 57-69). Buffalo, NY: Prometheus Books,
(Reprinted from The International Journal of
Ethics, 1927, 37, 173-188.)

8-036   Horowitz, L. (1972). The morality of suicide.
Journal of Critical Analysis, 3, 161-165.

It is argued that suicide is morally neutral
and is the choice of the individual.

8-037   Jacobs, J. (1982). The moral justification of
suicide. Springfield, IL: Charles C. Thomas.

A collection of 8 revised and abridged papers
published by Jacobs from 1966 to 1982,
including reference 8-110. Also included is a
previously unpublished Chapter 1, "On the
nature of moral justifications and their
relationship to suicide," pp. 3-16.

8-038   Kobler, A. L. (1980). Suicide: Right and reason.
Bioethics Quarterly, 2, 46-55.

8-039   Landsberg, P. L. (1953). The experience of death;
The moral problem of suicide (C. Rowland, Trans.)
(pp. 65-97). New York: Philosophical Library.
(Originally published, 1936.) (Reprinted, New
York: Arno Press, 1977.)

8-040   Lester, D. (1969). Suicide as a positive act.
Psychology, 6(3), 43-48.

8-041   Lester, D. (1977). Bereavement and suicide: A
positive perspective. In B. L. Danto &
A. H. Kutscher (Eds.), Suicide and bereavement
(pp. 194-198). New York: MSS Information
Corporation.

Lester argues that suicide may at times be
appropriate and that the bereavement of the
survivors may be an experience from which
growth and self-actualization may occur.

8-042 Litman, R. E. (1979). A suicide attempt and
emergency room ethics: Commentary. Hastings
Center Report, 9(4), 12-13.

8-043 Lum, D. (1974). Responding to suicidal crisis:
For church and community (pp. 61-82). Grand
Rapids, MI: William B. Eerdmans, Chapter 4,
"Formulating ethical guidelines on suicide."

Theological ethics regarding suicide are
discussed.

8-044 Maris, R. (1982). Rational suicide: An
impoverished self-transformation. Suicide and
Life-Threatening Behavior, 12, 4-16.

8-045 Maris, R. (1982). Review of Exit house [By
J. Roman, see reference 8-062 below]. Suicide
and Life-Threatening Behavior, 12, 123-126.

8-046 May, J. D. (1980). Paternalism and self-interest.
Journal of Value Inquiry, 14, 195-216.

The justifications of paternalistic suicide
prevention are discussed.

8-047 McCartney, J. R. (1978). Suicide vs. the right to
refuse treatment in the chronically ill.
Psychosomatics, 19, 548-551.

6-048 McCartney, J. R. (1979). Refusal of treatment:
Suicide or competent choice. General Hospital
Psychiatry, 1, 338-343.

8-049 McConnell, T. A. (1968). Suicide ethics in
cross-disciplinary perspective. Journal of
Religion and Health, 7, 7-25.

8-050 Moskop, J., & Engelhardt, H. T., Jr. (1979). The
ethics of suicide: A secular view. In
L. D. Hankoff & B. Einsidler (Eds.), Suicide:
Theory and clinical aspects (pp. 49-57).
Littleton, MA: PSG Publishing.

8-051 Motto, J. A. (1981). Rational suicide and medical
ethics. In M. D. Basson (Ed.), Rights and
responsibilities in modern medicine: The second
volume in a series on ethics, humanism, and
medicine (pp. 201-209). New York: Liss.
[Published also as part of volume 50 of Progress
in Clinical and Biological Research, see

reference 8-060.]

8-052   Murphy, G. E. (1973). Suicide and the right to
        die. American Journal of Psychiatry, 130,
        472-473. (Reprinted in S. Gorovitz,
        A. L. Jameton, R. Macklin, J. M. O'Connor,
        E. V. Perrin, B. P. St. Clair, & S. Sherwin
        (Eds.) (1976), Moral problems in medicine
        (pp. 387-388). Englewood Cliffs, NJ:
        Prentice-Hall.)

8-053   Nelson, F. L. (1978-79). Aggression and suicide:
        A critical evaluation of the suicide prevention
        ethic. Omega, 9, 167-174.

8-054   Nielsen, H. A. (1979). Margolis on rational
        suicide: An argument for case studies in ethics.
        Ethics, 89, 394-400.

8-055   O'Sullivan, R. (1956). The ethics of
        suicide--Aquinas and the common law. The
        Catholic Lawyer, 2, 146-148.

8-056   Portwood, D. (1978). Common-sense suicide: The
        final right. New York: Dodd, Mead. (Excerpt
        reprinted as "A right to suicide?" in Psychology
        Today, January 1978, pp. 66, 68, 71, 73-74, 76.
        See Bender, 1981, reference 8-008, above also.)

8-057   Pretzel, P. W. (1968, July). Philosophical and
        ethical considerations of suicide prevention.
        Bulletin of Suicidology, pp. 30-38. (Reprinted
        in B. Q. Hafen & E. J. Faux (Eds.) (1972),
        Self-destuctive behavior: A national crisis
        (pp. 269-284). Minneapolis, MN: Burgess.
        Reprinted in R. F. Weir (Ed.) (1977), Ethical
        issues in death and dying (pp. 387-400). New
        York: Columbia University Press.)

8-058   Pretzel, P. W. (1972). Understanding and
        counseling the suicidal person (pp. 200-225).
        Nashville, TN: Abingdon, Chapter 6, "The
        rational suicide."

8-059   Pretzel, P. W. (1977). Suicide prevention: A
        personal statement. In C. L. Hatton,
        S. M. Valente, & A. Rink (Eds.), Suicide:
        Assessment and intervention. New York:
        Appleton-Century-Crofts. (2nd ed., Hatton &
        Valente, 1984, pp. 249-256.)

        The right to suicide and the ethics of suicide
        prevention are discussed.

8-060   Rational suicide. (1981). Progress in Clinical and
        Biological Research, 50, 179-212.

The issue of rational suicide is considered in the context of medical ethics. Included are a case study and two divergent viewpoints regarding the case and rational suicide in general.

8-060.01 Basson, M. D. Introduction: Rational suicide. pp. 179-181.

8-060.02 The rational suicide: Case for discussion. pp. 183-184.

8-060.03 Hauerwas, S. Rational suicide and reasons for living. pp. 185-199.

8-060.04 Motto, J. A. Rational suicide and medical ethics. pp. 201-209.

8-060.05 Basson, M. D. Discussion summary: Rational suicide. pp. 211-212.

8-061 Rauscher, W. V. (1981). The case against suicide. New York: St. Martin's Press.

This book presents chapters on several ethical issues, including "The case for suicide?" (pp. 3-14), "The case against suicide" (pp. 67-78), "The philosophers and theologians" (pp. 79-91), and "The case against rational suicide" (pp. 92-102).

8-062 Roman, J. (1980). Exit house: Choosing suicide as an alternative. New York: Seaview Books.

A woman who later committed suicide describes her own feelings about rational suicide.

8-063 Schwyn, E. (1976). Ethical norms of suicide prevention and crisis intervention. Mental Health and Society, 3, 142-147.

8-064 Siegel, K. (1982). Rational suicide: Considerations for the clinician. Psychiatric Quarterly, 54, 77-84. (Abstract: PA, 1983, 69, No. 12961, pp. 1431-1432)

8-065 Siegel, K. (1982). Society, suicide, and social policy. Journal of Psychiatric Treatment & Evaluation, 4, 473-482. (Abstract: PA, 1983, 70, No. 8404, pp. 940-941)

8-066 Slater, E. (1976). Assisted suicide: Some ethical considerations. International Journal of Health Services, 6, 321-330.

8-067   Soble, A. (1982). Paternalism, liberal theory, and
        suicide. Canadian Journal of Philosophy, 12,
        335-352.

8-068   Szasz, T. L. (1976). The ethics of suicide. In
        B. B. Wolman (Ed.), Between survival and suicide
        (pp. 163-183). New York: Gardner Press.

8-069   Szasz, T. L. (1979). A critique of professional
        ethics. In L. D. Hankoff & B. Einsidler (Eds.),
        Suicide: Theory and clinical aspects
        (pp. 59-72). Littleton, MA: PSG Publishing.
        (Reprinted from Szasz, T. L. (1977). The
        theology of medicine: The political-
        philosophical foundations of medical ethics
        (pp. 68-85). New York: Harper & Row.)

8-070   Thaller, O. F. (1982). The ethics of suicide: A
        clinician's point of view. In D. Teichler-Zallen
        & C. D. Clements (Eds.), Science and morality:
        New directions in bioethics (pp. 233-238).
        Lexington, MA: Lexington Books.

8-071   Tolhurst, W. E. (1983). Suicide, self-sacrifice
        and coercion. Southern Journal of Philosophy,
        21, 109-122.

8-072   Tonne, H. A. (1974, November/December). The right
        to suicide. Humanist, 34(6), 33-34.

8-073   Victoroff, V. M. (1983). The suicidal patient:
        Recognition, intervention, management
        (pp. 163-172). Oradell, NJ: Medical Economics
        Books, Chapter 14, "The right to suicide."

8-074   Wallace, S. E., & Eser, A. (1981). Suicide and
        euthanasia: The rights of personhood.
        Knoxville: University of Tennessee Press.

        A collection of writings on suicide and
        euthanasia, including the following 3 which
        are appropriate here.

        8-074.01 Fletcher, J. (1976). In defense of
                  suicide. pp. 38-50. (Translated and
                  reprinted from "In verteidigung des
                  suizids." In A. Eser (Ed.), Suizid und
                  euthanasie. Stuttgart: Enke.)

        8-074.02 Graber, G. C. The rationality of
                  suicide. pp. 51-65.

        8-074.03 Wallace, S. E. The right to live and the
                  right to die. pp. 69-86.

8-075   Widiger, T. A., & Rinaldi, M. (1983). An

acceptance of suicide. <u>Psychotherapy: Theory,</u>
<u>Research and Practice,</u> <u>20</u>, 263-273.

8-076   Wrobleski, A. (1983). <u>Rational suicide: A</u>
<u>contradiction in terms.</u> An address given to the
First Unitarian Society, Minneapolis, MN,
February 27. (Copies available from the author
at 5124 Grove Street, Edina, MN 55436.)

8.3 <u>Philosophers and Suicide</u>

8-077   Beauchamp, T. L., & Perlin, S. (Eds.)   (1978).
<u>Ethical issues in death and dying.</u> Englewood
Cliffs, NJ: Prentice-Hall.

> This book includes a section on suicide where
> the following three articles appear. Aquinas
> discusses the morality (sinfulness) of suicide
> while Hume argues for a right to suicide.

8-077.01   Aquinas, T. Whether it is lawful to kill
oneself. pp. 102-105. (From <u>Summa</u>
<u>theologica</u>, 1925 trans.)

8-077.02   Hume, D. On suicide. pp. 105-110.
(Originally published, 1777.)

8-077.03   Beauchamp, T. L. (1976). An analysis of
Hume and Aquinas on suicide.
pp. 111-121. (Excerpted from "An
analysis of Hume's essay 'On suicide.'"
<u>Review of Metaphysics</u>, <u>30</u>, 73-95.)

8-078   Choron, J. (1972). <u>Suicide</u> (pp. 107-138). New
York: Scribner's, Chapter 13, "Philosophers on
suicide."

8-079   Choron, J. (1984). Philosophers on suicide. In
E. S. Shneidman (Ed.), <u>Death: Current</u>
<u>perspectives</u> (3rd ed.) (pp. 341-361). Palo Alto,
CA: Mayfield. (Reprinted from 8-078 above.)

8-080   Donne, J. (1982). <u>Biathanatos</u> (A modern spelling
edition). New York: Garland. (First printed,
1647; written, 1608.)

> Donne argues against suicide as a sin.

8-081a Dorter, K. (1976). Socrates on life, death and
suicide. <u>Laval Theologique et Philosophique</u>, <u>32</u>,
23-41.

8-081b Duff, R. A. (1982-83). Socratic suicide?
<u>Proceedings of the Aristotelian Society</u>, <u>83</u>,
35-48.

8-082   Fox, M. (1980).   Schopenhauer on death, suicide and
        self-renunciation.   In M. Fox (Ed.),
        Schopenhauer: His philosophical achievement
        (pp. 147-170).   Sussex: Harvester Press.

8-083   Frey, R. G. (1978).   Did Socrates commit suicide?
        Philosophy, 53, 106-108.   [Discussions of Frey's
        argument that Socrates did commit suicide are
        made: Lesser, H. (1980).   Suicide and
        self-murder. Philosophy, 55, 255-257.   Smith,
        M. (1980).   Did Socrates kill himself
        intentionally? Philosophy, 55, 253-254.] (Frey's
        article is reprinted in M. P. Battin & D. J. Mayo
        (Eds.) (1980), Suicide: The philosophical issues
        (pp. 35-38). New York: St. Martins Press.)

8-084   Hume, D. (1963).   Essay on suicide. In R. Abelson
        (Ed.), Ethics and metaethics (pp. 108-116). New
        York: St. Martin's Press. (Reprinted in
        S. Gorovitz, A. L. Jameton, R. Macklin,
        J. M. O'Connor, E. V. Perrin, B. P. St. Clair, &
        S. Sherwin (Eds.) (1976), Moral problems in
        medicine (pp. 381-387). Englewood Cliffs, NJ:
        Prentice-Hall.)

8-085   Kant, I. (1976).   Duties toward the body in regard
        to life. In S. Gorovitz, A. L. Jameton,
        R. Macklin, J. M. O'Connor, E. V. Perrin,
        B. P. St. Clair, & S. Sherwin (Eds.), Moral
        problems in medicine (pp. 376-377). Englewood
        Cliffs, NJ: Prentice-Hall. (Reprinted from
        Kant, I. (1963). Lectures on ethics (L. Infield,
        Trans.) (pp.147-148). New York: Harper & Row.)

8-086   Kant, I. (1976).   Suicide. In S. Gorovitz,
        A. L. Jameton, R. Macklin, J. M. O'Connor,
        E. V. Perrin, B. P. St. Clair, & S. Sherwin
        (Eds.), Moral problems in medicine (pp. 377-381).
        Englewood Cliffs, NJ: Prentice-Hall. (Reprinted
        from Kant, I. (1963). Lectures on ethics
        (L. Infield, Trans.) (pp. 148-154). New York:
        Harper & Row. Reprinted also in T. A. Mappes &
        J. S. Zembaty (Eds.) (1981). Biomedical ethics
        (pp. 309-312). New York: McGraw-Hill.)

8-087   Mijuskovic, B. (1980, January).   Loneliness and
        suicide. Journal of Social Philosophy, 11(1),
        11-17.

8-088   Noon, G. (1978).   On suicide. Journal of the
        History of Ideas, 39, 371-386.

        A discussion of views of suicide by various
        philosophers and others through history is
        presented.

8-089   Novak, D. (1976). Suicide and morality: The
        theories of Plato, Aquinas, and Kant and their
        relevance for suicidology. New York: Scholars
        Studies Press.

        After separate discussions of Plato
        (pp. 17-41), Aquinas (pp. 43-82), and Kant
        (pp. 83-113), Novak presents a unified
        resolution and its potential for suicidology
        (pp. 115-128).

8-090   O'Donohoe, B. P. (1981). Sarte's theories on
        death, murder, and suicide. Philosophy Today,
        25, 334-356.

8-091   Pepper, S. C. (1967). Can a philosophy make one
        philosophical? In E. S. Shneidman (Ed.), Essays
        on self-destruction (pp. 114-128). New York:
        Science House.

8-092   Pretzel, P. W. (1972). Understanding and
        counseling the suicidal person (pp. 175-199).
        Nashville, TN: Abingdon, Chapter 5,
        "Philosophical foundations."

        Pretzel discusses the view of philosophers and
        religious groups regarding suicide.

8-093   Sacharoff, M. (1972). Suicide and Brutus'
        philosophy in 'Julius Caesar.' Journal of the
        History of Ideas, 33, 115-122.

8-094   Seidler, M. J. (1983). Kant and the Stoics on
        suicide. Journal of the History of Ideas, 44,
        429-453.

8-095   Seneca. (1976). On suicide. In S. Gorovitz,
        A. L. Jameton, R. Macklin, J. M. O'Connor,
        E. V. Perrin, B. P. St. Clair, & S. Sherwin
        (Eds.), Moral problems in medicine (p. 376).
        Englewood Cliffs, NJ: Prentice-Hall. (Reprinted
        from R. N. Beck & J. B. Orr (Eds.) (1970),
        Ethical choice (p. 54). New York: Free Press.
        Originally from Epistula Morales Volume 2
        (R. M. Gumere, Trans.). Cambridge, MA: Harvard
        University Press, 1920.)

8-096   Sprott, S. E. (1961). The English debate on
        suicide: From Donne to Hume. LaSalle, IL: Open
        Court.

8-097   Walton, R. E. (1980). Socrates' alleged suicide.
        Journal of Value Inquiry, 14, 287-299.

8-098   Windstrup,G. (1980). Locke on suicide. Political
        Theory, 8, 169-182.

See also Lum (1974, reference 3-015); Battin & Maris (1983, reference 8-006 above).

8.4 Religious Aspects/Viewpoints Regarding Suicide

8-099   Al-Najjar, S. Y. (1976). Suicide and Islamic law. Mental Health and Society, 3, 137-141.

8-100   Baelz, P. R. (1980). Suicide: Some theological reflections. In M. P. Battin & D. J. Mayo (Eds.), Suicide: The philosophical issues (pp. 71-83). New York: St. Martin's Press. (Adapted from "Voluntary euthanasia: Some theological reflections." Theology, 1972, 75, 238-251.)

* 8-101   Battin, M. P. (1982). Ethical issues in suicide (pp. 27-75). Englewood Cliffs, NJ: Prentice-Hall, Chapter 1, "Religious views of suicide."

8-102   Blocher, H. (1981). Suicide is sinful. In D. L. Bender (Ed.), Problems of death: Opposing viewpoints (2nd ed.) (pp. 112-116). St. Paul, MN: Greenhaven Press. (Excerpted from Suicide. Inter-Varsity Christian Fellowship of the U.S.A., 1972.)

8-103   Cassidy, J. P., & Russo, P. M. (1979). Religion: A Catholic view. In L. D. Hankoff & B. Einsidler (Eds.), Suicide: Theory and clinical aspects (pp. 73-81). Littleton, MA: PSG Publishing.

8-104   Close, H. T. (1973). Suicide: A theological perspective. Journal of Pastoral Care, 27, 18-20.

8-105   Demopoulos, A. H. (1970). Suicide and church canon law (Doctoral dissertation, Claremont School of Theology, 1968). Dissertation Abstracts International, 31, 1876-1877A. (University Microfilms No. 70-19,082)

8-106   Dubois, M. J. (1976). Theological reflections on suicide. Mental Health and Society, 3, 148-153.

8-107   Ferracuti, F. (1957). Suicide in a Catholic country. In E. S. Shneidman & N. L. Farberow (Eds.), Clues to suicide (pp. 70-78). New York: McGraw-Hill.

8-108   Heard, G. (1967). Buddha and self-destruction. In E. S. Shneidman (Ed.), Essays in self-destruction (pp. 78-90). New York: Science House.

8-109   Hewett, J. H. (1980). After suicide (pp. 84-98).
        Philadelphia: Westminster Press, Chapter 5,
        "Suicide and your faith."

        A Christian minister speaks to survivors of
        suicide about reconciling the suicidal death
        with their religious beliefs and dealing with
        their faith afterward.

8-110   Jacobs, J. (1970). The use of religion in
        constructing the moral justification of suicide.
        In J. D. Douglas (Ed.), Deviance and
        respectability: The social construction of moral
        meaning (pp. 229-251). New York: Basic Books.
        (Revised and abridged version in Jacobs,
        J. (1982). The moral justification of suicide
        (pp. 43-66). Springfield, IL: Charles
        C. Thomas.)

8-111   Lepp, I. (1981). Christianity rejects suicide. In
        D. L. Bender (Ed.), Problems of death: Opposing
        viewpoints (2nd ed.) (pp. 123-127). St. Paul,
        MN: Greenhaven Press. (Appears also in Bender's
        (1974) 1st ed., as "A Catholic view of suicide,"
        pp. 120-125. Reprinted from Lepp, I. (1968).
        Death and its mysteries (pp. 101-105). New York:
        Macmillan.)

8-112   Lum, D. (1968). Suicide: Theological ethics and
        pastoral counseling (Doctoral dissertation,
        Claremont School of Theology, 1967).
        Dissertation Abstracts International, 29, 374B.
        (University Microfilms No. 68-9428)

8-113   McCaughley, J. D. (1967). Suicide: Some
        theological considerations. Theology, 70, 63-68.

8-114   Portwood, D. (1978). Common-sense suicide: The
        final right (pp. 60-74). New York: Dodd, Mead,
        Chapter 5, "Suicide and the churches."

8-115   Pretzel, P. W. (1972). Understanding and
        counseling the suicidal person (pp. 226-242).
        Nashville, TN: Abingdon, Chapter 7, "Religion
        and suicide."

8-116   Pretzel, P. W. (1973). Suicide and religion: A
        preliminary study (Doctoral dissertation,
        Claremont School of Theology, 1966).
        Dissertation Abstracts International, 34,
        2948-2949B. (University Microfilms
        No. 73-28,779)

8-117   Siegel, S. (1979). Religion: A Jewish view. In
        L. D. Hankoff & B. Einsidler (Eds.), Suicide:
        Theory and clinical aspects (pp. 83-90).

Littleton, MA: PSG Publishing.

8-118   Van Der Horst, P. W. (1971).   A pagan Platonist and
        a Christian Platonist on suicide.   Vigilae
        Christianae, 25, 282-288.

        Van Der Horst presents writings against
        suicide of Augustine, a Christian, and
        Macrobius and compares their arguments.

8-119   Whalley, J. D. (1964).   Religion and suicide.
        Review of Religious Research, 5, 91-110.

See also Chapter 3, especially Dublin (1963, reference
3-007);   Grollman (1971, reference 3-013);   Guernesy (1963,
reference 3-014);   Lum (1974, reference 3-015);   Cohn (1976,
reference 3-024);   Hankoff (1979, 1979, references 3-027 and
3-028);   Speijer (1948, reference 3-032).

Chapter 5, Section 5.10e presents religion as a demographic
variable in suicidal behavior.

8.5 Legal Aspects of Suicide

8-120   Berman, A. L., & Cohen-Sandler, R. (1982).   Suicide
        and the standard of care: Optimal
        vs. acceptable.   Suicide and Life-Threatening
        Behavior, 12, 114-122.   (Abstracts: PA, 1983,
        69, No. 3880, pp. 419-420.   CPA, 1982, 22,
        No. 2719, p. 580.)

8-121   Berman, A. L., & Cohen-Sandler, R. (1983).   Suicide
        and malpractice: Expert testimony and the
        standard of care.   Professional Psychology, 14,
        6-19.   (Abstract: PA, 1983, 70, No. 8840,
        p. 986)

8-122   Beyer, H. A. (1982).   Suicide: A legal
        perspective.   In E. L. Bassuk, S. C. Schoonover,
        & A. D. Gill (Eds.), Lifelines: Clinical
        perspectives on suicide (pp. 225-228).   New York:
        Plenum Press.

8-123   Breger, M. (1979).   Law, technology, and public
        policy: Suicide and euthanasia.   In R. M. Veatch
        (Ed.), Life span: Values and life-extending
        technologies (pp. 248-272).   New York: Harper &
        Row.

8-124   Brushwood, D. B. (1983).   Pharmacist liability for
        suicide by drug overdose.   American Journal of
        Hospital Pharmacy, 40, 439-443.

8-125   Cooper, T. R., Jr. (1975).   Medical treatment
        facility liability for patient suicide and other
        self-injury.   Journal of Legal Medicine, 3,

20-25, 28-29.

8-126   Curran, W. J. (1970). Public health and the law.
         Suicide: Civil right or punishable crime.
         American Journal of Public Health, 60, 163-164.

8-127   Davidson, H. (1969). Suicide in the hospital.
         Hospitals: Journal of the American Hospital
         Association, 43, 55-59. (Reprinted as "Liability
         and malpractice in relation to suicide," in
         M. Miller (Ed.) (1982), Suicide intervention by
         nurses (pp. 183-197). New York: Springer.)

8-128a   Dean, M. M. (1957). The judicial interpretation of
         suicide. University of Pennsylvania Law Review,
         105, 391-410. (Reprinted in J. Gibbs (Ed.)
         (1968), Suicide (pp. 266-283). New York: Harper
         & Row.)

8-128b   Deschamps, P. (1983). Suicides and attempted
         suicides based on the medical care provided:
         Study of attempted lawsuits in Quebec between
         1968 and 1977. Canadian Journal of Psychiatry,
         28, 475-483.

8-129a   Dublin, L. I. (1963). Suicide: A sociological and
         statistical study (pp. 136-149). New York:
         Ronald Press, Chapter 17, "Suicide and the law."

* 8-129b Engelhardt, H. T., Jr., & Malloy, M. (1982).
         Suicide and assisting suicide: A critique of
         legal sanctions. Southwestern Law Journal, 36,
         1003-1037.

8-129c   Feinsilver, D. L. (1983). The suicidal patient:
         Clinical and legal issues. Hospital Practice,
         18(10), 48E-48F, 48J-48L.

8-130   Francis, L. P. (1980). Assisting suicide: A
         problem for the criminal law. In M. P. Battin &
         D. J. Mayo (Eds.), Suicide: The philosophical
         issues (pp. 254-266). New York: St. Martin's
         Press.

8-131   Frederic v. United States. 246 F. Supp. 1078
         (D. La., 1965). (Reprinted in E. S. Shneidman,
         N. L. Farberow, & R. E. Litman (Eds.) (1970),
         The psychology of suicide (pp. 531-540). New
         York: Science House.)

         A case in which a Veterans Administration
         hospital was accused of negligence when a
         patient committed suicide by jumping from a
         window.

8-132   Goldberg, F. D. (1970). Suicide and the

physician's liability. Medical Legal Bulletin, 205, 1-3.

8-133   Grisez, G., & Boyle, J. M., Jr. (1979). Life and death with liberty and justice: A contribution to the euthanasia debate (pp. 121-138). Notre Dame, IN: University of Notre Dame Press, Chapter 5, "Suicide and liberty."

8-134   Hoffman, D. E., & Webb, V. J. (1981). Suicide as murder at common law: Another chapter in the falsification of consensus theory. Criminology, 19, 372-384.

An historical look at laws regarding suicide and their enforcement in the U.S. and Great Britain and the implications for the criminological theory of consensus.

8-135   Horty, J. F. (1977). Liability depends on anticipation of suicide. Modern Health Care, 7(6), 56, 58.

8-136   Knapp, S., & Vandecreek, L. (1983). Malpractice risks with suicidal patients. Psychotherapy: Theory, Research and Practice, 20, 274-280.

8-137   Larsson, T. (1972). Suicide and insurance. In J. Waldenstrom, T. Larsson, & N. Ljungstedt (Eds.), Suicide and attempted suicide (pp. 127-143). Stockholm: Nordiska Bokhandlens Forlag.

8-138   Litman, R. E. (1967). Medical-legal aspects of suicide. Washburn Law Journal, 8, 395-401.

8-139   Litman, R. E. (1970). Medical-legal aspects of suicide. In E. S Shneidman, N. L. Farberow, & R. E. Litman (Eds.), The psychology of suicide (pp. 511-518). New York: Science House.

8-140   Litman, R. E. (1980). Psycholegal aspects of suicide. In W. J. Curran A. L. McGarry, & C. S. Petty (Eds.), Modern legal medicine: Psychiatry and forensic science (pp. 841-853). Philadelphia: Davis.

8-141   Litman, R. E. (1982). Hospital suicides: Lawsuits and standards. Suicide and Life-Threatening Behavior, 12, 212-220. (Abstracts: CPA, 1983, 23, No. 1251, p. 264; PA, 1983, 70, No. 13367, p. 1502)

8-142   Lonsdorf, R. G. (1968). Legal aspects of suicide. In H. L. P. Resnik (Ed.), Suicidal behaviors: Diagnosis and management (pp. 135-143). Boston:

Little Brown.

8-143   Markson, D. S. (1969). Punishment of suicide: A
        need for change. Villanova Law Review, 14,
        463-483.

8-144   Muhr, E. (1964, January/February). Life insurance
        and suicide: History and the Colorado statute.
        Denver Law Center Journal, 41, 51.

8-145   Murphy, G. E. (1975). The physician's
        responsibility for suicide: I. An error of
        commission. Annals of Internal Medicine, 82,
        301-304.

8-146   Murphy, G. E. (1975). The physician's
        responsibility for suicide: II. Errors of
        omission. Annals of Internal Medicine, 82,
        305-309.

8-147   Parry-Jones, W. L. (1973). Criminal law and
        complicity in suicide and attempted suicide.
        Medicine, Science, and the Law, 13, 110-119.

        A review of legal cases of complicity in the
        suicide of another person are presented from
        Great Britain, 1961-70.

8-148   Perr, I. N. (1965). Liability of hospital and
        physician in suicide. American Journal of
        Psychiatry, 122, 631-638.

8-149   Perr, I. N. (1974). Suicide and civil litigation.
        Journal of Forensic Sciences, 19, 261-266.

8-150   Perr, I. N. (1978, January). Legal aspects of
        suicide. Legal Aspects of Medical Practice,
        6(1), 49-55. (Reprinted in L. D. Hankoff &
        B. Einsidler (Eds.) (1979), Suicide: Theory and
        clinical aspects (pp. 91-101). Littleton, MA:
        PSG Publishing.)

8-151   Podgers, J. (1980, December). 'Rational suicide'
        raises patient rights issues. American Bar
        Association Journal, 66, 1499-1501.

8-152   Portwood, D. (1978). Common-sense suicide: The
        final right (pp. 48-59). New York: Dodd, Mead,
        Chapter 4, "Suicide and the law."

8-153   Resnik, H. L. P., Sullivan, F. J., & Wilkie,
        C. H. (1972). Insurability and suicidal
        behaviors: Issues for the seventies.
        Transactions of the Association of Life Insurance
        Medical Directors of America, 55, 132-148.

8-154   Schwartz, V. E. (1971). Civil liability for causing suicide: A synthesis of law and psychiatry. Vanderbilt Law Review, 24, 217-256.

8-155   Schoonover, S. C. (1982). Clinical comment [on legal issues]. In E. L. Bassuk, S. C. Schnoover, & A. D. Gill (Eds.), Lifelines: Clinical perspectives on suicide (pp. 229-230). New York: Plenum Press.

8-156   Schroeder, O. C., Jr. (1973). Suicide: A dilemma for medicine, law, and society. Postgraduate Medicine, 53, 55-57.

8-157   Schulman, R. E. (1968). Suicide and suicide prevention: A legal analysis. American Bar Association Journal, 54, 855-862.

        Schulman presents historical background on suicide, statistics, psychological conceptions, the legal status of U.S. suicide, and legal aspects of suicide prevention.

8-158   Shaffer, T. L. (1976). Legal views of suicide. In E. S. Shneidman (Ed.), Suicidology: Contemporary developments (pp. 404-419). New York: Grune & Stratton.

8-159   Silving, H. (1957). Suicide and the law. In E. S. Shneidman & N. L. Farberow (Eds.), Clues to suicide (pp. 79-95). New York: McGraw-Hill.

8-160   Slawson, P. F., Flinn, D. E., & Schwartz, D. A. (1974). Legal responsibility for suicide. Psychiatric Quarterly, 48, 50-64.

        A review of court decisions from 1927-1962.

8-161a Slawson, P. F., & Flinn, D. E. (1977). Hospital liability for suicide: A regional survey. Bulletin of the American Academy of Psychiatry and the Law, 5, 29-33.

8-161b Smith, K. J. M. (1983, September). Assisting in suicide--The Attorney-General and the Voluntary Euthanasia Society. Criminal Law Review, pp. 579-586.

8-162   Soubrier, J.-P. (1972). Legal aspects on suicide and attempted suicide. In J. Waldenstrom, T. Larsson, & N. Ljungstedt (Eds.), Suicide and attempted suicide (pp. 148-159). Stockholm: Nordiska Bokhandlens Forlag.

8-163   Speaker, F. (1980, March). Malpractice liability case results from suicide attempt. Pennsylvania

Medicine, 83(3), 10.

8-164   St. John-Stevas, N. (1961).   Life, death and the
         law: Law and Christian morals in England and the
         United States (pp. 232-261). Bloomington:
         Indiana University Press, Chapter 6, "Suicide."

8-165   Victoroff, V. M. (1983).   The suicidal patient:
         Recognition, intervention, management. Oradell,
         NJ: Medical Economics Books.

         Suicide and the law (pp. 173-193; chapter
         co-authored with G. T. Victoroff), the
         liability of physicians (pp. 194-200), are
         discussed and a table of state laws regarding
         suicide (pp. 229-232) is included.

8-166   Waltzer, H. (1980).   Malpractice liability in a
         patient's suicide. American Journal of
         Psychotherapy, 34, 89-98.

8-167   Woolf-Brenner, S. (1982). Undue influence in the
         criminal law: A proposed analysis of the
         criminal offense of 'causing suicide.' Albany Law
         Review, 47, 62-95. (Abstract: CPA, 1983, 23,
         No. 760, pp. 157-158)

8-168   Wright, D. M. (1975). Criminal aspects of suicide
         in the United States. North Carolina Central Law
         Journal, 7, 156-163.

See also Guernesy (1963, reference 3-014).

See also Hipple and Cimbolic (1979, reference 8-033).

Chapter 9
AFTER SUICIDE: POSTVENTION

While much has been written about suicide prevention and intervention, little attention until recently (see the section below on papers recently presented at professional meetings) has been focused upon "postvention," Shneidman's third level of suicide prevention efforts. When one commits suicide, it has been suggested that this "puts his psychological skeleton in the survivor's emotional closet" (Shneidman, 1969, p. 22, reference 9-195). Shneidman labeled this set of surviving individuals "survivor-victims."

The number of survivor-victims of suicide is uncertain, but it is likely that they number in the millions (Andress & Corey, 1978, reference 9-003) and estimates are that their rolls are increased annually by between 200,00 (Shneidman, 1972, reference 9-196) and 300,000 (Shneidman, 1969, reference 9-195). Such a significant number of people represents a major mental health population. However, few empirical considerations have been conducted of the family members and friends of the person who committed suicide and the effects the suicide had and perhaps continues to have upon them. A recent review of these studies (Calhoun, Selby, & Selby, 1982, reference 9-017) concluded that survivors of suicide 1) feel a need to understand the death, 2) may experience less social support than in other types of deaths and often experience social interaction difficulties, and 3) may experience more feelings of guilt than do survivors of other causes of death. Calhoun et al. also point out the great need for better and more research in this area.

The primary therapeutic regimen for survivors of suicide has consisted chiefly of support groups comprised of other survivors of suicide. Such groups have developed across the U.S. and a directory is maintained and available from the American Association of Suicidology (see Chapter 1 for address). Informal networks of these groups have begun but no coordinated effort has yet been initiated. A quarterly newsletter (Afterwords: A Letter for and about

<u>Suicide Survivors</u>) is compiled and distributed by Adina
Wrobleski of Minnesota (for subscription information write
to: 5124 Grove Street, Minneapolis, MN 55436-2481).

A comprehensive rather than a selective bibliography is
included here for several reasons. First, there is much
less literature on the topic of suicide survivors than most
other topics in suicidology. Relatedly, this topic has been
a neglected area of research and concern in suicidology.
Third, no one has previously compiled a comprehensive
bibliography on survivors of suicide. Fourth, as noted
above, interest has increased in recent years, and finally
previous bibliographies have listed few or no references on
this topic (e.g., Farberow, 1972, reference 1-003, lists
only 15 from 1897 to 1970; Lester et al., 1980, reference
1-009, list 4; Miller, 1979, reference 1-010, lists 9;
Poteet & Santora, 1978, reference 1-012, list only 2;
Prentice, 1974, reference 1-013, lists 4).

Another post-suicide issue is that of "psychological
autopsies." A psychological autopsy is a procedure
conducted primarily in the case of "equivocal deaths," i.e.,
deaths in which the cause is uncertain or unclear. Much
more than simply a case study, such psychological autopsies
attempt to determine the individual's role in the death by
reconstructing in great detail the events, climate, and
feelings of the deceased during the period immediately
preceding the death. This reconstruction is performed
primarily by interviewing the survivors of the dead
individual (relatives, friends, employers, physicians,
etc.). In some cases, these detailed data are presented to
a panel or team of multidisciplinary professionals (e.g.,
psychologists, psychiatrists, social workers, medical
examiners/coroners, etc.) and when possible, a decision is
made as to the cause of death. Such a procedure often has
therapeutic or positive outcomes for the grieving survivors,
but the primary purpose of the psychological autopsy remains
as a tool to investigate equivocal deaths.

A final aspect of the post-suicide situation is that of
suicide notes. Communication of suicidal intent (see
section 7.6) occurs prior to most suicidal acts but suicide
notes are discovered in no more than perhaps 15 to 25% of
all suicides.

A large number of studies of suicide notes have been
conducted. These investigations have attempted to derive an
understanding of the motivation and thoughts of the suicidal
person immediately before their death. As Shneidman (1973,
reference 9-162) observed, however, the mental state of the
suicidal individual disallows great explanatory revelations
and results in notes that are often "dull." The notes are
felt to be useful in understanding individual cases but not
to aid in the general comprehension of suicidal persons.

9.1 Suicide Survivors: Bibliographies

9-001 Miller, M. Survivors of suicide [Non-annotated
       bibliography]. San Diego: Center for
       Information on Suicide, Bibliography No. R-28.
       (Listed in the 1984 catalog.) See also reference
       1-010.

9-002 McIntosh, J. L. (in press). Survivors of suicide:
       A comprehensive bibliography. Omega.

       An earlier, less complete version of the
       references on survivors in this chapter is
       included.

9.2 Suicide Survivors: Family Members

9-003 Andress, V. R., & Corey, D. M. (1978).
       Survivor-victims: Who discovers or witnesses
       suicide? Psychological Reports, 42, 759-764.

9-004 Backer, B. A., Hannon, N., & Russell, N. A. (1982).
       Death and dying: individuals and institutions
       (pp. 205-225, esp. pp. 218-219, "Impact on
       survivors"). New York: Wiley, Chapter 7,
       "Suicide."

9-005 Barraclough, B. M., & Shepherd, D. M. (1976).
       Public interest: Private grief. British Journal
       of Psychiatry, 129, 109-113.

       A study of the spouses of suicides with a
       focus on the distress resulting from the
       coroners' inquest following the suicides.

9-006 Barraclough, B. M., & Shepherd, D. M. (1977). The
       immediate and enduring effects of the inquest on
       relatives of suicides. British Journal of
       Psychiatry, 131, 400-404.

9-007 Bowlby, J. (1980). Loss: Sadness and depression:
       Attachment and loss: Volume III (pp. 381-389).
       New York: Basic Books, Chapter 22, "Effects of a
       parent's suicide."

9-008 Buksbazen, C. (1976). Legacy of a suicide.
       Suicide and Life-Threatening Behavior, 6(2),
       106-122.

       A student essay presenting a case study of a
       suicide survivor--a brother of the young woman
       interviewed had committed suicide three years
       earlier.

* 9-009   Cain, A. C. (1972).   <u>Survivors of suicide</u>.
Springfield, IL: Thomas.

A collection of articles on families and
suicide, children of suicides, the impact of
suicide on other family members, and case
studies. Of the 19 articles included, 13 are
clearly related to survivors and are listed
below.

9-009.01 Lindemann, E., & Greer, I. M. (1953).   A
study of grief: Emotional responses to
suicide. pp. 63-69. (Reprinted from
<u>Pastoral Psychology</u>, <u>4</u>, 9-13.)

9-009.02 Lindemann, E., Vaughan, W. T., Jr., &
McGinnis, M. (1955). Preventive
intervention in a four-year-old child
whose father committed suicide.
pp. 70-92. (Reprinted from G. Caplan
(Ed.), <u>Emotional problems of early</u>
<u>childhood</u> (pp. 5-30). New York: Basic
Books.)

9-009.03 Cain, A. C., & Fast, I. (1966, 1969).
Children's disturbed reactions to
parent suicide: Distortions of guilt,
communication, and identification.
pp. 93-111. (Revised integration of
two papers: 1) Children's disturbed
reactions to parent suicide. <u>American</u>
<u>Journal of Orthopsychiatry</u>, <u>36</u>(5),
873-880 (1966a also Reprinted in
G. C. Morrison (Ed.) (1975),
<u>Emergencies in child psychiatry:</u>
<u>Emotional crises of children, youths,</u>
<u>and their families</u> (pp. 193-203).
Springfield, IL: Thomas.); and 2)
<u>Parent suicide and suicide prevention:</u>
<u>Implications and opportunities</u>. Paper
presented at the Fifth International
Conference for Suicide Prevention,
London, 1969 (Abstract in the
proceedings of that conference, R. Fox
(Ed.) (1970, pp. 187-190), Vienna:
International Association for Suicide
Prevention.).

9-009.04 Warren, M. Some psychological sequelae
of parental suicide in surviving
children. pp. 112-120.

9-009.05 Dorpat, T. L. Psychological effects of
parental suicide on surviving children.
pp. 121-142.

9-009.06   Cain, A. C., & Fast, I. (1966). The
            legacy of suicide: Observations on the
            pathogenic impact of suicide upon
            marital partners. pp. 145-154.
            (Reprinted from Psychiatry, 29,
            406-411.)

9-009.07   Whitis, P. R. (1968). The legacy of a
            child's suicide. pp. 155-166.
            (Reprinted from Family Process, 7,
            159-169.)

9-009.08   Resnik, H. L. P. (1969). Psychological
            resynthesis: A clinical approach to
            the survivors of a death by suicide.
            pp. 167-177. (Reprinted from
            E. S. Shneidman & M. J. Ortega (Eds.),
            Aspects of depression (pp. 213-224).
            Boston: Little, Brown (International
            Psychiatry Clinics, 6(2)).)

9-009.09   Augenbraun, B., & Neuringer, C. Helping
            survivors with the impact of a suicide.
            pp. 178-185.

9-009.10   Silverman, P. R. Intervention with the
            widow of a suicide. pp. 186-214.

9-009.11   Henslin, J. M. Strategies of adjustment:
            An ethnomethodological approach to the
            study of guilt and suicide.
            pp. 215-227.

9-009.12   Arthur, B. Parent suicide: A family
            affair. pp. 256-273.

9-009.13   Tooley, K. The meaning of maternal
            suicide as reflected in the treatment
            of a late adolescent girl.
            pp. 274-303.

9-010   Cain, A. (1977). Survivors of suicide. In
        S. Wilcox & M. Sutton (Eds.), Understanding death
        and dying: An interdisciplinary approach
        (pp. 229-233). Port Washington, NY: Alfred
        Publishing. (Excerpt from Cain, 1972, reference
        9-009 above.)

9-011   Cain, A. C. (1978). Impact of a parent suicide on
        children. In O. J. Z. Sahler (Ed.), Child and
        death (pp. 202-210). St. Louis: C. V. Mosby.

9-012   Cain, A. C., & Fast, I. (1965). A clinical study
        of some aspects of the psychological impact of
        parent suicide upon children. American Journal
        of Orthopsychiatry, 35(2), 318-319. [Abstract of

a paper presented at the 42nd annual meeting of
the American Orthopsychiatric Association, New
York, March 1965.]

9-013   Calhoun, L. G., Selby, J. W., & Gribble,
C. M. (1979). Reactions to the family of the
suicide. American Journal of Community
Psychology, 7(5), 571-575. (Abstract: PA, 1981,
65, No. 1475, p. 164)

An experimental study to determine how
differing characteristics of suicides in
newspaper accounts affect the responses of
readers to the surviving family members.

9-014   Calhoun, L. G., Selby, J. W., & Faulstich,
M. E. (1980). Reactions to the parents of the
child suicide: A study of social impressions.
Journal of Consulting and Clinical Psychology,
48(4), 535-536. (Abstract: PA, 1981, 65,
No. 1259, p. 139)

9-015   Calhoun, L. G., Selby, J. W., & Faulstich,
M. E. (1982). The aftermath of childhood
suicide: Influences on the perception of the
parent. Journal of Community Psychology, 10(3),
250-254. (Abstract: PA, 1983, 69, No. 7897,
p. 865)

9-016   Calhoun, L. G., Selby, J. W., & King, H. E. (1976).
Dealing with crisis: A guide to critical life
problems (pp. 220-239; esp. pp. 232-235, "The
aftermath of suicide"). Englewood Cliffs, NJ:
Prentice-Hall, Chapter 11, "The critical problem
of suicide."

* 9-017   Calhoun, L. G., Selby, J. W., & Selby,
L. E. (1982). The psychological aftermath of
suicide: An analysis of current evidence.
Clinical Psychology Review, 2, 409-420.
(Abstract: PA, 1983, 69, No. 10607, p. 1164)

A survey of the literature regarding
affective, cognitive, behavioral, and physical
reactions by survivors of suicide as well as
family interaction and social reactions to the
survivors. Findings regarding survivors of
parental suicide are excluded.

9-018   Calhoun, L. G., Selby, J. W., Tedeschi, R. G., &
Davis, B. (1981). The aftermath of suicide: An
instrument for measuring reactions to the
surviving family. Journal of Psychiatric
Treatment and Evaluation, 3(1), 99-104.
(Abstract: Biological Abstracts, 1983, 75(3),
No. 21783)

9-019   Cantor, P. (1975, July).   The effects of youthful
        suicide on the family.   Psychiatric Opinion,
        12(6), 6-11.

9-020   Charmaz, K. (1980).   The social reality of death:
        Death in contemporaty America (pp. 233-279;
        esp. pp. 271-274, "Effects of suicide on
        survivors").   Reading, MA: Addison-Wesley,
        Chapter 8, "The social context of suicide."

9-021   Coleman, W. L. (1979).   Understanding suicide.
        Elgin, IL: David C. Cook.

        A book written primarily to and for survivors
        of suicide which discusses how to face and
        deal with the situation.

* 9-022   Danto, B. L., & Kutscher, A. H.   (Eds.)   (1977).
        Suicide and bereavement.   New York: MSS
        Information Corporation.

        A collection of 25 separate articles on
        suicidal behavior.   Of these 25, 11 clearly
        relate to survivors of suicide and are listed
        below.

        9-022.01   Danto, B. L.   Family survivors of
                   suicide.   pp. 11-20.

        9-022.02   Fliegel, M. L.   Bereavement as a cause of
                   suicide.   pp. 32-38 (esp. pp. 36-38).

        9-022.03   Neuringer, C.   Bereavement reactions in
                   survivors of suicide.   pp. 39-43.

        9-022.04   Wallace, S. E.   On the atypicality of
                   suicide bereavement.   pp. 44-53.

        9-022.05   Simon, W.   Reflections on suicide and
                   bereavement among veterans.   pp. 54-60.

        9-022.06   Shneidman, E. S. (1975).   To the bereaved
                   of a suicide.   pp. 67-69.   (Reprinted
                   from A. H. Kutscher, D. Peretz,
                   S. Klagsbrun, D. Cherico, &
                   L. G. Kutscher (Eds.), But not to lose:
                   A book of comfort for those bereaved
                   (2nd ed.)   (pp. 168-169).   New York:
                   MSS Information Corporation.   Appears
                   also in For those bereaved (rev. ed. of
                   But not to lose) (pp. 166-168).   New
                   York: Arno Press, 1980.)

        9-022.07   Achte, K.   Perspectives on death and
                   suicide.   pp. 73-89 (esp. pp. 77-79).

9-022.08   Flesch, R. Mental health and bereavement
           by accident or suicide: A preliminary
           report. pp. 128-137.

9-022.09   Welu, T. C. (1975). Pathological
           bereavement: A plan for its
           prevention. pp. 201-210. (Reprinted
           from B. Schoenberg, I. Gerber,
           A. Weiner, A. H. Kutscher, D. Peretz, &
           A. C. Carr (Eds.), Bereavement: Its
           psychosocial aspects (pp. 139-149).
           New York: Columbia University Press.)

9-022.10   Doyle, P. Grief counseling for children.
           pp. 211-221.

9-022.11   Danto, B. L. Project SOS: Volunteers in
           action with survivors of suicide.
           pp. 222-239.

9-023   Davis, P. A. (1983). Suicidal adolescents
        (pp. 62-66). Springfield, IL: Thomas, Chapter
        9, "Postvention."

9-024   Demi, A. M. (1978). Adjustment to widowhood after
        a sudden death: Suicide and non-suicide
        survivors compared (Doctoral dissertation,
        University of California, San Francisco, 1978).
        Dissertation Abstracts International, 38,
        5847-5848B. (University Microfilms No. 7809192)

9-025   Demi, A. M. (1978). Adjustment to widowhood after
        a sudden death: Suicide and non-suicide
        survivors compared. Community Nursing Research,
        11, 91-99.

9-026   Doyle, P. (1980). Grief counseling and sudden
        death: A manual and guide (pp. 166-172).
        Springfield, IL: Thomas, Chapter 12, "The
        anniversary interview."

        Discussion of and suggestions for an interview
        of survivors of suicide on the anniversary
        date of the suicide as a part of grief
        counseling.

9-027   Farberow, N. L. (1968). Suicide: Psychological
        aspects (2). In D. L. Sills (Ed.), International
        encyclopedia of the social sciences Volume 15
        (pp. 390-394, esp. p. 394, "Psychology of the
        survivors"). New York: Macmillan & Free Press.

9-028   Fisher, J. V., Barnett, B. C., & Collins,
        J. (1976). The post-suicide family and the
        family physician. Journal of Family Practice, 3,
        263-267.

* 9-029 Foglia, B. B. (1977). Survivor-victims of suicide:
         Review of the literature. In C. L. Hatton,
         S. M. Valente, & A. Rink (Eds.), Suicide:
         Assessment and intervention (pp. 113-124). New
         York: Appleton-Century-Crofts. (2nd ed., Hatton
         & Valente, 1984, pp. 149-162.)

  9-030 Giffin, M., & Felsenthal, C. (1983). A cry for
         help (pp. 286-299). Garden City, NY: Doubleday,
         Chapter 13, "Helping the survivors."

         A popular literature consideration of teen
         suicide, written primarily as a guide for the
         parents of teenagers.

  9-031 Goldberg, M., & Mudd, E. H. (1968). The effects of
         suicidal behavior upon marriage and the family.
         In H. L. P. Resnik (Ed.), Suicidal behaviors:
         Diagnosis and management (pp. 348-356;
         esp. pp. 352-354). Boston: Little, Brown.

  9-032 Grollman, E. A. (1971). Suicide: Prevention,
         intervention, postvention (pp. 109-117). Boston:
         Beacon Press, Chapter 7, "When a suicide is
         committed: Postvention."

  9-033 Hajal, F. (1977, April). Post-suicide grief work
         in family therapy. Journal of Marriage and
         Family Counseling, 3(2), 35-42. (Abstract: PA,
         1978, 59, No. 3826, p. 416)

  9-034 Hammond, J. M. (1980). A parent's suicide:
         Counseling the children. The School Counselor,
         27(5), 385-388.

  9-035 Hatton, C. L., & Valente, S. M. (1981).
         Bereavement group for parents who suffered a
         suicidal loss of a child. Suicide and
         Life-Threatening Behavior, 11(3), 141-150.
         (Reprinted in C. L. Hatton & S. M. Valente
         (Eds.) (1984), Suicide: Assessment and
         intervention (2nd ed.) (pp. 163-173). Norwalk,
         CT: Appleton-Century-Crofts.) (Abstract: PA,
         1982, 67, No. 10352, p. 1113.)

  9-036 Henley, S. H. A. (in press). Bereavement following
         suicide: A review of the literature. Current
         Psychological Research & Reviews.

  9-037 Henslin, J. M. (1970). Guilt and guilt
         neutralization: Response and adjustment to
         suicide. In J. D. Douglas (Ed.), Deviance and
         respectability: The social construction of moral
         meaning (pp. 192-228). New York: Basic Books.

  9-038 Henslin, J. M. (1971, Fall). Problems and

prospects in studying significant others of
suicides. Bulletin of Suicidology, No. 8, 81-84.

The author relates the purpose of a study
conducted with 58 survivors of suicides, the
problems encountered, and suggestions for
further research.

9-039   Herzog, A., & Resnik, H. L. P. (1969). A clinical
study of parental response to adolescent death by
suicide with recommendations for approaching the
survivors. British Journal of Social Psychiatry,
3(3), 144-152. (Abstract: ACP, 1971, 11,
No. 772, p. 247)

9-040   Hewett, J. (1980). After suicide. Philadelphia:
Westminister Press.

Written for survivors of suicide, this
sensitive book discusses grief, the family,
helping children after the suicide, and living
as a suicide survivor.

9-041   Ilan, E. (1973). The impact of a father's suicide
on his latency son. In E. J. Anthony &
C. Koupernik (Eds.), The child in his family:
The impact of disease and death, Volume 2
(pp. 299-306). New York: Wiley.

9-042   Impact of a suicide inquest [Editorial] (1978,
September 23). Lancet, 2(8091), 666-667. A
reply, Barraclough, B. M., & Shepherd,
D. M. (1978, October 7). Impact of a suicide
inquest [Letter]. Lancet, 2(8093), 795.

This editorial is directed toward the research
of Barraclough and Shepherd (references 9-005,
9-006, 9-062, 9-063) listed in this section on
suicide survivors and the implications of
those articles for coroners.

9-043   Jakab, I., & Howard, M. C. (1969). Art therapy
with a 12-year-old girl who witnessed suicide and
developed school phobia. Psychotherapy and
Psychosomatics, 17(5-6), 309-324.

9-044   Junghardt, D. Z. (1977). Survivors of suicide: A
program in postvention. In C. L. Hatton,
S. M. Valente, & A. Rink (Eds.), Suicide:
Assessment and intervention (pp. 124-132). New
York: Appleton-Century-Crofts.

9-045   Klagsbrun, F. (1977). Too young to die: Youth and
suicide (pp. 98-110). New York: Pocket Books,
Chapter 7, "Friends and relatives: How suicide
can destroy more than one." (Originally

published, 1976, Boston: Houghton Mifflin.)

9-046   Krementz, J. (1981).   How it feels when a parent dies (pp. 9-15, 85-87).   New York: Knopf.

This book presents the feelings and thoughts of 18 children and teenagers whose parents died.   Among these personal accounts are two by children whose parents committed suicide.

9-047   Lum, D. (1974).   Responding to suicidal crisis: For church and community (pp. 142-154).   Grand Rapids, MI: Eerdmans, Chapter 8, "Opening avenues to after-care."

A discussion of the research on suicide bereavement and pastoral counseling at and after the funeral are included in this chapter.

9-048   Maris, R. W. (1981).   Pathways to suicide: A survey of self-destructive behaviors (pp. 279-285, "Consequences of suicide attempts").   Baltimore: John Hopkins University Press.

Survivors of suicides were interviewed about the suicide victims as a data collection method.   The interview conducted also asked for the reactions of the survivors.   These responses were compared to those close to non-fatal suicide attempters and to survivors of natural death victims.

9-049   Masserman, J. H. (1954, November).   Emotional reactions to death and suicide.   American Practitioner and Digest of Treatment, 5, 41-46.

9-050   Miller, M. (1982).   Surviving the loss of a loved one: An inside look at grief counseling.   In J. A. Fruehling (Ed.), Sourcebook on death and dying (pp. 189-192; esp. pp. 191-192, "Surviving a suicide").   Chicago: Marquis Professional Publications.   (Reprinted from Michigan Funeral Directors Association Journal, February 1980.)

9-051   Pfeffer, C. R. (1981).   Parental suicide: An organizing event in the development of latency age children.   Suicide and Life-Threatening Behavior, 11(1), 43-50.

9-052   Pretzel, P. W. (1972).   Understanding and counseling the suicidal person (pp. 136-174).   Nashville, TN: Abingdon, Chapter 4, "The aftermath of suicide."

9-053   Prophit, P. (1979). The enigma of adolescent
        suicide. In R. T. Mercer (Ed.), Perspectives on
        adolescent health care (pp. 226-242;
        esp. pp. 237-241, "Postvention: The
        survivor-victims of suicide."). Philadelphia:
        Lippincott.

9-054   Raphael, B. (1983). The anatomy of bereavement
        (pp. 120-122, "Special bereavements: Suicide").
        New York: Basic Books.

9-055   Roberts, A. R. (1975). Self-destruction by one's
        own hand: Suicide and suicide prevention. In
        A. R. Roberts (Ed.), Self-destructive behavior
        (pp. 21-77, esp. pp. 46-49, "Survivors of
        suicide"). Springfield, IL: Thomas. (A portion
        of this chapter is adapted from "Suicide and
        suicide prevention: An overview." Public Health
        Reviews, 1973, 2, 4-24.)

9-056   Rogers, J., Sheldon, A., Barwick, C., Letofsky, K.,
        & Lancee, W. (1982). Help for families of
        suicide: Survivors Support Group. Canadian
        Journal of Psychiatry, 27(6), 444-449.
        (Abstract: PA, 1983, 69, No. 13202, p. 1459)

9-057   Rudestam, K. E. (1977). Physical and psychological
        responses to suicide in the family. Journal of
        Consulting and Clinical Psychology, 45(2),
        162-170.

9-058   Rudestam, K. E. (1977). The impact of suicide
        among the young. Essence, 1, 221-224.
        (Abstract: PA, 1978, 60, No. 5442, p. 600)

9-059   Rudestam, K. E., & Imbroll, D. (1983). Societal
        reactions to a child's death by suicide. Journal
        of Consulting and Clinical Psychology, 51(3),
        461-462. (Abstract: PA, 1983, 70, No. 5467,
        pp. 613-614)

        A study of the reactions of members of the
        community to the surviving family of children
        who had died by various methods, including
        suicide. Responding to newspaper accounts,
        subjects felt the child and the family were
        more disturbed in the case of suicide and the
        parents were seen as more to blame.

9-060a Saunders, J. M. (1981). A process of bereavement
        resolution: Uncoupled identity. Western Journal
        of Nursing Research, 3, 319-332.

        Saunders investigates the bereavement process
        in young widows whose husbands died from
        natural deaths, accidents, homicide, or

suicide.

9-060b Scholz, J. A. (1971). The aftermath of suicide:
        Reactions of the family. Life-Threatening
        Behavior, 2, 86-91.

9-061   Schuyler, D. (1973). Counseling suicide survivors:
        Issues and answers. Omega, 4, 313-321.

9-062   Shepherd, D. M., & Barraclough, B. M. (1974, June
        15). The aftermath of suicide. British Medical
        Journal, 2, 600-603.

9-063   Shepherd, D. M., & Barraclough, B. M. (1976). The
        aftermath of parental suicide for children.
        British Journal of Psychiatry, 129, 267-276.
        (Abstracts: PA, 1977, 57, No. 8420, p. 953.
        ACP, 1977, 17, No. 294, p. 70.)

9-064   Sheskin, A., & Wallace, S. E. (1976). Differing
        bereavements: Suicide, natural and accidental
        deaths. Omega, 7(3), 229-242.

9-065   Shneidman, E. S. (1971). Prevention, intervention
        and postvention of suicide. Annals of Internal
        Medicine, 75, 453-458 (esp. pp. 455-457).

            One of six papers in this issue of the journal
            (pp. 441-458). The papers were presented at a
            conference on suicide at UCLA. In Shneidman's
            paper, the definition of suicide as well as
            the prevention, intervention, and postvention
            are discussed.

* 9-066 Shneidman, E. S. (1973). Deaths of man
        (pp. 33-41). New York: Quandrangle, Chapter 3,
        "Postvention and the survivor-victim."
        (Reprinted in E. S. Shneidman (Ed.) (1976),
        Death: Current perspectives (pp. 347-356) (2nd
        ed., 1980, pp. 233-240; 3rd ed., 1984,
        pp. 412-419.). Palo Alto, CA: Mayfield
        Publishing.)

9-067   Shneidman, E. S. (1975). Postvention: The care of
        the bereaved. In R. O. Pasnau (Ed.),
        Consultation-Laison Psychiatry (pp. 245-256).
        New York: Grune & Stratton. (Reprinted in
        Suicide and Life-Threatening Behavior, 1981,
        11(4), 349-359.)

9-068   Sickel, R. Z. (1979, May/June). Children who
        experience parental suicide. Pediatric Nursing,
        5(3), 37-39.

9-069   Simpson, M. A. (1979). The facts of death: A

complete guide for being prepared (pp. 202-221;
esp. pp. 219-220, "The survivor-victims.").
Englewood Cliffs, NJ: Prentice-Hall, Chapter 10,
"Suicide."

The feelings of survivors of suicide and
suggestions of how to aid and interact with
them are discussed.

9-070   Solomon, M. I. (1982-83). The bereaved and the
stigma of suicide. Omega, 13(4), 377-387.
(Abstract: PA, 1983, 70, No. 10505, p. 1176)

9-071   Stone, H. W. (1972). Suicide and grief.
Philadelphia: Fortress Press.

Based on research conducted by the author,
presentations are made of grief in general and
among suicide and non-suicide survivors.

9-072   Todd, S. H. (1981). Sibling survivors of suicide:
A qualitative study of the experience of
adolescent siblings whose brother or sister
completed suicide (Doctoral dissertation, Boston
University School of Education, 1980).
Dissertation Abstracts International, 41,
3164-3165B. (University Microfilms No. 8101918)

9-073   Victoroff, V. M. (1983). The suicidal patient:
Recognition, intervention, management
(pp. 203-212). Oradell, NJ: Medical Economics
Books, Chapter 17, "Survivors."

The effects of a suicide on the survivors as
well as therapy for suicide survivors are
covered.

9-074   Vorkoper, C. F., & Petty, C. S. (1980). Suicide
investigation. In W. J. Curran, A. L. McGarry, &
C. S. Petty (Eds.), Modern legal medicine,
psychiatry, and forensic science (pp. 171-185,
esp. pp. 181-184). Philadelphia: Davis.

Suggestions and guidelines are made in dealing
with family survivors of suicides when
conducting an investigation of a suicide
death.

9-075   Wallace, S. (1973). After suicide. New York:
Wiley.

Information and the case studies of 12 women
whose husbands committed suicide are
presented.

9-076   Warren, M. (1966). Psychological effects of

parental suicide in surviving children. Excerpta
Medica, Series 117, 433.

9-077   Wekstein, L. (1979). Handbook of suicidology:
Principles, problems and practice (pp. 123-127,
"Treatment of the survivor-victim"). New York:
Brunner/Mazel.

9-078   Wetherill, P. S. (1975). Predictability, failure,
and guilt in suicide: A personal account.
Family Process, 14, 339-370.

An in-depth consideration of the life and
suicide of the son of the author (the latter
is a marriage and family counselor). A brief
discussion of the feelings of various
survivors (mother, father, wife) after the
suicide is also included.

9-079   Worden, J. W. (1981). Coping with suicide in the
family. In A. Milunsky (Ed.), Coping with crisis
and handicap (National Symposium on Coping with
Crisis and Handicap, Boston, September 1979)
(pp. 103-114, esp. pp. 107-108). New York:
Plenum.

Worden discusses suicide in children and
children as survivors of suicide.

9-080   Worden, J. W. (1982). Grief counseling and grief
therapy: A handbook for the mental health
practitioner (pp. 79-83). New York: Springer,
Chapter 6, "Grieving special types of losses:
Suicide."

9-081   Wrobleski, A. (in press). The Suicide Survivors
Grief Group. Omega.

9-082   Wrobleski, A. (1983). Suicide. In H. C. Raether &
R. C. Slater (Eds.), Advocating understanding: A
manual for funeral directors relating to
caregiving groups (pp. V1-V27). Milwaukee:
National Funeral Directors Association.

A brief overview of the field of suicide
focusing predominantly on reactions of and aid
to survivors.

See also American Association of Suicidology (1977,
reference 7-082), Session 4, "After the suicide," Workshops
12-14, pp. 26-30, and reprinted in Wekstein (1979, reference
9-077), pp. 178-180, for educational workshop experiences to
help in dealing with the survivors of suicide.

9.3 Papers Published in Proceedings of Professional Meetings

9-083   International Association for Suicide Prevention
         (IASP), 4th International Conference for Suicide
         Prevention, Los Angeles, CA, October 18-21, 1967.
         Abstracts published in N. L. Farberow (Ed.)
         (1968), Proceedings. Los Angeles: Delmar
         Publishing.

     9-083.01   Herzog, A., & Resnik, H. L. P. A
                 clinical study of parental response to
                 adolescent death by suicide with
                 recommendations for approaching the
                 survivors. pp. 381-390.

9-084   International Association for Suicide Prevention,
         5th International Conference for Suicide
         Prevention, London, September 24-27, 1969.
         Abstracts published in R. Fox (Ed.) (1970),
         Proceedings. Vienna: IASP.

     9-084.01   Cain, A. C., & Fast, I. Parent suicide
                 and suicide prevention. pp. 187-190.

     9-084.02   Gorceix, A. L. First clinical encounters
                 with the survivor. pp. 36-37.

9-085   International Association for Suicide Prevention,
         6th International Conference for Suicide
         Prevention, Mexico City. Abstracts appeared in
         Proceedings (1972). Ann Arbor, MI: Edward
         Brothers.

     9-085.01   Cain, A. C. Survivors of suicide:
                 Current findings and future directions.
                 pp. 192-198.

     9-085.02   Shneidman, E. S. Postvention and the
                 survivor-victim. pp. 31-39.

9-086   International Association for Suicide Prevention,
         7th International Conference for Suicide
         Prevention, Amsterdam, The Netherlands, August
         27-30, 1973. Abstracts published in N. Speyer
         (Ed.) (1974), Proceedings. Amsterdam: Swets &
         Zeitlinger.

     9-086.01   Johnson, B. M. Psychological services
                 for relatives of suicide victims.
                 pp. 372-375.

9-087   International Association for Suicide Prevention,
         8th International Conference for Suicide
         Prevention and Crisis Intervention, Jerusalem,
         October 1975. Papers appear in H. Z. Winnick &

L. Miller (Eds.) (1978), Aspects of suicide in modern civilization (Proceedings of the 8th conference). Jerusalem: Jerusalem Academic Press.

9-087.01 Doyle, P. Grief counseling for the survivors of suicide: A volunteer project. pp. 155-164.

9-088 International Association for Suicide Prevention, 10th International Conference for Suicide Prevention and Crisis Intervention, Ottawa, Canada, June 17-20, 1979. Abstracts appear in Proceedings (1979). Ottawa: IASP.

9-088.01 Demi, A. S. Mental health of widows after a sudden death: Suicide and non-suicide survivors compared. pp. 230-237.

9-089 American Association of Suicidology (AAS), 8th annual meeting, St. Louis, April 1975. Abstracts appear in B. S. Comstock & R. Maris (Eds.) (1976), Proceedings. Houston: AAS.

9-089.01 Doyle, P. The anniversary interview in grief counseling for the survivors of suicide. pp. 27-31.

9-089.02 Lynd, J. G. Helping survivors with the impact of suicide through grief counseling: With the cooperation of coroner's deputies. pp. 33-35.

9-089.03 Rudestam, K. E. Effects of suicide on survivors. pp. 15-19.

9-090 American Association of Suicidology, 15th annual meeting, New York City, April 15-18, 1982. Abstracts appear in C. R. Pfeffer & J. Richman (Eds.) (1984), Proceedings. Denver: AAS.

9-090.01 Bolton, I. When your child has died of suicide. pp. 102-103.

9-090.02 Conley, B. H.. The funeral as "first aid" for the suicide survivor. pp. 96-98.

9-090.03 Ross, E. After suicide: A Ray of Hope. pp. 99-101.

9-090.04 Wrightman, C., & Langley-Hamby, P. The staff needs attention too--Management issues post patient suicide. pp. 104-106.

9-091   American Association of Suicidology, 16th annual
         meeting, Dallas, April 21-24, 1983. Abstracts
         appear in C. F. Vorkoper & K. Smith (Eds.)
         (1984), _Proceedings_. Denver: AAS.

    9-091.01   Bess, D., & White, S. B. Care for the
               caregivers. p. 70.

    9-091.02   Giuliani, J. L. Parent-child bonding: A
               factor in the grief processing of
               survivors. p. 65.

    9-091.03   Heilig, S. Reactions of a therapist to
               the suicide of a patient. pp. 73-74.

    9-091.04   Leonhardi, M. Similarities and
               differences between survivors of
               suicide and survivors of homicide.
               p. 66.

    9-091.05   Ross, E. Survivorship following suicide.
               p. 69.

    9-091.06   Wrobleski, A. A Suicide Survivors Grief
               Group. pp. 67-68.

See also reference 1-097.

9.4 Survivors: Presentations at Recent Professional Meetings

9-092a American Orthopsychiatric Association, annual
        meeting, Boston, MA, April, 1983. Panel 106:
        The Survivors of Suicides: Family Members and
        Therapists:

        Presented also at:

        American Association for Marriage and Family
        Therapy, Washington, D.C., October 1983.
        Workshop 233: Surviving a suicide: Family
        members and therapists:

    9-092a.01 Dunne, E. J. _Surviving suicide_.

    9-092a.02 Hauser, M. J. _Treatment and prevention
              considerations_.

    9-092a.03 Jones, F. A., Jr. _Implications for
              treatment when the therapist survives
              client suicide_.

    9-092a.04 Maxim, K. A. _Postvention issues in
              family functioning_.

    9-092a.05 Weiss, W., & Borowka, C. _Reverberations
              through the generations_.

9-092a.06 Wrobleski, A. Evolution of survivor
          self-help groups.

9-092b American Association of Suicidology, 17th annual
       meeting, Anchorage, Alaska, May 2-5, 1984.
       (Abstracts to appear in R. Cohen-Sandler &
       J. MacClarence (Eds.) (in preparation),
       Proceedings. Denver: AAS.):

       9-092b.01 Archibald, L. Permission to grieve:
                 Educating clergy toward reinforcement
                 of survivors of suicide.

       9-092b.02 Dunne, E. J. Double jeopardy: Suicide
                 survivors and the mental health system.

       9-092b.03 Hatton, C. L. Grief work of a suicide
                 bereavement revisted.

       9-092b.04 Maxim, K. D. Survivors and the press: A
                 synergistic partnership.

       9-092b.05 O'Brien, P. Impact of a patient's
                 suicide on treating clinicians.

9.5 Survivors: Pamphlets, Popular Media

   9-093 After suicide: A unique grief process. Write to:
          Elnora Ross, Ray of Hope, Inc., 1518 Derwen
          Drive, Iowa City, IA 52240.

   9-094 Grief after suicide. Write to: Mental Health
          Association, Room 101, 414 Moreland Boulevard,
          Waukesha, WI 53186.

   9-095 Help for families of suicide: Suicide Survivors
          Program. Write to: Joy Rogers, Clarke Institute
          of Psychiatry, 250 College Street, Toronto,
          Ontario M5T 1R8, Canada.

   9-096 Suicide Prevention Center, Dayton, Ohio.:
          9-096.01 Johnson, W. Y. (1982). The care of the
                    suicide survivor: A model for funeral
                    home personnel.
          9-096.02 Heller, J. (1982). The care of the
                    suicide survivor: A model for clergy.
          9-096.03 Heller, J. (1982). The care of the
                    suicide survivor: A model for coroners
                    and medical examiners.
          (3 separate pamphlets). Write to: Suicide
          Prevention Center, Inc., 184 Salem Avenue,
          Dayton, OH 45406.

   9-097 Rubey, C. (1979, September). Chicago archdiocese
          aids survivors of young suicides. Thanatology
          Today, 1(6), 2.

9-098   Scheinin, A.-G. (1983, February 7).   The burden of
        suicide. Newsweek, p. 13.

9-099   Valente, S. (1980, March).   Suicides' families:
        Structures more normal than believed.
        Thanatology Today, 1(12), 2.

9-100   When reason fails...Understanding bereavement by
        suicide...A pamphlet for friends. Write to:
        Creative Marketing, P. O. Box 2423, Springfield,
        IL 62705.

9.6 Suicide Survivors: Non-Family Members

9-101   Ables, B. S. (1974).   The loss of a therapist
        through suicide. Journal of the American Academy
        of Child Psychiatry, 13, 143-152.

9-102   Albert, R., Jr. (1972).   Attitudes and reactions
        evoked by a suicide.   In E. S. Shneidman (Ed.),
        Death and the college student: A collection of
        brief essays on death and suicide by Harvard
        youth (pp. 103-109). New York: Behavioral
        Publications.

        A student essay recording the responses and
        feelings of the author and four other students
        to the recent suicide of a fellow student.
        Two of those interviewed knew the deceased
        well.

9-103   Alexander, P. (1977).   A psychotherapist's reaction
        to his patient's death. Suicide and
        Life-Threatening Behavior, 7, 203-210.

        A therapist's reflections on the suicide of a
        patient, the effects of client suicide on the
        therapist, and the need on the part of the
        therapist to mourn the dead person are
        presented.

9-104   Backer, B. A., Hannon, N., & Russell, N. A. (1982).
        Death and dying: Individuals and institutions
        (pp. 205-225, esp. pp. 219-220, "The health care
        professional's response to suicide"). New York:
        Wiley, Chapter 7, "Suicide."

9-105   Ballenger, J. C. (1978).   Patients' reactions to
        the suicide of their psychiatrist. Journal of
        Nervous and Mental Disease, 166(12), 859-867.

9-106   Binder, R. (1978).   Dealing with patients' suicides
        [Letter]. American Journal of Psychiatry, 135,
        1113.

9-107   Bray, D. (1976).   When prevention fails. Journal

of Practical Nursing, 26, 19-20. (Reprinted in
M. Miller (Ed.) (1982b), Suicide intervention by
nurses (pp. 175-180). New York: Springer.)

A recognition that health care professionals
must also come to grips with their feelings
regarding the suicide of a patient.

9-108   Carter, R. E. (1971). Some effects of client
suicide on the therapist. Psychotherapy:
Theory, Research, and Practice, 8, 287-289.

9-109   Chiles, J. A. (1974). Patient reactions to the
suicide of a therapist. American Journal of
Psychotherapy, 28, 115-121.

9-110   Cotton, P. G., Drake, R. E., Whitaker, A., &
Potter, J. (1983). Dealing with suicide on a
psychiatric inpatient unit. Hospital and
Community Psychiatry, 34, 55-58. (Abstract: PA,
1983, 70, No. 8717, p. 973)

9-111   Getz, W. L., Allen, D. B., Myers, R. K., & Lindner,
K. C. (1983). Brief counseling with suicidal
persons (pp. 145-159). Lexington, MA: Lexington
Books, Chapter 12, "When a client commits
suicide."

Primarily written for the crisis intervention
worker, this chapter deals with when a client
commits suicide, the feelings of survivors,
and survivors as clients of the crisis
intervention service.

9-112   Graves, J. S. (1978). Adolescents and their
psychiatrist's suicide: A study of shared grief
and mourning. Journal of the American Academy of
Child Psychiatry, 17(3), 521-532.

9-113   Henn, R. F. (1978). Patient suicides as part of
psychiatric residency. American Journal of
Psychiatry, 135, 745-747.

9-114   Holden, L. D. (1978, May). Therapist response to
patient suicide: Professional and personal.
Journal of Continuing Education in Psychiatry,
39(5), 23-32.

9-115   Kayton, L., & Freed, F. (1967). Effects of a
suicide in a psychiatric hospital. Archives of
General Psychiatry, 17, 187-194.

9-116   Kibel, H. D. (1973). A group member's suicide:
Treating collective trauma. International
Journal of Group Psychotherapy, 23, 42-53.

9-117   Kirtley, D. D., & Sacks, J. M. (1969). Reactions
        of a psychotherapy group to ambiguous
        circumstances surrounding the death of a group
        member. Journal of Consulting and Clinical
        Psychology, 33, 195-199.

9-118   Kolodny, S., Binder, R., Bronstein, A., & Friend,
        R. (1979). The working through of patients'
        suicides by four therapists. Suicide and
        Life-Threatening Behavior, 9, 33-46.

9-119   Krueger, D. W. (1979). Patient suicide: Model for
        medical student teaching and mourning. General
        Hospital Psychiatry, 1(3), 229-233.

9-120   Litman, R. (1965). When patients commit suicide.
        American Journal of Psychotherapy, 19, 570-576.
        (Reprinted in E. S. Shneidman, N. L. Farberow, &
        R. E. Litman (Eds.) (1970), The psychology of
        suicide (pp. 475-482). New York: Science
        House.)

9-121   Marshall, K. (1980). When a patient commits
        suicide. Suicide and Life-Threatening Behavior,
        10, 29-40.

9-122   Olin, H. S. (1980). Management precautions for
        surviving patients after a ward suicide.
        Hospital & Community Psychiatry, 31(5), 348-349.

9-123   Soreff, S. M. (1975). The impact of staff suicide
        on a psychiatric inpatient unit. Journal of
        Nervous and Mental Disorders, 161, 130-133.

        The effect of a nurse's suicide on patients
        and staff are studied and discussed.

See also Fuchs (1982, reference 6-228.04).

9.7 Psychological Autopsies: Bibliographies

9-124   American Association of Suicidology. Psychological
        autopsies [Annotated bibliography]. Denver, CO:
        AAS.

9-125   Miller, M. Psychological autopsies [Non-annotated
        bibliography]. San Diego: Center for
        Information on Suicide, Bibliography No. R-13.
        (Listed in the 1984 catalog.) See also reference
        1-010.

9.8 Psychological Autopsies: Description and Applications

9-126   Choron, J. (1972). Suicide (pp. 86-90). New York:
        Scribner's, Chapter 9, "The psychological
        autopsy."

9-127   Curphy, T. (1967). The forensic pathologist and
         the multidisciplinary approach to death. In
         E. S. Shneidman (Ed.), Essays in self-destruction
         (pp. 463-474). New York: Science House.

9-128   Curphy, T. (1968, July). The psychological
         autopsy: The role of the forensic pathologist in
         the muti-disciplinary approach to death.
         Bulletin of Suicidology, No. 3, pp. 39-45.

9-129   Diller, J. (1979). The psychological autopsy in
         equivocal deaths. Perspectives in Psychiatric
         Care, 17(4), 156-161.

9-130   Hatton, C. L., Valente, S. M., & Rink, A. (1977).
         Variables in suicide statistics. In
         C. L. Hatton, S. M. Valente, & A. Rink (Eds.),
         Suicide: Assessment and intervention
         (pp. 133-138; esp. pp. 137-138, "The
         psychological autopsy"). New York:
         Appleton-Century-Crofts.

9-131   Krieger, G. (1968). Psychological autopsies of
         hospital suicides. Hospital & Community
         Psychiatry, 19, 218-220.

9-132   Litman, R. E., Curphy, T., Shneidman, E. S.,
         Farberow, N. L., & Tabachnick, N. (1963).
         Investigations of equivocal suicides. Journal of
         the American Medical Association, 184, 924-929.
         (Reprinted in E. S. Shneidman, N. L. Farberow, &
         R. E. Litman (Eds.) (1970), The psychology of
         suicide (pp. 485-496). New York: Science House,
         under the title, "The psychological autopsy of
         equivocal deaths.")

9-133   Neill, K., Benensohn, H. S., Farber, A. N., &
         Resnik, H. L. P. (1974). The psychological
         autopsy: A technique for investigating a
         hospital suicide. Hospital & Community
         Psychiatry, 25, 33-36.

9-134   Rudestam, K. E. (1979). Some notes on conducting a
         psychological autopsy. Suicide and
         Life-Threatening Behavior, 9(3), 141-144.

9-135   Sanborn, D. E., III, & Sanborn, C. J. (1976). The
         psychological autopsy as a therapeutic tool.
         Diseases of the Nervous System, 37(1), 5-8.

9-136   Shneidman, E. S. (1969). Suicide, lethality and
         the psychological autopsy. In E. S. Shneidman &
         M. Ortega (Eds.), Aspects of depression
         (pp. 225-250; esp. pp. 239-249). Boston:
         Little, Brown. (International Psychiatry
         Clinics, 6(2).)

9-137   Shneidman, E. S. (1973). Deaths of man
         (pp. 131-149). New York: Quandrangle, Chapter
         12, "The psychological autopsy."

9-138   Shneidman, E. S. (1977). The psychological
         autopsy. In L. I. Gottschalk, F. L. McGuire,
         E. C. Dinovo, H. Birch, & J. F. Heiser (Eds.),
         Guide to the investigation and reporting of drug
         abuse deaths: Problems and methods (pp. 42-56).
         Washington, D.C.: USGPO, DHEW Publication
         No. (ADM) 77-386. (Reprinted in Suicide and
         Life-Threatening Behavior, 1981, 11(4), 325-340.)

9-139   Victoroff, V. M. (1983). The suicidal patient:
         Recognition, intervention, management
         (pp. 210-212, "The psychological autopsy").
         Oradell, NJ: Medical Economics Books.

9-140   Weisman, A. (1967, December). The psychological
         autopsy and the potential suicide. Bulletin of
         Suicidology, No. 2, 15-24.

9-141   Weisman, A. (1974). The realization of death: A
         guide for the psychological autopsy. New York:
         Jason Aronson.

9-142   Weisman, A. D., & Kastenbaum, R. (1968). The
         psychological autopsy: A study of the terminal
         phase of life. (Community Mental Health Journal
         Monograph No. 4). New York: Behavioral
         Publications.

9-143   Wekstein, L. (1979). Handbook of suicidology:
         Principles, problems and practice (pp. 121-123,
         "The psychological autopsy"). New York:
         Brunner/Mazel.

9.9 Psychological Autopsies Appearing in the Literature

9-144   Blanchard, J. D., Blanchard, E. L., & Roll,
         S. (1976). A psychological autopsy of an Indian
         adolescent suicide with implications for
         community services. Suicide and Life-Threatening
         Behavior, 6(1), 3-10.

9-145   Casey, T. M., Niswander, D., Sanborn, D. E., III, &
         Segal, B. (1971, Fall). Psychological autopsy:
         The life history of Kip. Bulletin of
         Suicidology, No. 8, 85-89. Case commentary by
         J. T. Ungerleider, 90-91.

9-146   Diekel, S. M. (1974). The life and death of Lenny
         Bruce: A psychological autopsy.
         Life-Threatening Behavior, 4, 176-192.

9-147   Grow, B. K., Jr., Schwartz, A. H., Grinder, D. H.,

& Lorensen, S. L.(1970). Psychological autopsy
in two cases of reported suicide in early
adolescence. American Journal of
Orthopsychiatry, 40(1), 339-340.

9-148   Kissin, G., & Laury, G. V. (1981). The
psychological autopsy: A life reconstruction.
Journal of Psychiatric Treatment and Evaluation,
3(4), 391-394. (Abstract: Biological Abstracts,
1983, 75, No. 21768)

9-149   Lester, G., & Lester, D. (1971). Suicide: The
gamble with death (pp. 149-158). Englewood
Cliffs, NJ: Prentice-Hall, Chapter 19, "A case
of suicide."

9-150   Lum, D. (1974). Responding to suicidal crisis:
For church and community (pp. 117-141,
esp. pp. 135-140, "A retrospective exercise,"
p. 203). Grand Rapids, MI: Eerdmans, Chapter 7,
"Coping with the suicidal crisis."

A case history is offered to readers along
with questions to consider in deciding for
themselves, in psychological autopsy fashion,
if there is evidence for the death to be
classified as a suicide. The professional
assessment of the case appears in an appendix
(p. 203).

9-151   Miller, M. (1978). A psychological autopsy of a
geriatric suicide. Journal of Geriatric
Psychiatry, 10, 229-242. (Abstract: PA, 1980,
64, No. 1284, p. 144) (Reprinted in Miller,
M. (1979). Suicide after sixty: The final
alternative (pp. 82-90). New York: Springer.)

9-152   Niswander, G. D., Casey, T. M., & Humphrey,
J. A. (1973). A panorama of suicide: A casebook
of psychological autopsies. Springfield, IL:
Thomas.

Psychological autopsies are presented of
individuals in various situations and
circumstances: child and adolescent,
mid-life, elderly, terminally ill, psychotic,
anniversary, impulsive, planned, minimum
signal.

9-153   Pretzel, P. W., Alexander, P. P., Peck, M. L.,
Klugman, D. J., Heilig, S. M., Marks, G. H.,
Farberow, N. L., Wold, C. I., Litman, R. E., &
Green, J. S. (1970, Fall). Psychological autopsy
No. 1: From the files of the Los Angeles Suicide
Prevention Center. Bulletin of Suicidology,
No. 7, 27-33. Case commentary by R. Kastenbaum,

33-35.

9-154   Salmon, J. A., Hajek, P. T., Rachut, E., Mackenzie,
        T. B., & Popkin, M. K. (1982). Mortality
        conference: Suicide of an "appropriately"
        depressed medical inpatient. General Hospital
        Psychiatry, 4, 307-313. (Abstract: PA, 1983,
        70, No. 5720, p. 642)

9-155   Shneidman, E. S., & Farberow, N. L. (1961). Sample
        investigations of equivocal suicidal deaths. In
        N. L. Farberow & E. S. Shneidman (Eds.), The cry
        for help (pp. 118-128). New York: McGraw-Hill.
        (Reprinted in E. S. Shneidman, N. L. Farberow, &
        R. E. Litman (Eds.) (1970), The psychology of
        suicide (pp. 497-510). New York: Science House,
        with the title of "Sample psychological
        autopsies.")

9.10 Suicide Notes: Bibliographies

9-156   Miller, M. Suicide notes [Non-annotated
        bibliography]. San Diego, CA: Suicide
        Information Center, Bibliography No. R-9.
        (Listed in the 1984 catalog.) See also reference
        1-010.

* 9-157   Shneidman, E. S. (1979). A bibliography of suicide
        notes: 1856-1979. Suicide and Life-Threatening
        Behavior, 9, 57-59.

        A non-annotated, chronologically arranged
        bibliography.

9.11 Suicide Notes: General Considerations and Overviews

* 9-158   Frederick, C. J. (1969, March). Suicide notes: A
        survey and evaluaton. Bulletin of Suicidology,
        No. 5, pp. 17-26.

        Frederick reviews in detail the methods and
        results of 18 studies on suicide notes from
        1945 to 1969.

* 9-159   Lester, D. (1972). Why people kill themselves: A
        summary of research findings on suicidal behavior
        (pp. 242-258). Springfield, IL: Thomas, Chapter
        22, "The suicide note."

9-160   Lester, D. (1983). Why people kill themselves: A
        1980's summary of research findings on suicidal
        behavior (2nd ed.) (pp. 101-105;
        esp. pp. 101-102). Springfield, IL: Thomas,
        Chapter 17, "Communication and the suicidal act."

        In these two chapters (9-159 and 9-160) Lester

reviews and presents a methodological critique
and the results of research on suicide notes.

9-161 Lester, G., & Lester, D. (1971). Suicide: The
gamble with death (pp. 74-81; esp. pp. 76-80).
Englewood Cliffs, NJ: Prentice-Hall, Chapter 10,
"Suicidal communications and the suicide note."

* 9-162 Shneidman, E. S. (1973). Suicide notes
reconsidered. Psychiatry, 36, 379-394.
(Reprinted in E. S. Shneidman (Ed.) (1976),
Suicidology: Contemporary developments
(pp. 257-278). New York: Grune & Stratton.)

Following his personal research of suicide
notes and that of others, Shneidman concludes
that they cannot generally help in our
understanding of why people kill themselves
and that they are not very revealing.

* 9-163 Shneidman, E. S. (1980). Voices of death
(pp. 41-76). New York: Harper & Row, Chapter 3,
"Self-destruction: Suicide notes and tragic
lives." (Reprinted in E. S. Shneidman (Ed.)
(1980), Death: Current perspectives (2nd ed.)
(pp. 467-491). Palo Alto, CA: Mayfield
Publishing. Reprinted in Suicide and
Life-Threatening Behavior, 11(4), 286-299.)

Shneidman contends, as in 1973 (reference
9-162), that suicide notes generally will not
be the explanatory documents we had hoped, but
in the context of the specific individual's
life they may be quite valuable.

9.12 Suicide Notes: Research Investigations

9-164 Atkinson, M. W., Kessel, N., & Dalgaard,
J. B. (1975). The comparability of suicide
notes. British Journal of Psychiatry, 127,
247-256. (Abstract: ACP, 1976, 16, No. 299,
p. 93)

9-165 Beck, R. W., Morris, J., & Lester, D. (1974).
Suicide notes and the risk of future suicide.
Journal of the American Medical Association, 228,
495-496.

Those in the samples who left suicide notes
(14% of attempters and 24% of the completed
suicides) displayed greater suicide intent
than those who did not leave notes.

9-166 Bjerg, K. (1967). The suicidal life space:
Attempts at a reconstruction from suicide notes.
In E. S. Shneidman (Ed.), Essays in

self-destruction (pp. 475-493). New York: Science House.

9-167   Chynoweth, R. (1977). The significance of suicide notes. Australian & New Zealand Journal of Psychiatry, 11, 197-200. (Abstracts: EM, 1978, Section 32, 38, No. 1150, pp. 210-211; PA, 1979, 61, No. 6205, p. 623)

9-168   Cohen, S. L., & Fiedler, J. E. (1974). Content analysis of multiple messages in suicide notes. Life-Threatening Behavior, 4, 75-95.

9-169   Darbonne, A. R. (1969). Suicide and age: A suicide note analysis. Journal of Consulting and Clinical Psychology, 33, 46-50.

9-170   Darbonne, A. R. (1969). Study of psychological content in the communications of suicidal individuals. Journal of Consulting and Clinical Psychology, 33, 590-596.

9-171   Edelman, A. M., & Renshaw, S. L. (1982). Genuine versus simulated suicide notes: An issue revisited through discourse analysis. Suicide and Life-Threatening Behavior, 12, 103-113. (Abstracts: CPA, 1982, 22, No. 2718, p. 580; PA, 1983, 69, No. 3666, p. 396)

9-172   Edland, J. F., & Duncan, C. E. (1973). Suicide notes in Monroe County: A 23 year look (1950-1972). Journal of Forensic Sciences, 18, 364-369.

9-173   Farberow, N. L., & Shneidman, E. S. (1957). Suicide and age. In E. S. Shneidman & N. L. Farberow (Eds.), Clues to suicide (pp. 41-49). New York: McGraw-Hill. (Reprinted in E. S. Shneidman, N. L. Farberow, & R. E. Litman (Eds.), The psychology of suicide (pp. 165-174). New York: Science House.)

        A study of 619 suicide notes revealed differences in motivation by age.

9-174   Frederick, C. J. (1968). An investigation of handwriting of suicide persons through suicide notes. Journal of Abnormal Psychology, 73, 263-267.

9-175   Gottschalk, L. A., & Gleser, G. C. (1960). An analysis of the verbal content of suicide notes. British Journal of Medical Psychology, 33, 195-204.

9-176   Henken, V. J. (1976). Banality reinvestigated: A

computer-based content analysis of suicidal and
forced death documents. Suicide and
Life-Threatening Behavior, 6, 36-43.

9-177   Hood, R. W. (1970). Effects of foreknowledge of
manner of death in the assessment from genuine
and simulated suicide notes of intent to die.
Journal of General Psychology, 82, 215-221.

9-178   Jacobs, J. (1967). Phenomenological study of
suicide notes. Social Problems, 15, 60-72.
(Reprinted in A. Giddens (Ed.) (1971), The
sociological of suicide: A selection of readings
(pp. 332-348). London: Cass. An abridged and
revised version is reprinted in Jacobs,
J. (1982). The moral justification of suicide
(pp. 25-42). Springfield, IL: Thomas.)

Jacobs categorized a set of 112 notes from
suicides in Los Angeles.

9-179   Leenaars, A. A., & Balance, W. D. G. (1981). A
predictive approach to the study of manifest
content in suicide notes. Journal of Clinical
Psychology, 37, 50-52.

9-180   Lester, D. (1971). Choice of method for suicide
and personality: A study of suicide notes.
Omega, 2, 76-80.

9-181   Lester, D. (1971). Need for affiliation in suicide
notes. Perceptual & Motor Skills, 33, 550.

9-182   Lester, D., & Hummel, H. (1980). Motives for
suicide in elderly people. Psychological
Reports, 47, 870.

A study of 52 suicide notes revealed different
results by age than Farberow and Shneidman
(1957, reference 9-173) had observed.

9-183   Lester, D., & Reeve, C. (1982). The suicide notes
of young and old people. Psychological Reports,
50, 334. (Abstract: CPA, 1982, 22, No. 2715,
pp. 579-580)

Further investigation of the 52 notes studied
by Lester and Hummel (1980, reference 9-182)
above, by sex and age.

9-184   Maris, R. W. (1981). Pathways to suicide: A
survey of self-destructive behaviors
(pp. 275-279, "Suicide notes"). Baltimore: John
Hopkins University Press.

Of the 330 suicide attempters and completers

Maris studied, 75 (23%) left notes. Some
examples are presented and the issue is
discussed.

9-185   Ogilvie, D. M., Stone, P. J., & Shneidman,
E. S. (1966). Some characteristics of genuine
and simulated suicide notes. In P. J. Stone,
D. C. Dunphy, M. S. Smith, & D. M. Ogilvie
(Eds.), The general inquirer: A computer
approach to content analysis (pp. 527-535).
Cambridge, MA: M.I.T. Press. (Reprinted,
Bulletin of Suicidology, March 1969, No. 5,
pp.27-32. Reprinted as "A computer analysis of
suicide notes." In E. S. Shneidman,
N. L. Farberow, & R. E. Litman (Eds.), The
psychology of suicide (pp. 249-256). New York:
Science House.)

9-186   Osgood, C. E., & Walker, E. G. (1959). Motivation
and language behavior: A content analysis of
suicide notes. Journal of Abnormal and Social
Psychology, 59, 58-67.

9-187   Shneidman, E. S., & Farberow, N. L. (1956). Clues
to suicide. Public Health Reports, 71, 109-114.
(Reprinted with minor changes in E. S. Shneidman
& N. L. Farberow (Eds.) (1957). Clues to
suicide (pp. 3-10). New York: McGraw-Hill.)

An investigation in which case histories,
psychological tests, and suicide notes are
studied to provide insight into the suicidal
individual.

9-188   Shneidman, E. S., & Farberow, N. L. (1957).
Appendix: Genuine and simulated suicide notes.
In E. S. Shneidman & N. L. Farberow (Eds.), Clues
to suicide (pp. 197-215). New York:
McGraw-Hill.

Thirty-three pairs of genuine and simulated
suicide notes are published here. This set of
notes has been the focus of a number of
studies: Edelman & Renshaw (1982, reference
9-171); Gottschalk & Gleser (1960, reference
9-175); Henken (1976, reference 9-176); Hood
(1970, reference 9-177); Leenaars & Balance
(1981, reference 9-179); Ogilvie, Stone, &
Shneidman (1966, reference 9-185); Osgood &
Walker (1959, reference 9-186); Shneidman &
Farberow (1956, reference 9-187); Shneidman &
Farberow (1957, reference 9-189); Spiegel &
Neuringer (1963, reference 9-190); Tripodes
(1976, reference 9-191); and Tuckman &
Ziegler (1966, reference 9-193).

9-189   Shneidman, E. S., & Farberow, N. L. (1957). Some
        comparisons between genuine and simulated suicide
        notes in terms of Mowrer's concepts of discomfort
        and relief. Journal of General Psychology, 56,
        251-256. (Reprinted as "A psychological approach
        to the study of suicide notes." In E. S.
        Shneidman, N. L. Farberow, & R. E. Litman (Eds.),
        The psychology of suicide (pp. 159-164). New
        York: Science House.)

9-190   Spiegel, D. E., & Neuringer, C. (1963). Role of
        dread in suicidal behavior. Journal of Abnormal
        and Social Psychology, 66, 507-511.

9-191   Tripodes, P. (1976). Reasoning patterns in suicide
        notes. In E. S. Shneidman (Ed.), Suicidology:
        Contemporary developments (pp. 207-228). New
        York: Grune & Stratton.

9-192   Tuckman, J., Kleiner, R. J., & Lavell, M. (1959).
        Emotional content of suicide notes. American
        Journal of Psychiatry, 116, 59-63.

9-193   Tuckman, J., & Ziegler, R. (1966). Language usage
        and social maturity as related to suicide notes.
        Journal of Social Psychology, 68, 139-142.

9-194   Tuckman, J., & Ziegler, R. (1968). A comparison of
        single and multiple note writers among suicides.
        Journal of Clinical Psychology, 24, 179-180.

9.13 Sources Cited in the Chapter Text But Not Listed Above

9-195   Shneidman, E. S. (1969). Prologue: Fifty-eight
        years. In E. S. Shneidman (Ed.), On the nature
        of suicide (pp. 1-30). San Francisco:
        Jossey-Bass.

9-196   Shneidman, E. S. (1972). Foreword. In A. C. Cain
        (Ed.), Survivors of suicide (pp. ix-xi).
        Springfield, IL: Thomas.

Chapter 10
SUICIDE LITERATURE DIRECTED TO SPECIFIC GATEKEEPERS
& SUICIDE AND ART

As pointed out in the introduction to this book, the field of suicidology is extremely multidisciplinary. Reflecting this diversity, the present chapter presents information and references specifically directed to audiences within a single discipline. Also included is a section on suicide and the arts.

10.1 Clergy

10-001   Anderson, D. A. (1972, February). A resurrection model for suicide prevention through the church. Pastoral Psychology, 23, 33-40.

10-002   Coleman, W. L. (1979). Understanding suicide. Elgin, IL: Cook Publishing.

         This book gives an overview of suicide as well as particular chapters which are especially relevant to clergy: Chapter 3, "From God's perspective," 15, "The role of the minister." This book contains much practical information on how to recognize and get help for the suicidal person as well as how to deal with personal feelings and the family.

10-003   Grollman, E. A. (1966, January). Pastoral counseling of the potential suicidal person. Pastoral Psychology, 16(160), 46-52.

10-004   Hewett, J. H. (1980). After suicide. Philadelphia: Westminster Press.

         The author, a Baptist pastor, wrote this book for those surviving a suicide. Included is a section on "Suicide and your faith," which includes chapters on "Suicide in Jewish tradition," "Suicide in Christian tradition," "Thinking straight about God," and "Your religious life in the aftermath." Also included is an example of an anniversary memorial service to aid in working through the grief and bereavement process.

10-005   Hiltner, S. (1966, January). The pastor and suicide prevention: An editorial. Pastoral Psychology, 16(160), 28-29.

10-006   Lum, D. (1974). Responding to suicidal crisis: For church and community. Grand Rapids, MI: Eerdmans Publishing.

Lum includes a survey of pastoral clinical experiences with suicide among Los Angeles clergy. Also presented is a chapter on "Involving the church in suicide prevention."

10-007   McGee, L. I., & Hiltner, S. (1968). The role of the clergy. In H. L. P. Resnik (Ed.), Suicide: Diagnosis and management (pp. 462-474). Boston: Little, Brown.

10-008   Pretzel, P. W. (1970, April). The role of the clergyman in suicide prevention. Pastoral Psychology, 21, 47-52.

10-009   Pretzel, P. W. (1972). Understanding and counseling the suicidal person. Nashville, TN: Abingdon.

In addition to presenting a broad coverage of suicide, Pretzel also presents a chapter "Religion and suicide," which elaborates the the place of religion and pastoral counseling of suicides.

10-010   Rauscher, W. V. (1981). The case against suicide. New York: St. Martin's Press.

Rauscher presents the pro and con arguments regarding suicide and includes especially a chapter entitled "What does the Bible say?"

10-011   Stone, H. W. (1972). Suicide and grief. Philadelphia: Fortress Press.

A Lutheran minister, Stone has written this book for ministers but also for the layperson who experiences a suicide among someone they know and love. The book centers on the grief experience and dealing with it. Especially important here are two chapters, "Pastoral care of the suicide survivor," and "Preventative pastoral care."

10-012   Strunk, O., & Jordan, M. R. (1972, March).

Experimental course for clergymen in suicidology
and crisis intervention. Journal of Pastoral
Care, 26, 50-54.

10-013 Vincent, M. O. (1970, January 16). Suicide and how
to prevent it. Christianity Today, 14(8), 10-12.

10-014 Vincent, M. O. (1973). Suicide--A Christian
perspective. Suicide prevention--Where there's
hope there is life. In C. A. Frazier (Ed.), Is
it moral to modify man? (pp. 129-149).
Springfield, IL: Thomas.

10-015 Warren, H. M. (1979). Pastoral counseling. In
L. D. Hankoff & B. Einsidler (Eds.), Suicide:
Theory and clinical aspects (pp. 383-389).
Littleton, MA: PSG Publishing.

See also sections on religion: Sections 5.10e & 8.4. See
also: Holmes & Howard (1980, reference 7-123).

10.2 Law Enforcement Personnel

Bibliography:

10-016 Martin, C. E. (1980). Readings in suicide for law
enforcement officers. Monticello, IL: Vance
Bibliographies, Public Administration Series
Bibliography P-635. (29 pages)

Other Sources:

10-017 Cesnik, B. I., Pierce, N., & Puls, M. (1977). Law
enforcement and crisis intervention services: A
critical relationship. Suicide and
Life-Threatening Behavior, 7, 211-215.

10-018 Cooke, G. (1979). Training police officers to
handle suicidal persons. Journal of Forensic
Science, 24, 227-233.

10-019 Danto, B. L. (1979). New frontiers in the
relationship between suicidology and law
enforcement. Suicide and Life-Threatening
Behavior, 9, 195-204.

10-020 Heiman, M. F. (1975). Police suicide. Journal of
Police Science Administration, 3, 267-273.

10-021 Heiman, M. F. (1975). Police suicides revisited.
Suicide, 5, 5-20.

10-022 Heiman, M. F. (1977). Suicide among police.
American Journal of Psychiatry, 134, 1286-1290.

10-023 Litman, R. E. (1966). Police aspects of suicide.

Police, 10, 14-18. (Reprinted in
E. S. Shneidman, N. L. Farberow, & R. E. Litman
(Eds.) (1970), The psychology of suicide
(pp. 519-530). New York: Science House.)

10-024   Murphy, G. E., Clendenin, W. W., Darvish, H. S., &
         Robins, E. (1971). The role of the police in
         suicide prevention. Life-Threatening Behavior,
         1, 96-105.

10-025   Nelson, Z., & Smith, W. (1970). The law
         enforcement profession: An incident of high
         suicide. Omega, 1, 293-299.

10-026   O'Connor, G. W. (1968). The role of
         law-enforcement agencies. In H. L. P. Resnik
         (Ed.), Suicide: Diagnosis and management
         (pp. 475-478). Boston: Little, Brown.

See also: Section 5.11h, for jail and prison suicides.

10.3 Medical Professions

Bibliographies:

10-027   Miller, M. Non-annotated bibliographies. San
         Diego, CA: The Information Center. The 1984
         catalog lists:

         10-027.01 Physician suicides. Bibliography R-3.

         10-027.02 Intervention by nurses. Bibliography
                    R-12.

Other Sources:

10-028   Bell, K. K. (1970, Spring). The nurse's role in
         suicide prevention: Some aspects. Bulletin of
         Suicidology, No. 6, pp. 60-65.

10-029   Bergman, J. (1979). The suicide rate among
         psychiatrists revisited: A review. Suicide and
         Life-Threatening Behavior, 9, 219-226.

10-030   Bressler, B. (1976). Suicide and drug abuse in the
         medical community. Suicide and Life-Threatening
         Behavior, 6, 169-178.

10-031   Busteed, E. L., & Johnstone, C. (1983, May). The
         development of suicide precautions for an
         inpatient psychiatric unit. Journal of
         Psychosocial Nursing and Mental Health Services,
         21(5), 15-19.

10-032   Catalan, J., Hewett, J., Kennard, C., & McPherson,
         J. (1980). The role of the nurse in the

management of deliberate self-poisoning in the general hospital. International Journal of Nursing Studies, 17, 275-282.

10-033 Davis, J. H., & Spelman, J. W. (1968). The role of the medical examiner or coroner. In H. L. P. Resnik (Ed.), Suicide: Diagnosis and management (pp. 453-461). Boston: Little, Brown.

10-034 Farberow, N. L. (1981). Suicide prevention in the hospital. Hospital & Community Psychiatry, 32, 99-104.

10-035 Frederick, C. J. (1973). The role of the nurse in crisis intervention and suicide prevention. Journal of Psychiatric Nursing and Mental Health Services, 11, 27-31. (Reprinted in B. A. Backer, P. M. Dubbert, & E. J. P. Eisenman (Eds.) (1978), Psychiatric/Mental health nursing: Contemporary readings (pp. 193-203). New York: Van Nostrand.)

10-036 Horvath, K. (1982). Nursing issues. In E. L. Bassuk, S. C. Schoonover, & A. D. Gill (Eds.), Lifelines: Clinical perspectives on suicide (pp. 155-167). New York: Plenum Press.

10-037 Miller, M. (1977). The physician and the older suicidal patient. Journal of Family Practice, 5, 1028-1029. (Reprinted as "The role of the physician in geriatric suicides," in M. Miller (Ed.) (1979), Suicide after sixty: The final alternative (pp. 69-75). New York: Springer.)

*10-038 Miller, M. (1982). Suicide intervention by nurses. New York: Springer.

This collection of articles reprinted from various nursing publications includes writings on management, assessment and recognition, treatment, suicidal colleagues, liability and malpractice among its collection.

10-039 Pfeffer, C. R. (1980). Unanswered questions about childhood suicidal behavior: Perspectives for the practicing physician. Journal of Developmental and Behavioral Pediatrics, 1, 11-14.

10-040 Pisetsky, J. E., & Brown, W. (1979). The general hospital patient. In L. D. Hankoff & B. Einsidler (Eds.), Suicide: Theory and clinical aspects (pp. 279-289). Littleton, MA: PSG Publishing.

10-041   Rebal, R. F. (1982). Identification of the
         psychiatric resident at risk for suicide.
         Journal of Psychiatric Education, 6, 160-165.
         (Abstract: PA, 1983, 70, No. 8901, pp. 991-992)

10-042   Reguero, C. (1979). Suicide: The ultimate cry for
         help--How nurses can answer. Journal of
         Practical Nursing, 24, 21-22.

10-043   Rich, C. L., & Pitts, F. N., Jr. (1980). Suicide
         by psychiatrists: A study of medical specialists
         among 18,730 consecutive physician deaths during
         a five-year period, 1967-72. Journal of Clinical
         Psychiatry, 4, 261-263.

10-044   Rosenbauer, A. (1978). Suicide prevention and the
         emergency room nurse. Heart & Lung, 7, 101-104.

*10-045 Victoroff, V. M. (1983). The suicidal patient:
         Recognition, intervention, management. Oradell,
         NJ: Medical Economics Books.

         This book presents an excellent overview of
         suicide and focuses particularly on issues of
         importance to the medical professions:
         physicians and patients suicides, clues,
         predictors, treatment, prevention in the
         hospital, suicide among physicians, ethical
         and legal issues, and survivors of suicide.

10-046   von Brauchitsch, H. (1976). The physician's
         suicide revisited. Journal of Nervous and Mental
         Disease, 162, 40-45.

10-047   Waltzer, H. (1979). Physicians. In L. D. Hankoff
         & B. Einsidler (Eds.), Suicide: Theory and
         clinical aspects (pp. 323-333). Littleton, MA:
         PSG Publishing.

See also: Section 5.11e on physical illness and suicide;
Section 6.4 for intervention, management and medical
treatment; Bedeian (1982, reference 5-734b) for a review of
suicide among medical personnel as well as other
occupations; Shneidman (1965, reference 7-093), for a
review of clues to suicide.

10.4 Suicide and the Military

10-048   Chaffee, R. B. (1982). Completed suicide in the
         Navy and Marine Corps. US Naval Health Research
         Center Report, No. 82-17, 8 pages. (Abstract:
         PA, 1983, 70, No. 10458, p. 1171)

10-049   Datel, W. E., & Johnson, A. W., Jr. (1979).
         Suicide in United States Army personnel,
         1975-1976. Military Medicine, 144, 239-244.

(Data for 1977-1978, Datel with Jones, F. D., &
Esposito, M. E.: 1981, 146, 387-392. Data for
1979-1980, Datel with Jones, F. D.: 1982, 147,
843-847.)

10-050   Flach, H. (1983). A social-psychological
investigation on suicide attempts in a military
population. Crisis, 4, 16-32. (Abstract: PA,
1984, 71, No. 9776, p. 1027)

10-051   Gaines, T., Jr., & Richmond, L. H. (1980).
Assessing suicidal potential in basic military
trainees. Military Medicine, 145, 263-266.

10-052   Hankoff, L. D. (1979). The armed forces. In
L. D. Hankoff & B. Einsidler (Eds.), Suicide:
Theory and clinical aspects (pp. 343-349).
Littleton, MA: PSG Publishing.

10-053   Johnston, J. H., Cantlay, L., & Cormack,
J. D. (1980). Self-poisoning in a military
community from 1976-1977. Journal of the Royal
Army Medical Corps, 126, 88-91.

10-054   Rosenbaum, M., & Richman, J. (1970). Suicide
prevention in the military. Military Medicine,
135, 500-501.

10-055   Smith, V. A., & Whitley, M. Q. (1981).
Self-destructive behavior and alcohol abuse
patterns among United States naval recruits in
training. Military Medicine, 146, 346-347.

10-056   Strange, R. E., & Brown, D. E. (1970). Home from
the war: A study of psychiatric problems in Viet
Nam returnees. American Journal of Psychiatry,
127, 488-492.

10-057   Wasileski, M., & Kelly, D. A. (1982).
Characteristics of suicide attempters in a Marine
recruit population. Military Medicine, 147,
818-819, 827-830.

See also: Flinn & Leonard (1972, reference 5-812);   Datel
(1979, reference 5-032).

10.5 School Personnel: Faculty & Counselors

10-058   Bagley, C. (1975). Suicidal behaviour and suicidal
ideation in adolescents: A problem for
counselors in education. British Journal of
Guidance and Counseling, 3, 190-208.

10-059   Baker, H. S. (1978). A nurses' guide to the acute
management of suicidal patients in the student

health center. _Journal of the American College Health Association_, 26 253-255.

10-060 Blomquist, K. B. (1974, January-February). Nurse, I need help: The school nurse's role in suicide prevention. _Journal of Psychiatric Nursing_, 12, 22-26. (Reprinted in M. Miller (Ed.) (1982). _Suicide intervention by nurses_ (pp. 133-142). New York: Springer.)

10-061 Finley, B., & Mynatt, S. (1981). Faculty intervention into suicidal crisis. _Nurse Educator_, 6, 12-16.

10-062 Fitchette, B. (1982). Suicide in youth: What counsellors can do about it. _School Guidance Worker_, 38(2), 23-26.

10-063 Frederick, C. J. (1970). The school guidance counselor as a preventive agent to self-destructive behavior. _New York State Personnel and Guidance Journal_, 5(1), 1-5.

10-064 Grob, M. C., Klein, A. A., & Eisen, S. V. (1983). The role of the high school professional in identifying and managing adolescent suicidal behavior. _Journal of Youth and Adolescence_, 12, 163-173. (Abstract: _PA_, 1984, 71, No. 7019, p. 742)

10-065 Hart, N. A. (1978, April). How teachers can help suicidal adolescents. _The Clearing House_, 51(8), 369-373.

10-066 Hipple, J. L., Cimbolic, P., & Peterson, J. (1980). Student services response to a suicide. _Journal of College Student Personnel_, 21, 457-458.

10-067 McBrien, R. J. (1983). Are you thinking about killing yourself?: Confronting students' suicidal thoughts. _School Counselor_, 31, 75-82.

10-068 McKenry, P. C., Tishler, C. L., & Christman, K. L. (1980). Adolescent suicide and the classroom teacher. _Journal of School Health_, 50, 130-132. (Condensed version reprinted in _Education Digest_, September 1980, pp. 43-45.)

10-069 Morgan, L. B. (1981). Counselor's role in suicide prevention. _Personnel & Guidance Journal_, 59, 284-286.

10-070 Powers, D. (1979).The teacher and the adolescent suicide threat. _Journal of School Health_, 49, 561-563.

10-071   Ross, C. P. (1980). Mobilizing schools for suicide
         prevention. Suicide and Life-Threatening
         Behavior, 10, 239-243.

10-072   Schuyler, D. (1973). Preventing suicides among
         children--What the schools can do. Social
         Science Record, 10(2), 25-29.

10-073   Schuyler, D. (1973). When was the last time you
         took a suicidal child to lunch? Journal of
         School Health, 43, 504-506.

10-074   Smith, E. J. (1981). Adolescent suicide: A
         growing problem for the school and family. Urban
         Education, 16, 279-296.

See Hendrickson & Cameron (1975, reference 5-227); Section
5.6d, college students; Section 5.6c children and
adolescents.

10.6 Social Workers & Family Therapists

10-075   Farmer, R. D. T., & Hirsch, S. R. (Eds.) (1980).
         The suicide syndrome. London: Croom Helm.

         10-075.01   Newson-Smith, J. G. B. The use of social
                     workers as alternatives to
                     psychiatrists in assessing parasuicide.
                     pp. 215-225. (see also: British
                     Journal of Psychiatry, 1979, 134,
                     335-342.)

         10-075.02   Gibbons, J. S. Management of
                     self-poisoning: Social work
                     intervention. pp. 237-245.

10-076   Gibbons, J. S., Elliot, J., Urwin, P., & Gibbons,
         J. L. (1978). Evaluation of a social work
         service for self-poisoning patients. British
         Journal of Psychiatry, 133, 111-118.

10-077   Kress, H. (1982). The role of the social worker.
         In E. L. Bassuk, S. C. Schoonover, & A. D. Gill
         (Eds.), Lifelines: Clinical perspectives on
         suicide (pp. 169-179). New York: Plenum.

10-078   Walker, B. A., & Mehr, M. (1983). Adolescent
         suicide--A family crisis: A model for effective
         intervention by family therapists. Adolescence,
         18(70), 285-292.

For family therapy, see also Section 6.6 on therapy,
especially references 6-225, 6-270.03, and 6-272--6-274.

10.7 Suicide in Art and Literature

Bibliographic Sources:

10-079   Trautmann, J., & Pollard, C. (1982).   Literature
         and medicine: An annotated bibliography
         (esp. pp. 225-226, "Suicide"). Pittsburgh:
         University of Pittsburgh Press.

         This book lists novels, poems, dramas,
         novellas, sonnets, and short stories dealing
         with the topic of suicide.

See also: Lester et al. (1980, reference 1-009), for a
section on "Suicide and literature," pp. 113-142. For art,
this is an excellent source, listing authors who have
completed suicide, literary works dealing with the theme of
suicide, and strategies for locating works of various types
(novels, short stories, poetry, etc.).

See also: Cutter (1983, reference 10-085 below) for
appendices which list artists who painted suicidal themes
and artists who committed suicide in addition to an
historical look at suicide in art.

See also: Prentice (1974, reference 1-013), for a section
on "Literary works," pp. 190-197, which includes novels,
plays, short stories, and poetry.

Other Works:

10-080   Adler, C. S., Stanford, G., & Adler,
         S. M. (Eds.) (1976). We are but a moment's
         sunlight: Understanding death (pp. 205-249,
         "'Unspeakable darkness': Suicide," 6 works).
         New York: Pocket Books.

10-081   Alvarez, A. (1972). The savage god: A study of
         suicide (pp. 139-264, Part 4, "Suicide and
         literature," an historical presentation). New
         York: Random House.

10-082   Alvarez, A. (1975). Literature in the nineteenth
         and twentieth centuries. In S. Perlin (Ed.), A
         handbook for the study of suicide (pp. 31-60).
         New York: Oxford University Press.

10-083   Chase, K. S. (1973). Subintentioned death in
         Tolstoy's The death of Ivan Ilych.
         Life-Threatening Behavior, 3, 225-233.

10-084   Cutter, F. (1972). Suicidal themes in visual art.
         Omega, 3, 1-22. [includes 15 illustrations]

*10-085 Cutter, F. (1983). Art and the wish to die.
         Chicago: Nelson-Hall.

10-086   Eisen, G. S. (1980). The suicide of Seymour Glass
         [character in Salinger's fiction]. Suicide and
         Life-Threatening Behavior, 10, 51-60.

10-087   Faber, M. D. (1967). Shakespeare's suicides: Some
         historic, dramatic and psychological reflections.
         In E. S. Shneidman (Ed.), Essays in
         self-destruction (pp. 30-58). New York: Science
         House.

10-088   Faber, M. D. (1970). Suicide and Greek tragedy.
         New York: Sphinx.

10-089   Faber, M. D. (1972). The adolescent suicides of
         Romeo and Juliet. Psychoanalytic Review, 59,
         169-181.

10-090   Feggetter, G. (1980). Suicide in opera. British
         Journal of Psychiatry, 136, 552-557.

10-091   Foy, J. L., & Rojcewicz, S. J., Jr. (1979).
         Dostoevsky and suicide. Confinia Psychiatrica,
         22, 65-80.

10-092   Heiman, M. (1976). Psychoanalytic observations on
         the last painting and suicide of Vincent van
         Gogh. International Journal of Psychoanalysis,
         57, 71-84.

10-093   Lester, D. (1972). Suicide in Ibsen's plays.
         Life-Threatening Behavior, 2, 35-41.

10-094   Lester, D. (1974). Comment on Faber's analysis of
         Jacosta's suicide in "Oedipus Rex."
         Psychological Reports, 34, 182.

10-095   Murray, H. A. (1967). Dead to the world: The
         passions of Herman Melville. In E. S. Shneidman
         (Ed.), Essays in self-destruction (pp. 7-29).
         New York: Science House.

10-096   Nigro, D. (1975). Death and suicide in modern
         lyrics. Suicide, 5, 232-245.

10-097   Norman, M. (1983). 'night mother. New York: Hill
         & Wang.

         A Broadway play which won the Pulitzer Prize
         for drama in 1983.

10-098   Ravin, J. G., Hartman, J. J., & Fried,
         R. I. (1978). Mark Rothko's paintings...suicide
         notes? Ohio State Medical Journal, 74(2), 78-79.

10-099   Shneidman, E. S. (1968). The deaths of Herman
         Melville. In H. P. Vincent (Ed.), Melville and

Hawthorne in the Berkshires (pp. 118-143). Kent, OH: Kent State University Press. (Reprinted in E. S. Shneidman, N. L. Farberow, & R. L. Litman (Eds.) (1970), The psychology of suicide (pp. 587-613). New York: Science House. Reprinted in edited version as "A literary example of partial death," in E. S. Shneidman (1973), Deaths of man (pp. 161-177). New York: Quandrangle.)

10-100   Shneidman, E. S. (1976). Some psychological reflections on the death of Malcolm Melville. Suicide and Life-Threatening Behavior, 6, 231-242.

10-101   Shneidman, E. S. (1979). Risk writing: A special note about Cesare Pavese and Joseph Conrad. Journal of the American Academy of Psychoanalysis, 7, 575-592.

10-102   Shneidman, E. S. (1982). The suicidal logic of Cesare Pavese. Journal of the American Academy of Psychoanalysis, 10, 547-563.

10-103   Simone, F., Felici, F., Valerio, P., & Montella, P. (1977). Suicide in the literary work of Cesare Pavese. Suicide and Life-Threatening Behavior, 7, 183-188.

10-104   Slochower, H. (1975). Suicides in literature: Their ego function. American Imago, 32, 389-416.

10-105   Walley, K. W., & Kalish, R. A. (1971). Suicide in opera: A brief analysis. Omega, 2, 191-194.

10-106   Weir, R. F. (Ed.) (1980). Death in literature (pp. 225-268, section on "Suicide," 12 works). New York: Columbia University Press.

10-107   Zito, G. V. (1973). Durkheimian suicides in Shakespeare. Omega, 4, 293-304.

See also: Schipkowensky et al. (1975, reference 5-430.11).

AUTHOR INDEX

Numbers are those of the citations (of the form: chapter number-reference number). Only the authors of the citations are listed, i.e., authors of edited books in which the citations occur and citations of authors in text are not referenced in the index.

Draper, R., 6-189, 6-249,
    6-410
Dressler, D. M., 6-207,
    7-016
Droogas, A., 7-017
Drummond, H. P., 1-093
Dublin, L. I., 1-037,
    1-038, 3-007, 5-091,
    6-010, 6-294, 8-129a
Dubois, M. J., 8-106
Dubovsky, S. L., 5-690
Duff, R. A., 8-081b
Duncan, C. E., 9-172
Duncan-Jones, P., 2-015
Dunne, E. J., 9-092a.01,
    9-092b.02
Dunner, D. L., 5-676, 6-149
Durkheim, E., 1-039, 4-013,
    5-092
Duszynski, K. R., 6-153
Dwyer, P. M., 5-779
Dyer, J. A. T., 5-844a

Eastwood, M. R., 5-500,
    5-598, 6-295
Eaton, W. W., 5-138
Ebersole, E., 5-899
Eckert, W. G., 5-780
Eckman, T., 6-255
Eddy, J. M., 1-049c
Eddy, S., 6-143
Edelman, A. M., 9-171
Edington, B. M., 2-086.02
Edland, J. F., 5-045, 9-172
Edwards, D. E., 6-431
Einsidler, B., 1-066
Eisen, G. S., 10-086
Eisen, S. V., 10-064
Eisenthal, S., 6-128.07
Elkins, R. L., Jr., 6-296
Ellenson, G. M., 6-353
Elliott, J., 10-076
Elliott, T. N., 6-237
Ellner, M., 5-405
Emery, G. D., 5-844b, 6-229
Emery, P. E., 5-172
Engelhardt, H. T., Jr.,
    8-050, 8-129b
Engelsmann, F., 6-064
Enright, M. F., 5-396
Epstein, L. C., 6-065,
    7-009
Erbaugh, J., 6-043
Erdman, H., 6-079
Eser, A., 8-074

Esposito, M. E., 10-049
Esveldt-Dawson, K., 6-090
Ettlinger, R., 6-403,
    6-404a
Evans, D. L., 5-173
Evenson, R. C., 2-049,
    5-054, 5-646, 6-404b
Exner, J. E., 6-066

Faber, M. D., 10-087,
    10-088, 10-089
Fabsitz, R., 5-517
Fagg, J., 5-698, 6-055,
    7-024
Faheem, A. D., 5-403
Faigel, H. C., 5-174
Farber, A. N., 9-133
Farber, M. L., 4-076,
    5-369, 5-429, 5-430.09,
    6-011
Farberow, N. L., 1-003,
    1-004, 1-049d, 1-060.03,
    1-061, 1-075, 1-076,
    2-029, 2-048, 2-055,
    2-055.05, 2-056, 2-057,
    2-057.01, 2-057.05,
    2-058, 2-059, 2-060,
    2-063, 2-082, 2-083,
    3-008, 3-009, 4-051,
    5-035, 5-053, 5-071,
    5-072, 5-080, 5-081,
    5-256, 5-430, 5-430.01,
    5-430.10, 5-877, 6-012,
    6-042.08, 6-067, 6-068,
    6-069, 6-070, 6-113,
    6-114, 6-128.11, 6-150,
    6-178, 6-179, 6-198,
    6-238, 6-239a, 6-239b,
    6-241, 6-270.02,
    6-291.10, 6-297, 6-298,
    6-310, 6-346.01, 6-347,
    6-348, 6-349, 7-018,
    7-028, 7-062, 7-067,
    9-027, 9-132, 9-153,
    9-155, 9-173, 9-187,
    9-188, 9-189, 10-034
Farmer, R. D. T., 1-062,
    2-037, 5-443, 5-462,
    5-463, 5-626, 5-626.03,
    10-075
Fast, I., 9-009.03,
    9-009.06, 9-012, 9-084.01
Faulstich, M. E., 9-014,
    9-015
Faux, E. J., 1-065

10-073
Schwab, J. J., 5-829, 5-830
Schwartz, A. H., 9-147
Schwartz, A. J., 5-063,
  5-235
Schwartz, D. A., 5-605,
  6-278a, 8-160
Schwartz, M. L., 5-714
Schwartz, V. E., 8-154
Schwartzberg, A. Z., 5-175
Schwyn, E., 8-063
Scott, K. F., Jr., 6-434
Segal, B. E., 2-047, 5-246,
  5-370, 9-145
Seibert, D. J., 5-713
Seiden, R. H., 2-004,
  5-162, 5-212, 5-236,
  5-237, 5-276, 5-296,
  5-297, 5-300.04, 5-321,
  5-322, 5-485, 5-783,
  6-056, 6-430b
Seidler, M. J., 8-094
Selby, J. W., 5-777, 7-046,
  9-013, 9-014, 9-015,
  9-016, 9-017, 9-018
Selby, L. E., 9-017
Selkin, J., 5-732, 6-261,
  6-278b
Sell, B. H., 1-009
Sell, K. D., 1-009
Selvin, H. C., 5-082
Selzer, M. L., 2-057.18
Sendbuehler, J. M., 5-277,
  5-875, 6-145, 6-160
Seneca, 8-095
Senter, R. J., 5-811
Shaffer, D., 5-213,
  5-220.05
Shaffer, J. W., 2-088,
  6-065, 6-146
Shaffer, T. L., 8-158
Shapiro, D. L., 6-207,
  7-016
Sharma, P. C., 1-017
Shaw, B. F., 6-229
Shea, M., 6-364, 6-378
Shein, H., 7-081
Sheldon, A., 9-056
Shepherd, D. M., 5-492,
  5-748, 5-911, 5-929,
  9-005, 9-006, 9-042,
  9-062, 9-063
Sheran, T. J., 6-050
Sherick, R. B., 6-090
Shershow, J. C., 5-083
Sheskin, A., 9-064

Shichor, D., 5-449
Shin, Y., 5-315
Shneidman, E. S., 1-004,
  1-057, 1-058, 1-060.02,
  1-061, 1-071, 1-072,
  1-073, 1-074, 1-075,
  1-076, 2-025, 2-026,
  2-027, 2-028, 2-029,
  2-048, 2-089, 2-090,
  4-067, 5-702, 5-804,
  5-876, 5-877, 6-030,
  6-031, 6-279, 6-280,
  6-298, 6-310, 6-346,
  6-347, 6-348, 6-349,
  7-005, 7-047, 7-062,
  7-093, 9-022.06, 9-065,
  9-066, 9-067, 9-085.02,
  9-132, 9-136, 9-137,
  9-138, 9-155, 9-157,
  9-162, 9-163, 9-173,
  9-185, 9-187, 9-188,
  9-189, 9-195, 9-196,
  10-099, 10-100, 10-101,
  10-102
Shochet, B. R., 7-127
Shore, J. H., 5-343, 6-350
Short, J. F., Jr., 4-019,
  4-020, 5-096, 5-251,
  5-310
Shulman, K., 5-278
Shulman, M. D., 5-529
Siani, R., 6-074, 6-147
Sickel, R. Z., 9-068
Sider, R. C., 8-018, 8-019
Siegel, K., 8-064, 8-065
Siegel, S., 8-117
Siegler, M., 8-016b
Siiter, R., 7-017
Silbowitz, M., 5-853, 6-098
Silver, J. R., 5-708
Silverman, D., 6-174.04
Silverman, P. R., 9-009.10
Silving, H., 8-159
Simkin, S., 5-222
Simon, J. L., 5-749
Simon, M. D., 5-430.10
Simon, W., 5-384, 9-022.05
Simone, F., 10-103
Simpson, G., 5-084
Simpson, M. A., 2-057.17,
  9-069
Sims, L., 5-238
Sims, M., 5-486
Singer, R. G., 7-094
Singh, A. N., 6-211, 6-392
Singh, B. K., 7-048

SUBJECT INDEX

Numbers are those of the citations (of the form: chapter number-reference number).

Adolescents, See Children
Africa, 5-424, 5-434.02, 5-434.03, 5-444, 5-553, 6-006
Age, 5-005, 5-146--5-283, 5-409, 5-412, 5-419, 5-486, 5-512, 5-734a, 9-169, 9-173, 9-182, 9-183, See also specific age groups: Aged, Children, & Middle Aged
Aged (Elderly, Old), 2-069, 2-070, 2-078, 2-082, 2-085, 5-005, 5-050, 5-141, 5-146.01, 5-148, 5-150, 5-151.04, 5-192, 5-244, 5-245, 5-247--5-283, 5-360, 5-377, 5-449, 5-479, 5-492, 5-582, 5-771, 6-109, 6-282, 7-011, 7-092, 7-119, 8-008.03, 8-014b, 8-056, 9-169, 9-173, 9-151, 9-152, 9-182, 9-183, 10-037
Alcohol & Alcoholism, 1-097, 2-055.03, 2-057.13, 2-057.14, 2-057.18, 2-086.03, 5-330, 5-331, 5-622, 5-640.01, 5-645, 5-649, 5-660, 5-675, 5-696, 5-809, 5-837, 5-838, 7-009, 10-055
Anniversaries, 5-498, 5-611, 9-026, 9-089.01, 9-152, 10-004
Asian/Oriental-Americans,

5-289, 5-295, 5-360, See also Chinese, Japanese-, and Filipino-Americans
Assessment & Prediction & Evaluations (including scales, tests, MMPI, Rorschach, etc.), 1-097, 2-087, 5-184.01, 5-192, 5-196, 5-203.02, 5-220.01, 5-231, 5-633, 5-660, 5-661, 5-668, 5-676, 5-890, 5-895, 5-899, 5-906, 6-038--6-172, 7-015, 7-026, 7-035, 7-044, 7-047, 7-056, 7-058, 7-118, 9-018, 9-174, 10-051
Attempted Suicide ("Parasuicide," "Non-Fatal Deliberate Self-Harm"), 1-045, 1-051, 1-077, 1-093, 2-006, 2-009, 2-013, 2-015, 2-016, 2-017, 2-022, 2-023, 2-035--2-050, 4-077, 5-095, 5-099, 5-100, 5-101, 5-112, 5-113, 5-115, 5-120, 5-125, 5-127, 5-130, 5-131, 5-137, 5-159, 5-160, 5-168, 5-200, 5-210, 5-216, 5-220.03, 5-222, 5-240, 5-248, 5-270, 5-277, 5-278, 5-302, 5-318, 5-324, 5-325, 5-355, 5-358, 5-391,

About the Compiler

JOHN L. MCINTOSH is Assistant Professor of Psychology at Indiana University at South Bend. He is the author of *Suicide Among U.S. Racial Minorities, Suicide Among Children, Adolescents, and Students,* and *Suicide Among the Elderly,* and articles in *Omega, Suicide and Life-Threatening Behavior,* and *Journal of Gerontological Social Work.*